LAB MANUAL AND WORKBOOK

The Pharmacy Technician

Foundations and Practices,
2nd edition

MIKE JOHNSTON, CPhT
Chairman & CEO, National Pharmacy Technician Association
Houston, TX

PEARSON

Boston Columbus Indianapolis New York San Francisco Upper Saddle River
Amsterdam Cape Town Dubai London Madrid Milan Munich Paris Montréal Toronto
Delhi Mexico City São Paulo Sydney Hong Kong Seoul Singapore Taipei Tokyo

Publisher: Julie Levin Alexander
Publisher's Assistant: Regina Bruno
Editor-in-Chief: Marlene McHugh Pratt
Executive Editor: Joan Gill
Program Manager: Faye Gemmellaro
Editorial Assistant: Stephanie Kiel
Development Editor: Jill Rembetski, iD8-TripleSSS Media Development, LLC
Director of Marketing: David Gesell
Marketing Manager: Katrin Beacom
Senior Marketing Coordinator: Alicia Wozniak
Marketing Specialist: Michael Sirinides
Project Management Team Lead: Cynthia Zonneveld
Project Manager: Yagnesh Jani
Full-Service Project Management: Sneha Pant
Senior Operations Specialist: Nancy Maneri-Miller
Senior Media Editor: Matt Norris
Media Project Manager: Lorena Cerisano
Creative Director: Andrea Nix
Art Director: Maria Guglielmo Walsh
Composition: PreMediaGlobal Inc.
Printing and Binding: R.R. Donnelley/Harrisonburg
Cover Printer: R.R. Donnelley/Harrisonburg

Notice: Care has been taken to confirm the accuracy of information presented in this book. The authors, editors, and the publisher, however, cannot accept any responsibility for errors or omissions or for consequences from application of the information in this book and make no warranty, express or implied, with respect to its contents.

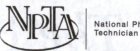

The NPTA logo is a trademark of the National Pharmacy Technician Association

straden-schaden, inc.®

RxPRESS
PUBLICATIONS®

The Straden-Schaden and RxPress logos are both trademarks of Straden-Schaden, Inc.

PEARSON

ISBN 10: 0-13-289809-8
ISBN 13: 978-0-13-289809-6

8 2019

*This workbook is dedicated to the memory of
Emily Jerry. Emily passed away, at the age of 2, as a result of a medication error made by a
pharmacy technician. I hope that this workbook, along with more stringent regulations, will
help prevent such tragedies in the future.*

To Eric
*Thank you for your constant support, patience, and understanding. I am a better man for
having met you and blessed to have you by my side.*

Contents

Preface

The Pharmacy Technician: Foundations and Practices, 2nd edition addresses today's comprehensive educational needs for one of the fastest growing jobs in the United States—that of the pharmacy technician. The pharmacy technician career is ranked number 19 among the 100 fastest-growing jobs in the United States. According to the U.S. Bureau of Labor Statistics, the pharmacy technician career is growing at approximately 32%, a much higher rate than other jobs in the health professions. This equates to an anticipated net increase in employment opportunities of 108,300 between 2010 and 2020.

In addition to the tremendous workforce demand for pharmacy technicians, professional regulations and requirements are being established for pharmacy technicians across the United States. With many state boards of pharmacy either considering, or having already enacted, requirements for mandatory registration, certification, and/or formal education, the need for a comprehensive and up-to-date pharmacy technician textbook such as *The Pharmacy Technician: Foundations and Practices, 2nd edition* has never been greater.

This *Workbook/Lab Manual to Accompany The Pharmacy Technician: Fundamentals of Practice, 2nd edition* is designed to give you additional practice in mastering the varied skills that will be required of you as a pharmacy technician. It is organized to correspond with the 38 chapters in the textbook. Each workbook/lab manual chapter includes:

- Learning objectives from the textbook, with references to related activities within the workbook/lab manual.

- An introduction that summarizes the main themes from the textbook chapter.

- Review Questions that evaluate your comprehension of the textbook chapter content. Question types include multiple choice, fill-in-the-blank, matching, and true/false.

- Pharmacy Calculation Problems that will give you additional practice and help increase your comfort level in using the math skills you will need on a daily basis as a practicing pharmacy technician.

- PTCB Exam Practice Questions related to the chapter's specific content will help you prepare for the Pharmacy Technician Certification Exam.

- Activities in each chapter challenge you to explore facets of the chapter material more thoroughly and offer a variety of exercises, including anatomy worksheets, case studies with critical thinking questions, Web research problems, and role-playing scenarios.

- Hands-on Lab activities in certain chapters give you the chance to practice procedures, work with equipment, or perform additional research.

MyHealthProfessionsLab for The Pharmacy Technician

The ultimate personalized learning tool is available at www.myhealthprofessionslab.com. This online course correlates with the textbook and is available for purchase separately or for a discount when packaged with the book. MyHealthProfessionsLab for the Pharmacy Technician is an immersive study experience that includes pretests and posttests to asses the skills the student learns in each chapter. Videos focused on math and other special topics, games, and anatomy & physiology activities round out the experience.

Learners track their own progess through the course and use a personalized study plan to achieve success. Visit www.myhealthprofessionslab.com to log into the course or purchase access. Instructors seeking more information about discount bundle options or for a demonstration should contact their Pearson sales representative.

About the Author

Mike Johnston is one of the most recognized and influential pharmacy technician leaders in the world. In 1999, Mike founded the National Pharmacy Technician Association (NPTA) and led the association from 3 members to more than 20,000 in less than two years, and now more than 60,000 members. Today, as chairman/CEO of NPTA and publisher of *Today's Technician* magazine, he spends the majority of his time meeting with and speaking to employers, manufacturers, industry leaders, and elected officials on issues related to pharmacy technicians, both across the United States and internationally.

Mike serves as the sole pharmacy technician delegate to the *United States Pharmacopeia* (USP) and is the only North American representative member of the European Association of Pharmacy Technicians (EAPT). He is also a CPE administrator and field reviewer approved by the Accreditation Council on Pharmacy Education (ACPE).

Mike's background includes experience in community-based pharmacy practice, health-system pharmacy practice, extemporaneous compounding, and as a pharmacy technician instructor. Mike has been nationally certified since 1997 (CPhT) and is also certified in IV/sterile products, chemotherapy, and extemporaneous compounding.

In 2013, Mike opened his own pharmacy—SCRIPTS Compounding Pharmacy—located in the suburbs of Houston, Texas. In addition, he is the author of eight previous textbooks on pharmacy technician education and *Rx for Success—A Career Enhancement Guide for Pharmacy Technicians*.

Mike holds a B.S. with honors in business management and ethics from Dallas Christian College and is currently working on his MBA at Dallas Baptist University.

About NPTA

The NPTA is the world's largest professional organization specifically for pharmacy technicians. The association is dedicated to advancing the value of pharmacy technicians and the vital roles they play in pharmaceutical care. In a society of countless associations, we believe that it takes much more than just a mission statement to meet the professional needs of and provide the necessary leadership for the pharmacy technician profession—it takes action and results.

The organization is composed of pharmacy technicians practicing in a variety of practice settings, such as retail, independent, hospital, mail-order, home care, long-term care, nuclear, military, correctional facilities, formal education, training, management, sales, and many more. NPTA is a reflection of this diverse profession and provides unparalleled support and resources to members.

NPTA is the foundation of the pharmacy technician profession; we have an unprecedented past, a strong present, and a promising future. We are dedicated to improving our profession while remaining focused on our members.

Pharmacy technician students are welcome to join more than 60,000 practicing pharmacy technicians as members of NPTA.

For more information:
call 888-247-8706
visit www.pharmacytechnician.org

Acknowledgments

The author wishes to give special acknowledgment and thanks to the following individuals who represent the greatest contributors to this text.

Joan Gill —for your strong leadership, guidance, and insight on this project as an executive editor. It is an honor and privilege to work with you.

Jill Rembetski —for your persistence, dedication, and amazing talent as a developmental editor. Thank you for keeping me on track with all of the overlapping deadlines and the intense schedule. You are the best in the business and it is a blessing to work with you.

Stephanie Kiel —for your ability to keep everything organized and on track as an editorial assistant.

Bronwen Glowacki —for all of your assistance and responsiveness as an associate editor over the years.

Julie Alexander —for your ongoing commitment and support as a publisher.

Mark Cohen —for your initial efforts in signing me with Pearson Education.

PreMediaGlobal —for your attention to detail and editing contributions.

Sandy Andrews, Jennifer Susan O'Reilly, Paul Sabatini , and Robin Luke—for being the most amazing team of researchers and assistant writers.

Reviewers

I would like to thank the following reviewers for their assistance.

Susan Fisher, CPhT
Pharmacy Technician Program Head
Anthem Career College—Memphis
Memphis, TN

Joshua Kramer, BS, CPhT
Director of Technology
Pharmacy Technician Program Director
Arizona College
Glendale, AZ

Shelby L. Newberry, MCPhT
Pharmacy Technician Program Director
Externship Coordinator
Vatterott College
Kansas City, MO

Jennifer Preuss, M.Ed
Program Manager
YTI Career Institute
Altoona, PA

Laura Skinner, BS
Program Director of Pharmacy Technology
Wayne Community College
Goldsboro, NC

Reviewers and Contributors from 1E

Clifford Frank, CPhT
Instructor
RxTech Training, Inc.
Chugiak, AK

Michelle Goeking, BM, CPhT
Instructor
Black Hawk College
Moline, IL

Michael M. Hayter, PharmD, MBA
Adjunct Instructor Pharmacy Technology and
Health Information
Virginia Highlands Community College
Abingdon, VA

Robin Luke, CPhT
Editorial Manager
Today's Technician Magazine
Vancouver, WA

CHAPTER 1
History of Pharmacy Practice

After completing Chapter 1 from the textbook, you should be able to:	Related Activity in the Workbook/Lab Manual
1. Describe the origins of pharmacy practice from the Age of Antiquity.	Review Questions, PTCB Exam Practice Questions, Lab 1-2
2. Discuss changes in pharmacy practice during the Middle Ages.	Review Questions, PTCB Exam Practice Questions, Lab 1-2
3. Describe changes in pharmacy practice during the Renaissance.	Review Questions, PTCB Exam Practice Questions, Lab 1-2
4. List significant milestones for pharmacy practice from the 18th, 19th, 20th, and 21st centuries.	Review Questions, PTCB Exam Practice Questions, Activity 1-1, Lab 1-1, Lab 1-2
5. Discuss the role biotechnology and genetic engineering could have on the future of pharmacy practice.	Review Questions, Activity 1-2

INTRODUCTION

The practice of pharmacy has ancient roots. The word *pharmacy* comes from the Greek word *pharmakon*, meaning "drug," and the origin of pharmacy practice goes back to ancient times, more than 7,000 years ago. The role of a pharmacy technician can be traced back to 2900 BCE, in ancient Egypt, where echelons were gatherers and preparers of drugs, similar to the modern-day pharmacy technician; chiefs of fabrication were the head pharmacists.

The history of pharmacy practice may seem to be unnecessary to you as you prepare to become a pharmacy technician. However, if you are to understand many of the concepts, theories, and practices covered in this workbook/laboratory manual and the textbook, you need to understand the evolution of the pharmacy profession. Many of the principles used in pharmacy thousands of years ago are still practiced today. Understanding the historic roots will also help you appreciate the areas in which the profession has evolved and how professional guidelines and regulations have developed. As you will discover, the responsibilities of and opportunities for pharmacy technicians continue to evolve, along with the profession of pharmacy itself.

REVIEW QUESTIONS

Match the following.

1. _____ pharmacogenomics
2. _____ pharmacy
3. _____ prescription
4. _____ apothecary
5. _____ biotechnology
6. _____ pharmacopoeia
7. _____ compounding

a. Latin term for pharmacist
b. Producing, mixing, or preparing a drug by combining ingredients
c. Use of living things to make or modify a product
d. An order to prepare/dispense
e. Study of genetic differences in responses to drug therapy
f. Art/science of preparing and dispensing medication
g. Book of products, formulae, and directions for preparation

Choose the best answer.

8. The word *pharmacy* comes from which ancient Greek word for drug?
   a. pharmakos
   b. pharmakopeia
   c. pharmakon
   d. pharmakot

9. The Latin word *recipere* or recipe means _____.
   a. Heal, Thou
   b. To Heal
   c. To Make
   d. Take, Thou

10. The Age of Antiquity refers to which time period?
    a. 8000 BCE up through 699 CE
    b. 5000 BCE up through 499 CE
    c. 3000 BCE up through 899 CE
    d. 4000 BCE up through 599 CE

11. The "father of botany" is considered to be:
    a. Shen Nung.
    b. Echelon.
    c. Theophrastus.
    d. Charaka Samhita.

Match the following scientists with their accomplishments.

12. _____ Fleming
13. _____ Mithridates
14. _____ Hippocrates
15. _____ Pedanios Dioscorides
16. _____ Galen

a. developed the theory of humors
b. poisons and poison preventatives
c. rules for drug collection, storage, and use
d. established principles of compounding
e. discovered penicillin

Choose the best answer.

17. The first apothecaries, or privately owned drugstores, were established in the late 8th century by the:
    a. Arabs.
    b. Greeks.
    c. Romans.
    d. Italians.

18. The first pharmacy technicians in ancient Egypt were known as:
    a. slaves.
    b. ebers.
    c. echelons.
    d. chiefs of fabrication.

19. The _____ is an ancient Indian manuscript, originating in approximately 1000 BCE, which records over 2,000 drugs.
    a. *De Materia Medica*
    b. *Charaka Samhita*
    c. *Pen T-Sao*
    d. *Corpus Hippocraticum*

20. The first school of pharmacy was:
    a. the Philadelphia College of Pharmacy.
    b. the University of Pennsylvania Pharmacy College.
    c. Boston University.
    d. the Massachusetts School of Pharmacology.

21. John Winthrop established the first apothecary in the American colonies in:
    a. 1617.
    b. 1729.
    c. 1640.
    d. 1751.

22. The *United States Pharmacopoeia* (USP) was first published in:
    a. 1820.
    b. 1877.
    c. 1822.
    d. 1869.

23. Gregor Mendel is known as the Father of Modern Genetics. He was an Austrian:
    a. pharmacist and scientist.
    b. priest and pharmacist.
    c. scientist and priest.
    d. priest and author.

24. The practice of pharmacy began to be regulated by the federal government:
    a. in the early 1900s.
    b. in the late 1800s.
    c. in the late 1900s.
    d. pharmacy has always been heavily regulated by the federal government.

25. Pharmacogenomics is the use of:
    a. genomic or genetic information to predict a drug's efficacy.
    b. personal DNA information to track patients.
    c. gene splicing to produce effective medications.
    d. a study of future drugs and their possible uses.

26. Colonial America's first hospital was established in:
    a. Boston.
    b. Jamestown.
    c. New York City.
    d. Philadelphia.

Match the following.

27. _____ Clinical Era
28. _____ Pharmaceutical Care Era
29. _____ Traditional Era
30. _____ Scientific Era

a. formulating and dispensing drugs
b. developing and testing drugs
c. dispensing information, warnings, and advice
d. positive outcomes of therapies

PHARMACY CALCULATION PROBLEMS

Calculate the following.

1. $12.7 + 58.3 + 91.2 + 0.4 =$

2. $120\ mL + 60\ mL + 80\ mL + 40\ mL =$

3. $750\ mg - 150\ mg - 75\ mg =$

4. $14.25\ oz. + 11.5\ oz. - 3.25\ oz. =$

5. $9.8\ mL - 5.4\ mL + 12.9\ mL =$

PTCB EXAM PRACTICE QUESTIONS

1. Which ancient civilization provides the earliest record of apothecary practice?
    a. Babylonian
    b. Chinese
    c. Indian
    d. Aztec

2. Who is credited with developing the polio vaccine?
    a. Wilson
    b. Marshall
    c. Fleming
    d. Salk

3. In what city was the first American school of pharmacy founded?
    a. Boston
    b. Baltimore
    c. Providence
    d. Philadelphia

4. Which organization is responsible for setting standards for pharmacy education and continuing pharmacy education?
    a. APHA
    b. NABP
    c. ASHP
    d. ACPE

5. Hippocrates, often referred to as the "Father of Medicine," was part of which ancient culture?
    a. Egyptian
    b. Greek
    c. Roman
    d. Chinese

ACTIVITY 1-1: History of Medicine Timeline

Instructions: List 10 major events in the history of pharmacy practice in its appropriate place on the timeline.

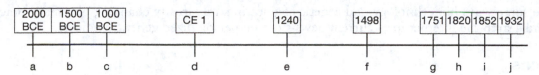

a. _____

b. _____

c. _____

d. _____

e. _____

f. _____

g. _____

h. _____

i. _____

j. _____

ACTIVITY 1-2: The Continuing Evolution of Pharmacy Practice

Chapter 1 touches on the role biotechnology and genetic engineering will play in the future of pharmacy practice, and you will learn more about these areas in Chapter 38 of the text.

What are some ways biotechnology and genetic engineering are already changing pharmacy practice? Go online and search the Internet for a current news story on personalized genetic medicine.

Questions

1. What is the topic and main point(s) of the news story you found online?

   _____

   _____

2. Was the story's coverage positive or negative in regard to biotechnology and/or genetic engineering?

   _____

   _____

3. What issues did the story raise?

   _____

   _____

   _____

   _____

4. Was the story from a credible source? Was there any potential bias from the author or publisher?

   _____

   _____

5. After reading the news story, what is your opinion of this topic?

   _____

   _____

   _____

   _____

6. Now research two to three other current stories on this same topic. Did the other stories raise new issues? If so, what are they?

   _____

   _____

   _____

   _____

7. After reading all the news stories on this topic, has your opinion changed from what you described in Question #4? If so, how? If not, discuss why.

   _____

   _____

   _____

   _____

LAB 1-1: Exploring the History of Pharmacy

Objective:

Visit an online pharmacy museum and explore the history of pharmacy as preserved in the museum exhibits.

Pre-Lab Information:

Visit the History of Pharmacy Museum at the University of Arizona College of Pharmacy's website: http://www.pharmacy.arizona.edu/visitors/pharmacy-museum/history-pharmacy-museum-photo-tour

Explanation:

The practice of pharmacy has a rich and very interesting history. It is important for you, a future pharmacy technician, to understand how pharmacy practice has evolved. This exercise will help you gain a historical perspective on the practice of pharmacy.

Activity:

Using the Internet, go to the History of Pharmacy Museum at the University of Arizona College of Pharmacy's website: http://www.pharmacy.arizona.edu/visitors/pharmacy-museum/history-pharmacy-museum-photo-tour. Take the virtual tour, then answer the following questions.

1. What time frame does the museum represent with the artifacts it has on display?

   _____

   _____

2. What is the significance of a red show globe?

   _____

   _____

3. What instrument was used to disinfect other instruments?

   _____

   _____

4. What was used to store the wet and dry ingredients used in pharmacy compounding?

   _____

   _____

5. What is the large box of natural products that were used in making prescriptions? (*Note*: It was produced by Parke-Davis and is one of the few remaining complete sets in the world.)

   _____

   _____

6. What is the box of homeopathic medicines called? (*Note*: A small amount was used to treat a particular malady and could be ordered by a number printed on the display box.)

   _____

   _____

7. What was the Lloyd continuous extraction apparatus used for from the 1940s through the 1970s?

_____

_____

8. What did you find most interesting?

_____

_____

_____

_____

9. What did you learn that you did not already know about pharmacy?

_____

_____

_____

_____

Student Name: _____

Lab Partner: _____

Grade/Comments: _____

_____

_____

Student Comments: _____

_____

_____

LAB 1-2: Pharmacy Pioneers

Objective:

To learn more about the origins of pharmacy practice by researching the achievements of a key pharmacy pioneer.

Pre-Lab Information:

- Review Chapter 1, History of Pharmacy Practice, in your textbook.
- Select a key pharmacy pioneer discussed in Chapter 1 of the text and presented in the following list, then perform additional online research to learn more about this person :

    Mithridates VI

    Emperor Shen Nung

    Hippocrates

    Theophrastus

    Pedanios Dioscorides

    Galen

    Savonarola

    John Winthrop

    Elizabeth Marshall

    Jonathan Roberts

    John Morgan

    Andrew Craigie

    Daniel B. Smith

    William Procter, Jr.

    Dr. Edward R. Squibb

    Gregor Mendel

    Alexander Fleming

    Jonas Salk

Explanation:

By focusing on the accomplishments of one key person in the history of pharmacy, you will gain a deeper understanding of that time period and an appreciation of how the practice of pharmacy has changed over time.

Activity:

Select a person from the preceding list, or choose another pharmacy pioneer who interests you. Go online or to the library to learn more about this person. Then answer the following questions.

1. What is the name of the pharmacy pioneer you researched?

   _____

   _____

2. In what time period did he or she live and work?

_____

_____

3. What was pharmacy practice like during this time period?

_____

_____

_____

_____

4. How is pharmacy practice today different from pharmacy practice in the time period in which the person you researched worked?

_____

_____

_____

_____

5. Why is the person you researched considered a pharmacy pioneer? What did he or she accomplish?

_____

_____

_____

_____

6. Are this person's accomplishments still important today? Why or why not?

_____

_____

_____

_____

7. What did you find most interesting about this person?

_____

_____

_____

_____

Student Name: _____

Lab Partner: _____

Grade/Comments: _____

_____

_____

Student Comments: _____

_____

_____

CHAPTER 2
The Professional Pharmacy Technician

After completing Chapter 2 from the textbook, you should be able to:	Related Activity in the Workbook/Lab Manual
1. Summarize the educational requirements and competencies of both pharmacists and pharmacy technicians.	Review Questions, PTCB Exam Practice Questions
2. Describe the two primary pharmacy practice settings and define the basic roles of pharmacists and pharmacy technicians working in each setting.	Review Questions Activity 2-1, Lab 1-2
3. Explain six specific characteristics of a good pharmacy technician.	Review Questions Activity 2-1, Activity 2-2, Lab 1-2
4. Demonstrate the behavior of a professional pharmacy technician.	Review Questions Activity 2-2, Lab 1-2
5. Explain the registration/licensure and certification process for becoming a pharmacy technician.	Review Questions, PTCB Exam Practice Questions, Lab 2-1

INTRODUCTION

Pharmacy is an industry consisting of professionals: pharmacists and .pharmacy technicians. Many claim—with good reason—that pharmacy is the most trusted profession in America. As with any profession, employment in this field requires you to be educated, trained, diligent, and ethical. You must maintain specific competencies, undergo specialized education and training, and exhibit key personal characteristics. The process of preparing for your future includes formal education and training, registration/licensure, national certification, and involvement with a professional organization. The benefits of your hard work and dedication are the tremendous career opportunities awaiting you as a future pharmacy technician.

REVIEW QUESTIONS

Match the following.

1. _____ certification
2. _____ licensing
3. _____ registration
4. _____ attitude

a. process of listing/being named to a list
b. government permission to do something
c. located on site where patients reside
d. common name for health system pharmacy

5. _____ compassion
    e. feelings of concern and understanding

6. _____ empathy
    f. deep awareness and sympathy

7. _____ ambulatory pharmacy
    g. retail pharmacy

8. _____ community pharmacy
    h. nongovernmental verification of competency

9. _____ health system pharmacy
    i. chain, drug/grocery store, mail-order, home health care pharmaci

10. _____ institutional pharmacy
    j. way of acting, thinking, or believing

True or False?

11. Historically, there were only two recognized professions: law and medicine.
    T   F

12. Pharmacy technicians must be licensed in all states.
    T   F

13. Today, pharmacy practice is based upon delivering direct patient care.
    T   F

14. Most institutional pharmacies are open 24 hours.
    T   F

15. Your body language can hide your true feelings and attitudes.
    T   F

Choose the best answer.

16. Which of the following tasks is most likely to be performed by a pharmacist?
    a. insurance billing
    b. patient private information maintenance
    c. patient counseling
    d. inventory ordering

17. Which of the following is considered an ambulatory pharmacy?
    a. hospitals
    b. extended-living facility
    c. home health care
    d. retirement home

18. The set of qualities and characteristics that represent perceptions of your competence and character, as judged by your constituents, is called your:
    a. attitude.
    b. professional image.
    c. professionalism.
    d. demeanor.

19. Which of the following attire would be unacceptable for a pharmacy technician?
    a. tie
    b. lab coat
    c. shorts
    d. scrubs

20. Since 2001, pharmacists are required to complete _____ years of college.
    a. 4
    b. 6
    c. 7
    d. 8

21. Which is an example of adapting to change?
    a. changing priorities, strategies, or methods
    b. maintaining effectiveness
    c. handling stress properly
    d. all of the above

22. _____ accredits pharmacy technician training programs.
   a. AAPT
   b. ACPE
   c. APhA
   d. ASHP

23. Which of the following is not a common eligibility requirement for technicians?
   a. no felony conviction(s)
   b. high school graduate or GED equivalent
   c. a two-year college degree
   d. certification

24. Pharmacy technicians are in the business of:
   a. selling drugs.
   b. patient care.
   c. patient consultations.
   d. making money.

25. Which of the following is considered an institutional pharmacy?
   a. retail drugstore
   b. home health care
   c. mail-order facility
   d. long-term care facility

List the four basic steps to problem solving.

26. _____

Name four sources of continuing education (CE) for pharmacy technicians.

27. _____
28. _____
29. _____
30. _____

PHARMACY CALCULATION PROBLEMS

Calculate the following.

1. Bobby has completed 16 hours of CE. How many more hours does he need to complete to meet the PTCB requirements?

2. If Judy worked 36.5 hours one week and 39 hours the next week, how much would her gross pay be for those two weeks if she were paid $13.05 per hour?

3. A customer has three prescriptions and owes a co-payment of $15.00 on each one. How much will the customer be charged for all three prescriptions?

4. A technician works the third shift at a hospital for seven days in a row, followed by seven days off. She is scheduled to work Sunday through Saturday from 10:00 P.M. till 8:00 A.M., every other week. If the pay period starts on Sunday, how many hours will she work in two consecutive weeks?

5. A medication order calls for a special mouthwash that the pharmacy must make. It contains 50% diphenhydramine syrup and 50% viscous lidocaine. The physician ordered 12 ounces. How much of each ingredient will you need to make this?

PTCB EXAM PRACTICE QUESTIONS

1. When a pharmacy student graduates from an accredited college of pharmacy in the United States, what degree does she or he receive?
   a. Bachelor of Science (BS)
   b. Bachelor of Arts (BA)
   c. Doctor of Pharmacy (PharmD)
   d. Master of Science (MS)

2. In the United States, pharmacy technicians are often required to be registered or licensed before they may perform the duties of a pharmacy technician. This requirement is mandated by which government agency?
   a. Food and Drug Administration (FDA)
   b. State Board of Pharmacy (SBOP)
   c. Drug Enforcement Agency (DEA)
   d. United States Pharmacopoeia (USP)

3. When a pharmacy technician successfully completes a certification examination to become a CPhT, this signifies to others that he or she is:
   a. smart.
   b. polite.
   c. empathetic.
   d. competent.

4. Which of the following statements is true about the PTCB Certification Exam (PTCE)?
   a. The exam consists of 100 questions, is computer-based, and is offered 4 times each year.
   b. The exam consists of 90 questions, is computer-based, and is offered year round.
   c. The exam consists of 90 questions, is paper-based, and is offered 4 times each year.
   d. The exam consists of 125 questions, is paper-based, and is offered year round.

5. An extended living facility is an example of a(n) _____ pharmacy.
   a. ambulatory
   b. institutional
   c. retail
   d. community

ACTIVITY 2-1: Case Study—Who Is Responsible?

Instructions: Read the following scenario and then answer the critical thinking questions that follow.

While processing a prescription for Bactrim DS, the pharmacy computer system notifies you that the patient has a recorded allergy to sulfur-based drugs. Bactrim DS is a sulfur-based antibiotic and could therefore pose a serious risk to the patient. You immediately alert the pharmacist to the situation; she determines that the prescriber has likely made a mistake and will need to select an alternative treatment.

The pharmacist explains that the pharmacy staff needs to:

- verify the allergy with the patient.
- upon confirmation of a sulfur allergy, explain to the patient that the pharmacy will have to call the prescriber to request a different prescription.
- call the doctor's office to explain the patient's allergy and to request a new, verbal prescription for the patient.

1. Who is responsible for verifying the drug allergy with the patient? Why?

   _____

   _____

   _____

   _____

2. Who is responsible for explaining to the patient that the pharmacy must call the doctor's office to request a different prescription? Why?

   _____

   _____

   _____

   _____

3. Who is responsible for calling the patient's doctor and requesting a new prescription? Why?

   _____

   _____

   _____

   _____

4. In what ways are the job functions of a pharmacist and pharmacy technician in an ambulatory setting different from those of a pharmacist and pharmacy technician in a health system pharmacy?

   _____

   _____

   _____

   _____

ACTIVITY 2-2: Case Study—Appropriate Behavior

Instructions: Read the following scenario and then answer the critical thinking questions that follow.

Regina is a certified pharmacy technician and has worked at a local community pharmacy for five years. She has the most seniority of the seven technicians who work in the pharmacy and she takes advantage of this.

When the pharmacy is busy, Regina takes charge and processes prescriptions with both speed and accuracy. She is typically able to have a prescription prepared for the pharmacist's review within 7 to 10 minutes, meaning that patients can generally expect only a 15-minute wait time. Regina is always dressed professionally and she is excellent at interacting with patients.

However, Regina refuses to help with receiving the weekly inventory order, stocking pharmacy supplies, or cleaning duties. She explains to the other technicians that those tasks are their jobs. In fact, Regina often takes personal calls on her cell phone during slow periods, rather than assisting with these tasks.

1. List Regina's appropriate behaviors and positive characteristics.

   _____

   _____

   _____

   _____

2. List Regina's inappropriate behaviors and unprofessional characteristics.

   _____

   _____

   _____

   _____

3. What role, or responsibility, does the pharmacy manager have in Regina's behavior?

   _____

   _____

   _____

   _____

4. What impact does Regina's behavior have on the pharmacy staff?

   _____

   _____

   _____

   _____

5. List six specific characteristics of a good pharmacy technician.

   _____

   _____

   _____

   _____

LAB 2-1: Becoming a Certified Pharmacy Technician

Objective:

Research the process involved in becoming a certified pharmacy technician, including the continuing education requirements required to maintain certification.

Pre-Lab Information:

Visit the Pharmacy Technician Certification Board website and other suggested online resources:

- https://www.ptcb.org
- http://www.pharmacytechnician.org/
- http://www.nhanow.com/pharmacy-technician/requirements.aspx

Explanation:

Certification is an important career step demonstrating that the pharmacy technician has met a set of standards. It is important for you to understand the exam process as well as the requirements for maintaining your certification.

Activity:

Using the Internet, visit the Pharmacy Technician Certification Board website at https://www.ptcb.org. Answer the following questions concerning technician certification.

1. What is the ATT letter and what does it mean?

   _____

   _____

2. What organization do you contact to schedule your certification exam?

   _____

   _____

3. What two requirements must you meet before registering for the PTCB certification exam?
   a. _____
   b. _____

4. How long is your initial certification valid (that is, how long before your initial certification must be renewed)?

   _____

   _____

5. How many hours of continuing education are required for each renewal period?

   _____

   _____

6. Continuing education programs must be approved by what organization?

_____

_____

7. When you successfully complete the Pharmacy Technician Certification Exam, what designation can you use after your name?

   a. _____

   Can you use this same designation if you take the National Technician Exam?

   b. _____

8. Visit the National Technician Exam website (http://www.nhanow.com/pharmacy-technician/requirements.aspx). Find your state and list its requirements for registration.

_____

_____

_____

_____

9. What is the cost to take the exam?

_____

_____

10. What testing site is located nearest to you?

_____

_____

Optional Activity:

Visit http://www.powerpak.com and complete one of the continuing education programs designated for "Pharmacy Technician."

Student Name: _____

Lab Partner: _____

Grade/Comments: _____

_____

_____

Student Comments: _____

_____

_____

LAB 2-2: Observing Professionalism in the Pharmacy

Objective:

Observe professionalism in a pharmacy setting.

Pre-Lab Information:

Review Chapter 2, "The Professional Pharmacy Technician," in your text.

Explanation:

Professionalism is a skill and a behavior. Although situations can sometimes be challenging, a pharmacy technician should always maintain a professional manner with both patients and coworkers.

Activity:

Go to a local pharmacy and take a seat in the pharmacy waiting area. Take a notebook with you and note your observations on the professionalism, or lack thereof, demonstrated by the pharmacy staff and the situations and challenges they encountered.

*It is important to first seek permission from the pharmacy staff before completing this activity. You should identify yourself as a pharmacy technician student who has been assigned to observe staff and patient interactions. However, specifically mentioning that you are assigned to observe the professionalism of the staff may result in altered behavior.

1. List the pharmacy, location, date, and time of your observation.

    _____

    _____

2. In what way(s) did you observe professionalism from your observation of the pharmacy staff?

    _____

    _____

3. In what way(s), if any, did you observe a lack of professionalism from your observation of the pharmacy staff?

    _____

    _____

4. Overall, how would you assess the professionalism of the pharmacy staff you observed?

    _____

    _____

5. List at least two ways in which the professionalism could have been improved:

    _____

    _____

6. List at least two "take aways" from your observational lab that will benefit your professionalism as a pharmacy technician.

    _____

    _____

Student Name: _____

Lab Partner: _____

Grade/Comments: _____

_____

_____

Student Comments: _____

_____

_____

CHAPTER 3
Communication and Customer Care

After completing Chapter 3 from the textbook, you should be able to:	Related Activity in the Workbook/Lab Manual
1. Describe and illustrate the communication process.	Review Questions, PTCB Exam Practice Questions, Activity 3-1
2. List and explain the three types of communication.	Review Questions, PTCB Exam Practice Questions, Activity 3-1, Lab 3-1
3. Summarize the various barriers to effective communication.	Review Questions, PTCB Exam Practice Questions, Activity 3-1, Lab 3-2
4. List and describe the primary defense mechanisms.	Review Questions, Activity 3-1, Lab 3-1, Lab 3-2
5. Describe specific strategies for eliminating barriers to communication.	Review Questions, PTCB Exam Practice Questions, Activity 3-1, Lab 3-2
6. Summarize the elements of and considerations in caring for patients.	Review Questions, PTCB Exam Practice Questions, Activity 3-2, Lab 3-2
7. List the Five Rights of medication administration.	Review Questions, Activity 3-2, Lab 3-2

INTRODUCTION

Communication is simply the process of transferring information, although it is not a simple process. You communicate to get your message across to others clearly and unambiguously. Communicating takes effort from everyone involved, including the sender (the person who initiates the communication) and the receiver (the person or group the sender is addressing). The communication process often breaks down, and errors may result in misunderstandings and confusion.

As a pharmacy technician, you will need to communicate effectively with a variety of people, including your immediate coworkers, customers or patients, health care personnel, suppliers, drug representatives, health insurance representatives, and many others. Pharmacy technicians work as frontline employees in the pharmacy, which means that both your management and your patients will rely on you to be an effective communicator and to identify and eliminate communication barriers as they arise. Remember that becoming an effective communicator is a lifelong process that gets easier with experience and time.

REVIEW QUESTIONS

Match the following.

1. _____ context
2. _____ projection
3. _____ inflection
4. _____ denial
5. _____ feedback
6. _____ channel
7. _____ kinesics
8. _____ defense mechanisms
9. _____ proxemics
10. _____ pitch

a. a change in the tone of voice

b. defense mechanism of refusing to acknowledge painful realities

c. body language

d. defense mechanism in which one's own attitudes are attributed to others

e. the situation or environment in which the message is delivered

f. the study of measurable distance between individuals as they interact

g. gesture, action, sound, written or spoken word used in transmitting information

h. how high or low the voice is in sound wave frequency

i. unconscious mental process used to protect the ego

j. the return of information back to the sender

Choose the best answer.

11. Directly related to the effectiveness of communication are:
    a. customer service and pharmaceutical care.
    b. speed of medication delivery and customer care.
    c. patient satisfaction and sales.
    d. pharmacy profitability and customer service.

12. The situation or environment in which a message is delivered is called:
    a. channel.
    b. feedback.
    c. context.
    d. verbal.

13. In communicating with patients, it is best to use a:
    a. monotone, impersonal tone.
    b. condescending patient tone.
    c. sympathetic caring tone.
    d. tone that mimics the patient's.

14. Effective communication will involve all of the following except:
    a. pleasantness.
    b. active listening.
    c. professional tones.
    d. aggressiveness

15. When leaving a voicemail for a patient, it is important not to:
    a. provide personal patient information.
    b. provide your name.
    c. provide your pharmacy's phone number.
    d. repeat information you have already given.

16. Facial expressions, eye contact, posture, and silence, are forms of:
    a. communication barriers.
    b. nonverbal communication.
    c. intimidation.
    d. not as effective as the spoken word.

17. Which of the following is not a barrier to communication?
    a. inaccurate information
    b. language
    c. overly lengthy message
    d. translators

18. If a patient does not speak good English, a technician should:
    a. see if a translator is available.
    b. speak the patient's native language if possible.
    c. provide instructions in the patient's native language.
    d. all of the above.

19. Defense mechanisms share two common properties:
    a. repression and sublimation.
    b. denial and displacement.
    c. unconscious trigger and distortion of reality.
    d. projection and rationalization.

20. When an individual transfers his or her own negative emotions to someone who is unrelated to those feelings, it is called:
    a. rationalization.
    b. displacement.
    c. denial.
    d. projection.

21. A patient who is prejudiced against minorities, and complains that an Asian-American technician showed him disrespect, may be using:
    a. regression.
    b. sublimation.
    c. projection.
    d. displacement.

22. The best strategy a technician can use for pharmacy conflict resolution is to:
    a. hold one's ground.
    b. demand respect.
    c. identify who has a problem.
    d. involve the supervisor.

23. In the Five Rights, the "right time" refers to the:
    a. pick-up time.
    b. drop-off time.
    c. time to fill the prescription.
    d. administration time(s).

24. The Patient's Bill of Rights includes being treated with courtesy and respect. It was passed by Congress in:
    a. 1905.
    b. 2005.
    c. 1995.
    d. 1955.

25. In various states, technicians may, with the approval of a pharmacist, do all the following except:
    a. read the instructions for a prescription to a patient.
    b. assist the patient with OTC selection.
    c. provide verbal advice and/or clinical information.
    d. assist the patient with medical devices.

List and describe five common defense mechanisms:

26. _____
    _____

27. _____
    _____

28. _____
    _____

29. _____
    _____

30. _____
    _____

PHARMACY CALCULATION PROBLEMS

Calculate the following.

1. At retail price, two prescriptions would cost $38.85 and $246.80, respectively. The customer has insurance and only pays $10 per prescription. How much money did the customer save with her insurance?

2. It costs the pharmacy $46.16 for 32 ounces of guaifenesin syrup. How much does it cost per ounce?

3. If a customer pays 30% of the retail price for a medication, how much would the customer pay for a prescription with a retail price of $200?

4. A technician gets paid $12 per hour for the first 40 hours worked in a week. He gets traditional overtime pay that is 1.5 times more than his regular pay for the hours he works over 40 hours. How much will he get paid if he works 48 hours in one week?

5. Jane works the second shift at a hospital. Her base pay is $13.25 per hour. The hospital gives a shift differential of $1.00 per hour for every hour worked on the second shift. How much will her weekly paycheck be if she works 32 hours?

PTCB EXAM PRACTICE QUESTIONS

1. Which of the following best describes the protection of a patient's privacy (identity and health information)?
   a. Compatibility
   b. Conformity
   c. Compliance
   d. Confidentiality

2. Some patients may feel uncomfortable if the pharmacist or technician stands too close or touches them. Other patients may initiate a handshake or pat on the back. These kinds of differences might be considered:
   a. genetic differences.
   b. cultural differences.
   c. physical differences.
   d. physiological differences.

3. You have a patient who is less than 12 years old. This patient would be categorized as what kind of patient?
   a. geriatric
   b. neonate
   c. pediatric
   d. ambulatory

4. An important communication concept, which refers to the situation, environment, or circumstance in which a message is communicated, is:
   a. projection.
   b. context.
   c. intellectualization.
   d. rationalization.

5. Which of the following is NOT one of the *Five Patient Rights*?
   a. Right Medication
   b. Right Price
   c. Right Strength
   d. Right Time

ACTIVITY 3-1: Case Study—Overcoming Communication Barriers

Instructions: Read the following scenario and then answer the critical thinking questions.

Mr. Hernandez arrives at your pharmacy with three prescriptions that he needs to have filled. You ask him, "Have you had any prescriptions filled here before?" He gets a puzzled look on his face, but says only, "No entiendo."

None of the staff currently working speaks Spanish, including yourself, and it is clear that Mr. Hernandez does not speak English. After you look for him in the computer's database, you find that Mr. Hernandez appears to be a new patient. You provide him with a New Patient Profile form, written in Spanish, and a pen, but he once again gets a puzzled look on his face and begins shaking his head and shrugging his shoulders.

Mr. Hernandez reaches into his pocket and presents you with an identity card, which has his address information, and his insurance card. It appears that Mr. Hernandez can only speak Spanish; he is unable to read or write.

You process his prescription using the information he has been able to provide with his ID card and insurance card. The label for his prescriptions is translated into Spanish, according to the pharmacist's instructions, even though he will not personally be able to read the label.

1. List the communication barriers present with Mr. Hernandez.

_____
_____
_____
_____

2. Describe the best method for explaining Mr. Hernandez's medications and how to take them properly, given the limitations on communication.

_____
_____
_____
_____

3. What additional steps can the pharmacy take to ensure that Mr. Hernandez fully understands his medications and administration instructions?

_____
_____
_____
_____

4. With the proliferation of bilingual individuals, it is not common for a pharmacy to have no staff members or employees from a different department available to translate for a patient such as Mr. Hernandez. How would your responses to questions 2 and 3 change, if at all, if the patient spoke Russian or Cantonese, and was unable to read or write?

_____
_____
_____
_____

5. In addition to language barriers, what are four other examples of barriers to communication? List and discuss how you might resolve each one.

_____
_____
_____
_____

Role Play: Find a partner and then select one of the other communication barriers you listed in question 5 of Activity 3-1. Role-play a scenario in which a customer demonstrates this communication barrier while coming to the pharmacy to have a prescription refilled. One person should assume the role of a customer, while the other plays the role of a pharmacy technician who uses strategies to communicate with this customer. After five minutes, switch roles. Discuss what worked and what didn't work effectively. What are some possible challenges of using the same strategies in a "real" situation with a customer?

Research: Research the Internet to discover other strategies people use to overcome communication barriers. Try searching under key terms like: "overcoming communication barriers," "types of communication barriers," or "how to communicate effectively," for example. How do the different strategies compare to those you learned in Chapter 3? Did you learn anything new that might also be helpful in your work as a pharmacy technician?

ACTIVITY 3-2: Case Study—Patient Care

Instructions: Read the following scenario and then answer the critical thinking questions.

Mr. Thomas, one of your regular customers who is in his mid-fifties, comes to the pharmacy visibly shaken and disturbed. He has just returned from his doctor's office, where he was diagnosed with diabetes.

Mr. Thomas is nervous at the mere thought of having to use a blood glucose monitor and testing his blood every day. He also shares the fact that his mother died of severe complications related to diabetes.

He has several new prescriptions to be filled. His doctor also instructed him to purchase a blood glucose meter, although there was not enough time to properly instruct him on how to use one.

1. What defense mechanisms might you potentially expect from Mr. Thomas? How would you overcome them?

   _____

   _____

   _____

   _____

2. What measures could you take to provide optimal patient care for Mr. Thomas? Explain.

   _____

   _____

   _____

   _____

3. What measures could the pharmacist take to provide optimal patient care for Mr. Thomas? Explain.

   _____

   _____

   _____

   _____

4. What rights does Mr. Thomas have as a patient?

   _____

   _____

   _____

   _____

5. What are the Five Patient Rights?

_____

_____

_____

_____

6. Why do you think the Five Rights you listed in question #5 are important? In your opinion, is any one more important than the others? Why or why not?

_____

_____

_____

_____

LAB 3-1: Leaving and Receiving Voicemail Messages

Objective:

To develop proper business telephone etiquette and communication skills.

Pre-Lab Information:

Review Chapter 3, "Communication and Customer Care," in your textbook.

Explanation:

As a pharmacy technician, you will spend a lot of time communicating with patients, vendors, health insurance representatives, and others on the telephone. Conducting business on the phone is different from making personal calls. Each time you make or answer a call, you are representing your pharmacy and yourself as an employee of that facility. Remember the following tips:

- Use a pleasant and professional tone of voice.
- State your name and place of business.
- If answering a phone call, ask how you can help the caller.
- If making a phone call, explain your need or objective.
- If taking a message, document important information from the caller (see lab activity for more details).
- When leaving a voicemail message, speak slowly and clearly, to allow the receiver time to write down the information.

Example of Correct Voicemail Message

"Hello, this is Lydia Smitts from Young's Pharmacy calling for Mr. Tom Lewis regarding your refill request. Please give me a call at your earliest convenience at 333-4455. Again, this is Lydia Smitts from Young's Pharmacy, and I may be reached at 222-333-4455. Thank you."

Example of Incorrect Voicemail Message

"This is Lydia Smitts calling about your refill for Prozac. Please give me a call back at 333-4455. Thank you."

Part One

Review the steps for leaving a voicemail.

1. Provide your full name and the name of the pharmacy.
2. Provide the pharmacy telephone number and hours of operation.
3. Indicate the purpose of your phone call.
4. Make any specific requests needed.
5. Provide your name and the pharmacy telephone number a second time.

Practice these steps with a partner.

Part Two: Role Play

Working with a partner, create a scenario in which you receive a patient's voicemail message, either a refill request or a question for the pharmacist. Write down the details you will provide and then compare your partner's accuracy in writing down the message after listening to the voicemail. Be creative.

Example

Patient's Name: Janice Meyers

Prescription Number or Drug Name: Rx 7786791-0245

Special Request: I need to have this refilled today before noon because I am going out of town tonight.

Part Three: Role Play

Working with a partner, state your message from Part Two. Be sure to include a date and time. As one partner leaves a "message," the other should record it on the following voicemail slip. Reverse roles so that each of you has the opportunity to leave a message and retrieve a message. Once you have both taken your turns, compare your voicemail slip against the written notes your partner made in Part One for accuracy.

MESSAGES

Date: _____ Time: _____

From: _____

To: _____

Message: _____

_____

_____

_____

Taken by: _____ Date: _____

---

1. How accurate were you in retrieving the voicemail message? Describe.

_____

_____

_____

_____

2. How accurate was your partner in retrieving your voicemail message? Describe.

_____

_____

_____

_____

3. What insight(s) has this lab provided in regard to leaving and retrieving messages?

_____

_____

_____

_____

Student Name: _____

Lab Partner: _____

Grade/Comments: _____

_____

_____

Student Comments: _____

_____

_____

LAB 3-2: Practicing Effective Communication and Customer Care

Objective:

To develop effective verbal and nonverbal communication skills.

Pre-Lab Information:

Review Chapter 3, "Communication and Customer Care," in your textbook.

Explanation:

As a pharmacy technician, you will be involved in face-to-face communication nearly all day long, excluding a few specialty practice settings. This face-to-face communication will be with your pharmacists, coworkers, patients, and customers. Communicating in person with another person involves both verbal and nonverbal communication. It is also a two-way process that involves both talking and listening. Effectively doing each is critical to successful communication. Here are some tips for effective face-to-face communication.

1. Smile. Be a pleasant individual to communicate with.
2. Speak clearly and at an appropriate volume.
3. Use professional and appropriate tones of voice, inflections, and diction. Never use slang.
4. Actively listen when someone is speaking to you, and acknowledge the speaker by nodding your head.
5. Do not interrupt someone while he or she is speaking. Wait until the speaker is finished.
6. Ask questions to ensure that you both completely understand the conversation.
7. Use appropriate eye contact.

Part One

Review the tips for effective face-to-face communication.

Practice these techniques with a partner for five minutes by discussing why you each decided to become a pharmacy technician. At the end of the five-minute period, take turns relaying back the information you have learned about each other. How much of it were you able to retain? Were you surprised at all by the results?

Part Two

Using the information provided, act out the following scenarios, and then reflect on the exercise through use of the discussion questions.

Scenario 1

Cast:

- Patient
- Pharmacy Technician
- Pharmacist (optional)

Scene:

The patient arrives at the pharmacy at 4:30 in the afternoon and requests a refill of the antidepressant Zoloft. Upon looking up the patient's prescription, the pharmacy technician realizes that there are no refills remaining and that the doctor's office will have to be called for refill authorization. The technician knows that it is too late to obtain a refill authorization, but on the patient's insistent demands explains that the supply of the medication is completely gone.

Discussion Questions:

1. Was the pharmacy technician effective in communicating with the patient? Why?

   _____

   _____

   _____

   _____

2. What defense mechanisms, if any, were evident in the patient and the pharmacy technician?

   _____

   _____

   _____

   _____

3. Was the situation resolved in the best manner possible? What other resolutions could have been attempted?

   _____

   _____

   _____

   _____

Scenario 2

Cast:

- Pharmacy Technician 1
- Pharmacy Technician 2
- Pharmacist

Scene:

The pharmacist requests that Pharmacy Technician 1 restock the prescription vials and take out the trash. Overloaded with inventory duties, Pharmacy Technician 1 asks Pharmacy Technician 2 to take care of these duties. Two hours later, the pharmacist is outraged to discover that the vials have not been restocked and that the trash is overflowing. The pharmacist reprimands Pharmacy Technician 1, who in turn blames Pharmacy Technician 2. A heated argument ensues.

Discussion Questions:

1. What is the root cause of this argument?

   _____

   _____

   _____

   _____

2. What defense mechanisms were evident in each individual?

   _____

   _____

   _____

   _____

3. How would you have handled the situation differently? Why?

   _____

   _____

   _____

   _____

Student Name: _____

Lab Partner: _____

Grade/Comments: _____

_____

_____

Student Comments: _____

_____

_____

CHAPTER 4
Pharmacy Law and Ethics

After completing Chapter 4 from the textbook, you should be able to:	Related Activity in the Workbook/Lab Manual
1. Classify the various categories of U.S. law.	Review Questions, Lab 4-1
2. List the regulatory agencies that oversee the practice of pharmacy and describe their function(s).	Review Questions, PTCB Exam Practice Questions, Lab 4-1, Lab 4-3
3. Summarize the significant laws and amendments that affect the practice of pharmacy.	Review Questions, PTCB Exam Practice Questions, Activity 4-1, Lab 4-1
4. Recognize and use a drug monograph.	Review Questions, Lab 4-2
5. Define ethics and moral philosophy.	Review Questions, Activity 4-1, Activity 4-2
6. List and explain the nine ethical theories.	Review Questions, Activity 4-3
7. Summarize the Pharmacy Technician Code of Ethics.	Review Questions, Activity 4-3

INTRODUCTION

Federal and state laws, as well as professional ethics, regulate the practice of pharmacy. The regulations on pharmacy practice in the United States have evolved over the past hundred or so years, and their number has increased as legislators responded to demands from citizens to serve and protect the public interest. The government began to take the initiative in regulating pharmacy practice toward the end of the 18th century. Over time, the profession of pharmacy has become increasingly more regulated. In the United States, a professional degree is a requirement for any individual who wishes to practice pharmacy. This requirement was established to protect the public and set minimum standards, so that citizens could rely on pharmacists having at least a standard level of education and competence.

Many of the regulations pertaining to practice as a pharmacy technician are established and enforced by your specific state's board of pharmacy. In general, federal laws govern the manufacturing of pharmaceutical products, and state laws govern the actual dispensing of those products. It is imperative that you familiarize yourself with both the federal laws and your state's laws pertaining to pharmacy practice. In addition, you should fully understand the basic ethical theories and *Code of Ethics for Pharmacy Technicians*, in preparation for ethical dilemmas and questions that will arise in the pharmacy setting.

REVIEW QUESTIONS

Choose the best answer.

1. The quality of keeping a promise is:
   a. beneficence.
   b. ethics.
   c. fidelity.
   d. veracity.

2. A drug that has been misleadingly or fraudulently labeled is referred to as:
   a. adulterated.
   b. a felony.
   c. a monograph.
   d. misbranded.

3. A system of principles often associated with a profession is:
   a. civil law.
   b. consequentialism.
   c. ethics.
   d. criminal law.

4. Most laws pertaining to pharmacy were enacted to:
   a. limit the scope and practice of pharmacy.
   b. protect the public interest.
   c. lower the number of drug addicts.
   d. protect drug manufacturers.

5. Which is not a type of law in the United States?
   a. legislative intent
   b. constitutional
   c. government policy
   d. statutes

6. Which set of laws would take priority?
   a. federal
   b. state
   c. municipality
   d. local codes

7. Statutes are laws that are passed by:
   a. the federal government.
   b. state governments.
   c. local governments.
   d. all of the above.

8. Legislative intent is often referred to as:
   a. common law.
   b. case law.
   c. civil law.
   d. all of the above.

9. Regulations:
   a. have the force of law.
   b. are guidelines.
   c. refine laws.
   d. are not connected to laws.

10. Crimes are classified as either _____ or _____.
    a. infractions, misdemeanors
    b. infractions, violations
    c. infractions, felonies
    d. felonies, misdemeanors

11. Professional liability insurance is:
    a. currently available only to pharmacists.
    b. available to both pharmacists and pharmacy technicians.
    c. required by most states.
    d. required by the federal government.

12. Which agency/administration is not involved in the practice of pharmacy?
    a. CMS
    b. HIPAA
    c. HCFA
    d. FEMA

13. Which agency/administration is responsible for protecting the privacy of patients?
    a. CLIA
    b. SCHIP
    c. HIPAA
    d. DEA

Match the following.

14. _____ Drug Enforcement Agency
15. _____ Food and Drug Administration
16. _____ Federal Bureau of Investigation
17. _____ State Board of Pharmacy
18. _____ Joint Commission
19. _____ Occupational Safety and Health Administration

    a. regulates and registers pharmacy technicians, pharmacists, and pharmacies

    b. establishes and enforces standards for health care organizations

    c. assures the safety, efficacy, and security of drugs

    d. regulates the legal trade in controlled drugs

    e. the administrator of the DEA reports to this chief

    f. assures the safety and health of American workers

Choose the best answer.

20. The Food and Drug Administration was created by the:
    a. Food, Drug, and Cosmetic Act of 1938.
    b. Pure Food and Drug Act of 1905.
    c. Controlled Substances Act of 1970.
    d. FBI's need to expand to combat prevalent drug abuse.

21. "A display of written, printed, or graphic matter upon the immediate container of an article" refers to the:
    a. label.
    b. labeling.
    c. package insert.
    d. patient information sheet.

22. Which of the following information is not a labeling requirement for a dispensed prescription?
    a. NDC
    b. serial number (Rx number)
    c. date of fill
    d. prescriber's name

23. Which of the following information is not required to be on the manufacturer's label of a prescription-only drug?
    a. route of administration
    b. name and quantity of active ingredients
    c. date of fill
    d. federal legend

24. Which of the following information is not required to be on the package insert?
    a. dosage
    b. indications and usage
    c. adverse reactions
    d. unique lot or control number

Fill in the blank.

25. The amendment signed in 1951 that required the "federal legend" to be printed on all prescription drugs was _____.

26. The Kefauver–Harris Amendment, signed in 1962, is also referred to as the _____.

Match the following.

27. _____ OBRA '90
28. _____ Pure Food and Drug Act of 1906
29. _____ Food, Drug, and Cosmetic Act
30. _____ Durham–Humphrey Amendment
31. _____ Schedule I
32. _____ Schedule II
33. _____ Schedule III
34. _____ Schedule IV
35. _____ Schedule V
36. _____ DEA Form 224
37. _____ DEA Form 225
38. _____ DEA Form 363
39. _____ DEA Form 222
40. _____ DEA Form 41

a. limits interstate commerce in drugs to those that are safe and effective
b. established "federal legend"
c. focused on funding Medicare and Medicaid
d. neglected to ban unsafe drugs
e. low abuse, limited dependence
f. lowest abuse potential, lowest dependency
g. no accepted medical use, high abuse potential and high dependency risk
h. high potential for abuse and dependency
i. mostly combination drugs, moderate dependency
j. needed to compound narcotics or conduct narcotic treatment
k. used to report lost or stolen C-II drugs
l. needed to order C-II drugs from distributor
m. needed to dispense
n. needed to manufacture or distribute

True or False?

41. A P.O. Box address is not permitted on a C-II prescription.

    T   F

42. C-II prescriptions must be kept separate from all other prescriptions.

    T   F

43. All prescription drugs must be distributed in childproof containers.

    T   F

Choose the best answer.

44. The NDC number identifies which of the following?
    a. drug
    b. manufacturer
    c. package size
    d. all of the above

45. Anabolic steroids (except estrogens, progestins, and corticosteroids) are classified in which schedule?
    a. C-I
    b. C-II
    c. C-III
    d. C-IV

46. A moral philosophy is a(n) _____ set of values or value system.
   a. individual
   b. professional
   c. community
   d. none of the above

47. Which agency/administration maintains a closed system for the distribution of controlled substances?
   a. CMS
   b. FDA
   c. DEA
   d. HHS

Match the following.

48. _____ indication
49. _____ warnings
50. _____ contraindications
51. _____ precautions

a. lists types of patient who should not use the drug
b. lists remaining possible side effects
c. specific conditions that the FDA has approved the drug to treat
d. serious side effects and what to do

Match the following.

52. _____ fidelity
53. _____ beneficence
54. _____ veracity
55. _____ justice
56. _____ autonomy
57. _____ ethics of care
58. _____ rights-based ethics
59. _____ principle-based ethics
60. _____ virtues-based ethics

a. acting with fairness or equity
b. acting with self-reliance
c. bringing about good
d. telling the truth
e. keeping a promise
f. the idealization of morals
g. more personal approach
h. democratic view of individuals
i. focus on kindness, tact, etc.

PHARMACY CALCULATION PROBLEMS

Calculate the following.

1. A prescription states that the patient is to take one tablet by mouth twice daily for 14 days. How many tablets will you need to dispense for a 14-day supply?

2. An antibiotic suspension is dispensed in a 150 mL bottle. If the patient takes 5 mL by mouth three times a day, how many days will the antibiotic last?

3. A customer gives herself one enoxaparin injection every day. If enoxaparin comes in a 10-count box (a box of 10 single-dose syringes), how many boxes will the customer need for 30 days?

4. A patient with a chronic pain condition applies one fentanyl patch every 72 hours for pain relief. How often does the patient need to apply a new patch?

5. If the patient in question #4 needs enough patches to last 30 days, how many patches should the pharmacy dispense?

PTCB EXAM PRACTICE QUESTIONS

1. Vicodin is an example of a Schedule _____ drug.
   a. II
   b. IV
   c. III
   d. V

2. HIPAA regulations were established to safeguard and maintain patient privacy. In the law, PHI stands for which of the following?
   a. personal health information
   b. protected health information
   c. private health information
   d. programmed health information

3. In response to incidents of fatal poisoning from liquid sulfanilamide, which of the following laws required proof that new drugs were safe before they could be marketed?
   a. Food and Drug Act of 1906
   b. 1938 Food, Drug, and Cosmetic Act
   c. 1951 Durham–Humphrey Amendment
   d. The Kefauver–Harris Amendment of 1962

4. The Combat Methamphetamine Epidemic Act requires that OTC cold and allergy medications that contain which of the following drugs be kept behind the counter?
   a. antihistamine
   b. methamphetamine
   c. ephedrine and pseudoephedrine
   d. dextromethorphan

5. Which law required childproof packaging for most prescription drugs?
   a. Food, Drug, and Cosmetic Act
   b. Poison Prevention Packaging Act
   c. Durham–Humphrey Amendment
   d. Kefauver–Harris Amendment

ACTIVITY 4-1: Case Study—Legal Matters and Patient Confidentiality

Instructions: Read the following scenarios and then answer the critical thinking questions.

You and your spouse are having dinner out one evening. As usual, you both discuss events from the day at work. Frustrated, you begin sharing with your spouse, "I had this one patient today, Sharon Eckels, who nearly put me over the edge. She came into the pharmacy and handed us her empty bottle for her antipsychotics, and demanded that we refill it right away. Why can't people call ahead before they run completely out?!"

"That's ridiculous," your spouse responds.

It just so happens that Mr. Eckels, a prominent attorney in the community, is having dinner with a client at a nearby table, and they both overhear your comments. Initially embarrassed, Mr. Eckels is now outraged by the breach of patient confidentiality.

1. What, if any, law or regulation was violated by your dinner conversation?

_____

_____

_____

2. Does Mr. Eckels have a legitimate lawsuit pertaining to patient confidentiality? Why?

_____

_____

_____

3. Could you be liable for your actions? Could the pharmacy be liable for your actions? Explain.

_____

_____

_____

_____

4. What would have been an appropriate way to express your frustration at dinner?

_____

_____

_____

_____

ACTIVITY 4-2: Case Study—Medication Errors and Liability

Instructions: Read the following scenario and then answer the critical thinking questions.

Note: Based on an actual event.

A pharmacy technician who worked at the inpatient pharmacy of a children's hospital made an error when preparing an IV bag. Instead of using a prepackaged saline solution containing 0.9% NaCl (salt), the technician prepared an IV bag with a solution that was 23.4% NaCl.

The IV was reviewed and verified by the staff pharmacist. Although the technician did raise several questions about the product, it was approved and dispensed for administration. The patient to whom it was given, who was two years old, died three days later.

1. Who is responsible for the medication error: the technician, the pharmacist, or both?

_____

_____

_____

_____

2. Who could be held liable for the medication error: the technician, the pharmacist, or both?

_____

_____

_____

_____

3. What do you think would be an appropriate judgment in this scenario: for the parents of the child, for the technician, for the pharmacist, and for the hospital?

_____

_____

_____

_____

4. Research online for a story containing a pharmacy-related medication error. Attach a copy of the article and answer questions 1–3, listed above, concerning this error.

_____

_____

_____

_____

_____

_____

_____

_____

_____

_____

ACTIVITY 4-3: Case Study—Ethical Considerations

Instructions: Read the following scenarios and then answer the critical thinking questions.

Scenario 1

A young man comes into the pharmacy and asks to purchase a box of syringes. When you inquire if he has a prescription for insulin or syringes on file at the pharmacy, he quickly says that he usually fills his prescription at another pharmacy. You also notice that he has not requested a specific size or gauge of syringe. Your intuition tells you that this young man wants to purchase syringes for recreational drug use. If you sell him the syringes, it could be argued that you are enabling his drug use. However, it could also be argued that if you do not sell him the syringes, he will likely still continue to abuse drugs, possibly with dirty or used syringes.

Scenario 2

During the peak of cold and flu season, the manufacturer of one of the best over-the-counter remedies is back-ordered on its products, with an expected delay of six weeks for shipments. You are aware that all the other pharmacies in town are already completely out of stock on this product, but your pharmacy has one package left. An elderly woman comes into the pharmacy, clearly suffering from a nasty cold, to ask if you have any of the medicine available. You promised your next-door-neighbor that you would hold the last package for his family; although they have not yet gotten sick, they want to have the medicine on hand.

1. In Scenario 1, would you sell the young man syringes as he is requesting? Why?

_____

_____

_____

_____

2. In Scenario 2, would you sell the last package of the cold remedy to the elderly woman, or would you reserve it for your neighbor as promised? Why?

_____

_____

_____

_____

3. What ethical theory or moral principle discussed in Chapter 4 of the text are you using as the basis of your decision in both questions? Explain.

_____

_____

_____

_____

4. Describe another ethical consideration, not discussed in the book, that you could imagine occurring in pharmacy practice. How would you handle the situation?

_____

_____

_____

_____

LAB 4-1: Creating a Pharmacy Law Timeline

Objective:

Review and remember the major laws that pertain to the practice of pharmacy in the United States.

Pre-Lab Information:

Review Chapter 4, "Pharmacy Law and Ethics," in your text.

Explanation:

It is important for pharmacy technicians to have an understanding of pharmacy law. Many of our current laws were enacted because of an injury to persons using medications. The progression of laws related to the practice of pharmacy through American history can give you a better perspective on current laws and regulations.

Activity:

Using the following chart, complete the timeline by filling in the correct year in which each law was passed.

Law	Timeline
The Pure Food and Drug Act	
The Prescription Drug Marketing Act	
The Occupational Safety and Health Act	
The Orphan Drug Act	
The Medical Device Amendment	
The Affordable Care Act	
The Poison Prevention Packaging Act	
The Omnibus Budget Reconciliation Act	
The Kefauver–Harris Amendment	
The Health Insurance Portability and Accountability Act	
The Controlled Substances Act	
The Combat Methamphetamine Epidemic Act	
The Medicare Modernization Act	
The Durham–Humphrey Amendment	
The Drug Listing Act	
The Anabolic Steroids Act	
The Food, Drug, and Cosmetic Act	
The Dietary Supplement Health and Education Act	
The Drug Price Competition and Patent Term Restoration Act	

1. Name four broad categories of law in the United States and provide a brief definition of each.

   _____

   _____

   _____

   _____

2. What is the difference between criminal and civil law?

_____

_____

_____

_____

3. Name six of the regulatory agencies that oversee the practice of pharmacy in the United States and describe their function(s).

_____

_____

_____

_____

_____

_____

Student Name: _____

Lab Partner: _____

Grade/Comments: _____

_____

Student Comments: _____

_____

LAB 4-2: Interpreting a Drug Monograph

Objective:

Recognize and use a drug monograph.

Pre-Lab Information:

- Review Chapter 4, "Pharmacy Law and Ethics," in your text.
- Gather the following materials:
- Drug monograph, either from home or supplied by your instructor

Explanation:

Drug monographs, also called *package inserts*, are a necessary component of a drug's labeling. They provide all the clinical information about a drug as required by the FDA. As a pharmacy technician, you need to be familiar with the format, components, and content of drug monographs.

Activity:

Review the drug monograph that you brought from home or received from your instructor. Then locate all of the components listed here and answer the questions.

Drug name: _____

Description

What is the dosage form of this drug?

_____

_____

Clinical Pharmacology

Does this drug include any notes relevant to specific patient populations? If so, what are they?

_____

_____

_____

_____

Indications and Usage

What specific conditions or symptoms has this drug been approved by the FDA to prevent or treat?

_____

_____

_____

_____

Contraindications

What types of patients should not use this medication?

_____

_____

_____

_____

Warnings

Does this drug include cautions about serious side effects that can be caused by the medication and instructions on what the patient should do if these effects are experienced? If so, describe them.

_____

_____

_____

_____

Precautions

Does the monograph list additional, possible, or potential side effects that the patient should be aware of? If so, what are they?

_____

_____

_____

_____

Drug Abuse and Dependence

Does this drug have a potential for abuse or dependence?

_____

_____

_____

Adverse Reactions

Does the monograph include a description of reactions that are unexpected and potentially life threatening? If so, what are they?

_____

_____

_____

_____

Dosage

What is the recommended dosage of this medication for an adult?

_____

_____

_____

_____

How Supplied

How is this medication supplied, including strengths, dosage formats, and storage requirements?

_____

_____

_____

_____

Student Name: _____

Lab Partner: _____

Grade/Comments: _____

_____

_____

Student Comments: _____

_____

_____

LAB 4-3: Selling Pseudoephedrine

Objective:

Demonstrate proper documentation of a pseudoephedrine product sale.

Pre-Lab Information:

- Review Chapter 4, "Pharmacy Law and Ethics," in your text.
- Gather the following materials:
- Pseudoephedrine-containing product package, such as Sudafed.
- Drivers Licenses
- Review state and federal regulations for the sale of pseudoephedrine, including daily and monthly limits.

Explanation:

The sale of products containing pseudoephedrine are regulated by the Combat Methamphetamine Epidemic Act of 2005, As a result, retail pharmacies are required to observe daily sales limits, monthly sales limits, direct customer access restrictions, and maintain documentation of sales.

Activity:

Although most chain retail pharmacies use technology-based platforms to comply with CMEA, hard copy log books are also an acceptable method for tracking and documenting the sale of products containing pseudoephedrine. With a lab partner, take turns as the patient and the pharmacy technician and complete a transaction for a product containing pseudoephedrine, including documentation on the log book form below.

1. Ensure that the request does not exceed daily or monthly limits.
2. Verify the customer's photo identification (e.g., driver's license).
3. Complete necessary paperwork and documentation of sale, including:
   - customer's name
   - customer's address and telephone number
   - customer's identification number (e.g., driver's license number)
   - product name
   - product strength
   - product quantity
   - date
   - customer's signature
   - your name and signature

4. Process the sales transaction at the pharmacy.

Pseudoephedrine Sales Log

ID Number	Date	Last Name	First Name	Phone	Street Address	City	State	Staff
Signature					Product & Qty		Strength	
ID Number	Date	Last Name	First Name	Phone	Street Address	City	State	Staff
Signature					Product & Qty		Strength	
ID Number	Date	Last Name	First Name	Phone	Street Address	City	State	Staff
Signature					Product & Qty		Strength	
ID Number	Date	Last Name	First Name	Phone	Street Address	City	State	Staff
Signature					Product & Qty		Strength	
ID Number	Date	Last Name	First Name	Phone	Street Address	City	State	Staff
Signature					Product & Qty		Strength	
ID Number	Date	Last Name	First Name	Phone	Street Address	City	State	Staff
Signature					Product & Qty		Strength	
ID Number	Date	Last Name	First Name	Phone	Street Address	City	State	Staff
Signature					Product & Qty		Strength	

Lab Partner: _____

Grade/Comments: _____

_____

_____

Student Comments: _____

_____

_____

CHAPTER 5
Terminology and Abbreviations

After completing Chapter 5 from the textbook, you should be able to:	Related Activity in the Workbook/Lab Manual
1. Identify selected root words used in pharmacy practice.	Review Questions, Activity 5-3, Lab 5-1, Lab 5-2, Lab 5-3
2. Identify and correctly use selected prefixes and suffixes in conjunction with root words.	Review Questions, Activity 5-3, Lab 5-1, Lab 5-2, Lab 5-3
3. Recognize and interpret common abbreviations used in pharmacy and medicine.	Review Questions, Pharmacy Calculation Problems, PTCB Exam Practice Questions, Activity 5-1, Activity 5-2, Lab 5-1, Lab 5-2, Lab 5-3
4. List abbreviations that are considered dangerous and explain why.	Review Questions, PTCB Exam Practice Questions
5. Recognize and list common drug names and their generic equivalents.	Review Questions, PTCB Exam Practice Questions, Lab 5-1, Lab 5-2, Lab 5-3
6. Recall and define common pharmacy and medical terminology.	Review Questions, Activity 5-3, Lab 5-1, Lab 5-2, Lab 5-3

INTRODUCTION

To understand the pharmacy industry and profession, you must learn its language, which consists of medical terminology, abbreviations, and drug names. Most medical terms derive from Greek and Latin and consist of a root word, prefix, and/or suffix. It is unlikely that you will remember all the information contained in Chapter 5 of the textbook, but by learning selected roots, prefixes, and suffixes, you will be able to understand words you may have never seen or heard before. Over time, with experience and practice, you will develop a strong working knowledge of medical terminology.

REVIEW QUESTIONS

Match the following.

1. _____ pneum
2. _____ arthr
3. _____ hemo
4. _____ my
5. _____ oste
6. _____ ectomy
7. _____ rhin
8. _____ ante
9. _____ dys
10. _____ hyper
11. _____ tachy
12. _____ itis
13. _____ cyte
14. _____ dipsia
15. _____ intra

a. fast
b. abnormal
c. nose
d. bone
e. blood
f. lung
g. muscle
h. too much
i. cell
j. inflammation
k. thirst
l. before
m. surgical removal
n. joint
o. within

Choose the best answer.

16. The part of a word that helps identify its major meaning is the:
    a. prefix.
    b. suffix.
    c. root.
    d. origin.

17. A part of a word that is attached at the beginning of the term is a:
    a. prefix.
    b. suffix.
    c. root.
    d. origin.

18. Which of the following are on the Joint Commission's "do not use" list?
    a. qhs
    b. SC
    c. QOD
    d. all of the above

19. ADR is the accepted abbreviation for:
    a. average drug response.
    b. adverse drug reaction.
    c. antibiotic-related dietary restriction.
    d. acute drug release.

Match the following.

20. _____ dispense as written
21. _____ after meals
22. _____ as needed
23. _____ before meals
24. _____ as directed
25. _____ left ear

a. AU
b. u.d.
c. apap
d. NPO
e. gtt
f. DAW

26. _____ twice daily
27. _____ both ears
28. _____ no known allergies
29. _____ drop
30. _____ milliliter
31. _____ aspirin
32. _____ potassium
33. _____ penicillin
34. _____ nothing by mouth
35. _____ acetaminophen
36. _____ sodium

g. NKA
h. pc
i. prn
j. bid
k. ac
l. AS
m. Na
n. ASA
o. K
p. PCN
q. mL

Match the following brand drugs with their generics.

37. _____ Accutane
38. _____ Zoloft
39. _____ Flexeril
40. _____ Toprol XL
41. _____ Allegra
42. _____ Zithromax
43. _____ Inderal
44. _____ Feldene
45. _____ Aldactone
46. _____ Coumadin
47. _____ Lodine
48. _____ Demerol
49. _____ Ambien
50. _____ Fastin
51. _____ Antivert
52. _____ Halcion
53. _____ Lamisil
54. _____ Aricept
55. _____ Catapres
56. _____ Phenergan
57. _____ Diovan
58. _____ Augmentin
59. _____ Plavix
60. _____ Biaxin

a. zolpidem tartrate
b. piroxicam
c. meperidine
d. warfarin
e. etodolac
f. propranolol HCl
g. fexofenadine HCl
h. azithromycin
i. clonidine HCl
j. donepezil HCl
k. spironolactone
l. meclizine
m. isotretinoin
n. phentermine
o. clarithromycin
p. triazolam
q. valsartan
r. sertraline
s. clopidogrel
t. amoxicillin and clavulanate potassium
u. promethazine HCl
v. metroprolol tartrate
w. terbinafine
x. cyclobenzaprine

PHARMACY CALCULATION PROBLEMS

Calculate the following.

1. A prescription reads: "Cephalexin 500 mg: 1 cap qid × 10d." How many capsules should you dispense?

2. If a patient takes 5 mL of albuterol syrup BID, how many mL should you dispense for a 10-day supply?

3. How many drops of timolol ophthalmic solution is a patient using per day if the instructions read: "2 gtts ou tid"?

4. A prescription reads: "Azithromycin 250 mg: Take two tablets by mouth once daily for the first day, then one tablet on days 2–5." How many tablets will you dispense?

5. A bottle of fluticasone nasal spray contains 120 metered doses. If the directions state: "Use 2 sprays in each nostril BID," how many days will the spray last?

PTCB EXAM PRACTICE QUESTIONS

1. Tobrex ophthalmic ung refers to:
   a. an ointment used for the eye.
   b. a solution used for the eye.
   c. a topical ointment for external use only.
   d. an ointment used for the ear.

2. If a medication is to be taken a.c., it should be taken:
   a. in the morning.
   b. around the clock.
   c. after meals.
   d. before meals.

3. Which of the following abbreviations is considered acceptable for use when writing medication orders?
   a. Q.D.
   b. Q.O.D.
   c. Q.I.D.
   d. U

4. What is the generic name for the drug Cataflam?
   a. cimetidine
   b. diltiazem HCl
   c. diclofenac sodium
   d. cytarabine

5. What health care accreditation organization has created a list of "do not use" abbreviations?
   a. APHA
   b. APA
   c. NABP
   d. Joint Commission

ACTIVITY 5-1: Case Study—Lost in Translation

Instructions: Read the following scenarios and then answer the critical thinking questions provided.

Scenario 1

A patient brings in a new prescription for Glucophage XR 500 mg. When you are processing the prescription into the pharmacy computer, you quickly select Glucophage 500 mg from the drop-down list of medications as you scroll down. The prescription is filled and dispensed, as neither you nor the pharmacist notice that the prescription was written for Glucophage XR (extended release) as opposed to Glucophage.

Scenario 2

When writing up a compounding formula sheet, you put down that .5 mg of active ingredient is to be used per dose. The following month, however, another technician is reviewing the formula to prepare the patient's refill. The refill is prepared using 5 mg of active ingredient per dose, as opposed to 0.5 mg.

1. What translation error occurred in Scenario 1?

   _____

   _____

   _____

   _____

2. What effect will the error in Scenario 1 have?

   _____

   _____

   _____

   _____

3. What translation error occurred in Scenario 2?

   _____

   _____

   _____

   _____

4. What effect will the error in Scenario 2 have?

   _____

   _____

   _____

   _____

5. Who is responsible for the mistake in Scenario 2? How could it most easily have been avoided?

   _____

   _____

   _____

   _____

6. What can you do to ensure that these types of errors are avoided?

_____

_____

_____

_____

ACTIVITY 5-2: Practice with Abbreviations

For each of the following, write the meaning next to the abbreviation.

1. p _____
2. pm _____
3. N/V _____
4. ac _____
5. po _____
6. DAW _____
7. NS _____
8. bid _____
9. u.d. _____
10. qd _____

11. s _____
12. AU _____
13. prn _____
14. qw _____
15. WA _____
16. disp. _____
17. fl. _____
18. D5W _____
19. DM _____
20. NKA _____

Now, write the appropriate abbreviation after its meaning.

21. suppository _____

22. every day at bedtime _____

23. microgram _____

24. with _____

25. right eye _____

26. intravenous _____

27. by mouth _____

28. left ear _____

29. otic _____

30. drops _____

ACTIVITY 5-3: Defining Medical Terms

Using a medical dictionary, your text, or an online medical resource, define the following medical terms. Then, break the term into its word parts and define each word part as well.

1. gynecologist

   Definition: _____

   Word parts: _____

2. rhinoplasty

   Definition: _____

   Word parts: _____

3. dermatologist

   Definition: _____

   Word parts: _____

4. arthritis

   Definition: _____

   Word parts: _____

5. polyurea

   Definition: _____

   Word parts: _____

6. erythrocytes

   Definition: _____

   Word parts: _____

7. leukocytes

   Definition: _____

   Word parts: _____

8. arteriosclerosis

   Definition: _____

   Word parts: _____

9. hematuria

   Definition: _____

   Word parts: _____

10. tachycardia

   Definition: _____

   Word parts: _____

LAB 5-1: Translating a Medical Record

Objective:

Reinforce your knowledge of terminology and abbreviations by completing this exercise based on a medical record entry.

Pre-Lab Information:

Review Chapter 5, "Terminology and Abbreviations," in your text.

Explanation:

It is important for pharmacy technicians to have a basic understanding of the language used in medicine. This exercise will help you gain experience by "translating" a medical record entry.

Activity:

Read the following pharmacist SOAP (Subjective, Objective, Assessment, Plan) note from a patient's pharmacist consultation and answer questions related to the content, using your knowledge of terminology and abbreviations.

S:	67 yo BF with Hx of arthritis, obesity, hyperlipidemia, hypertension. Several questions about medications and improving health status.	
O:	Type 2 DM	Morning BS 130–155+; does not test routinely, A1c 8.5% (6 mo ago)
	HTN	155/95 on ramipril 10 mg bid
	Hyperlipidemia	TC 219, LDL 143, TRG 185 (6 mo ago) on simvastatin 20 mg once daily
	Obesity	59'90" / 230 lb, BMI 34
	RA	Knee and hip pain with exercise, APAP prn only
	SCr	1.6 (6 mo ago)
	Vitals	P 78, R 19
		Not taking ASA for CVD prevention
A:	Diabetes	Poor compliance diet/meal planning; poor understanding of BS testing; above goal of A1c, 7%
	HTN	Above goal of BP 125/80 with Tx
	Hyperlipidemia	Above goal of LDL ≤ 100 with Tx
	Obesity	Above goal, 25 lb gain over last 6 mo, min exercise frequency; Initial goal 10% weight loss at 1–2 lb/wk (23 lb in 4 mo)
	RA	Still not well controlled

P:	Improve medication adherence and health outcomes.
	• HTN: Recommended changing ramipril 10 mg bid to lisinopril/HCTZ 20/12.5 bid
	• Hyperlipidemia: Recommended increasing simvastatin from 20 mg to 40 mg once daily
	• RA: Recommended diclofenac XR 100 mg once daily for RA
	• Cardiovascular health: Recommended adding lo-dose ASA daily
	• Provided and instructed pt with daily BS monitoring log
	• Provided and instructed pt with personal health tracking tool
	• Reviewed "ADA Dietary Guidelines" and shopping/meal planner guide
	• Suggested pt walk 30–60 min/day
	• Schedule for 90-day F/U appt.
	• Schedule for repeat of the following labs 2 weeks prior to 90-day FU appt: SCr, fasting lipid profile, A1c, BG

Duration of appt: 45 minutes

Pharmacist's signature: _____

Questions:

1. What does the abbreviation Hx mean?

   _____

   _____

2. What does APAP prn mean?

   _____

   _____

3. In the "Objective" section, which drug (generic and brand name) did the patient take to control cholesterol?

   _____

   _____

4. In the "Objective" section, which drug (generic and brand name) did the patient take to control blood pressure?

   _____

   _____

5. What does the abbreviation BS mean?

   _____

   _____

6. What does the abbreviation HTN mean?

   _____

   _____

7. In the "Plan" section, what drug (generic and brand) did the pharmacist recommend changing for the patient's HTN?

_____

_____

8. In the "Plan" section, what does the abbreviation ASA mean?

_____

_____

Student Name: _____

Lab Partner: _____

Grade/Comments: _____

_____

_____

Student Comments: _____

_____

_____

LAB 5-2: Translating a Prescription

Objective:

Reinforce your knowledge of terminology and abbreviations by completing this exercise based on a prescription.

Pre-Lab Information:

Review Chapter 5, "Terminology and Abbreviations," in your text.

Explanation:

It is critical for pharmacy technicians to have an understanding of the terminology and abbreviations used in pharmacy. This exercise will help you gain experience by "translating" the directions on prescriptions.

Activity:

Review and translate the following prescriptions, then either prepare an accurate prescription label for each prescription or write out the information requested below.

Rx #1

Towne Center Family Medicine
40 Towne Center Drive
Pleasantville, Texas 77248-0124
Phone 281-555-0134 Fax 281-555-0125

James L. Brook, MD BB1234563   Rebecca Smith, MD AS1234563   Walter Roberts, MD AR1234563
Sharon Ortiz, NP   Beth Matthews, NP   Terri King, NP

Name _Cindy Redding_____ Age _____

Address _____ Date _Aug 05_____

℞

Zoloft 50mg

#30

T po qam

Refill __2__ times

_Terri King_____
Signature

A generically equivalent drug product may be dispensed unless the practitioner hand writes the words
'Brand Necessary' or 'Brand Medically Necessary' on the face of the prescription.

6HUR133050

1. Patient name: _____
2. Prescriber: _____
3. Drug name and strength: _____
4. Is generic substitution permitted? _____
5. Quantity to dispense: _____
6. Directions: _____
7. Refills authorized: _____
8. Days Supply: _____

Rx #2

Towne Center Family Medicine
40 Towne Center Drive
Pleasantville, Texas 77248-0124
Phone 281-555-0134 Fax 281-555-0125

James L. Brook, MD BB1234563   Rebecca Smith, MD AS1234563   Walter Roberts, MD AR1234563
Sharon Ortiz, NP   Beth Matthews, NP   Terri King, NP

Name _Felix Ortiz_____ Age _____

Address _____ Date _Jan 20_____

℞

Glucophage 850mg

#30

T po qd c̄ food

Refill __1__ times

Rebecca Smith
Signature

A generically equivalent drug product may be dispensed unless the practitioner hand writes the words
'Brand Necessary' or 'Brand Medically Necessary' on the face of the prescription.

6HUR133050

1. Patient name: _____

2. Prescriber: _____

3. Drug name and strength: _____

4. Is generic substitution permitted? _____

5. Quantity to dispense: _____

6. Directions: _____

7. Refills authorized: _____

8. Days Supply: _____

Rx #3

James L. Brook, MD BB1234563   Rebecca Smith, MD AS1234563   Walter Roberts, MD AR1234563
Sharon Ortiz, NP   Beth Matthews, NP   Terri King, NP

Name _Nancy Nguyen_____ Age _____

Address _____ Date _Oct 12_____

Rx

Amoxil 500mg

#28

T po bid × 14d

Refill ___0___ times

J.L. Brooks (Signature)
Signature

6HUR133050

1. Patient name: _____
2. Prescriber: _____
3. Drug name and strength: _____
4. Is generic substitution permitted? _____
5. Quantity to dispense: _____
6. Directions: _____
7. Refills authorized: _____
8. Days Supply: _____

Student Name: _____
Lab Partner: _____
Grade/Comments: _____
_____
_____
Student Comments: _____
_____

LAB 5-3: Translating a Medication Order

Objective:

Reinforce your knowledge of terminology and abbreviations by completing this exercise based on a prescription.

Pre-Lab Information:

Review Chapter 5, "Terminology and Abbreviations," in your text.

Explanation:

It is critical for pharmacy technicians to have an understanding of the terminology and abbreviations used in pharmacy. This exercise will help you gain experience by "translating" the directions on medication orders.

Activity:

Review and translate the following medication orders, then either prepare an accurate prescription label for each prescription or write out the information requested below.

Medication Order #1

PHYSICIAN'S ORDER WORKSHEET

NOTE: *Person initiating entry should write legibly, date the form using (Mo/Day/Yr.), enter time, sign, and indicate their title.*

USE BALL POINT PEN (PRESS FIRMLY)

17325   220

04-06-1968

Dr. S. Turner

Date	Time	Treatment
5/15	18:30	*Merrem IV 500mg q 8hr*
		②

PHYSICIAN'S ORDER WORKSHEET

Distribution:
(Original) Medical Record Copy
(Plies 3, 2, & 1) Pharmacy

T-5

1. Patient name: _____
2. Prescriber: _____
3. Drug name and strength: _____
4. Is generic substitution permitted? _____
5. Quantity to dispense: _____
6. Directions: _____
7. Refills authorized: _____
8. Days Supply: _____

Medication Order #2

PHYSICIAN'S ORDER WORKSHEET

NOTE: *Person initiating entry should write legibly, date the form using (Mo/Day/Yr.), enter time, sign, and indicate their title.*

USE BALL POINT PEN (PRESS FIRMLY)

Date	Time	Treatment
9/4	10:15	*Morphine inj 3mg*
		②

	PHYSICIAN'S ORDER WORKSHEET	Distribution: (Original) Medical Record Copy (Plies 3, 2, & 1) Pharmacy	**T-5**

1. Patient name: _____
2. Prescriber: _____
3. Drug name and strength: _____
4. Is generic substitution permitted? _____
5. Quantity to dispense: _____
6. Directions: _____
7. Refills authorized: _____
8. Days Supply: _____

Medication Order #3

PHYSICIAN'S ORDER WORKSHEET

NOTE: *Person initiating entry should write legibly, date the form using (Mo/Day/Yr.), enter time, sign, and indicate their title.*

USE BALL POINT PEN (PRESS FIRMLY)

6702340   102

12-03-1949

Dr. R. Khan

Date	Time	Treatment
3/18	16.45	Zofran inj. 4mg
		②

PHYSICIAN'S ORDER WORKSHEET

Distribution:
(Original) Medical Record Copy
(Plies 3, 2, & 1) Pharmacy

T-5

1. Patient name: _____

2. Prescriber: _____

3. Drug name and strength: _____

4. Is generic substitution permitted? _____

5. Quantity to dispense: _____

6. Directions: _____

7. Refills authorized: _____

8. Days Supply: _____

Student Name: _____

Lab Partner: _____

Grade/Comments: _____

_____

_____

Student Comments: _____

_____

_____

CHAPTER 6
Dosage Formulations and Routes of Administration

After completing Chapter 6 from the textbook, you should be able to:	Related Activity in the Workbook/Lab Manual
1. Explain drug nomenclature.	Review Questions, Lab 6-1
2. Identify various dosage formulations.	Review Questions, PTCB Exam Practice Questions, Activity 6-4, Lab 6-2, Lab 6-3
3. Identify the advantages and disadvantages of solid and liquid medication dosage formulations.	Review Questions, PTCB Exam Practice Questions, Activity 6-4
4. Explain the differences between solutions, emulsions, and suspensions.	Review Questions, PTCB Exam Practice Questions, Activity 6-4
5. Explain the difference between ointments and creams.	Review Questions, PTCB Exam Practice Questions, Activity 6-4
6. Identify the various routes of administration and give examples of each.	Review Questions, PTCB Exam Practice Questions, Activity 6-2, Activity 6-4
7. Give examples of common medications for various routes of administration.	Review Questions, Activity 6-1, Activity 6-4, Lab 6-1
8. Identify the advantages and disadvantages of each route of administration.	Review Questions, Activity 6-4
9. Identify the parenteral routes of administration.	Review Questions, PTCB Exam Practice Questions, Activity 6-4
10. Explain the difference between transdermal and topical routes of administration.	Review Questions, PTCB Exam Practice Questions, Activity 6-4
11. Explain the difference between sublingual and buccal routes of administration.	Review Questions, PTCB Exam Practice Questions, Activity 6-4
12. Identify the abbreviations for the common routes of administration and dosage formulations.	Review Questions, Activity 6-4

INTRODUCTION

As a pharmacy technician, one of your many responsibilities is to work with the pharmacist to prepare and dispense medications to patients. You need to know that drugs can come from one of three sources: natural, synthetic, or genetically engineered.

You also need to understand the concept of drug nomenclature and how to recognize a drug's chemical, generic, and trade/brand names. Finally, you must be familiar with the meaning of and use for each dosage form and route. Most of the dosage forms do imply a certain route that is to be used. However, many dosage forms may be administered via several different routes. For example, a tablet is commonly administered orally, but it can be administered vaginally as well. Liquid medications can also be administered in a variety of ways. If the prescription order is not clear as to the dosage form and route, the pharmacy staff and medical staff must work together to determine what is best for the patient and to avoid medication errors.

REVIEW QUESTIONS

Match the following.

1. _____ anhydrous
2. _____ aromatic
3. _____ aqueous
4. _____ dosage form
5. _____ emollient
6. _____ emulsion
7. _____ formulary
8. _____ HMO
9. _____ homogenous
10. _____ hydrophobic
11. _____ nomenclature
12. _____ occlusive
13. _____ oleaginous
14. _____ route of administration
15. _____ synthesized
16. _____ semi-synthetic
17. _____ synthetic
18. _____ viscous
19. _____ volatile

a. actual form of the drug
b. listing of drugs approved for use
c. a group having all the same qualities
d. evaporates rapidly
e. set of names; way of naming
f. without water
g. thick; almost jelly-like
h. containing oil; has oil-like properties
i. having a fragrant aroma
j. a naturally occurring compound that has been chemically altered
k. drug produced in a laboratory to imitate a naturally occurring compound
l. contains water
m. health maintenance organization
n. liquid mixture of water and oil
o. how a drug is introduced into or on the body
p. closes off; keeps air away
q. repels water
r. softening and soothing to the skin
s. drugs that are not naturally occurring in the body

Choose the best answer.

20. Which is not one of the classifications of sources of drugs?
    a. genetically engineered
    b. synthetic
    c. natural
    d. manufactured

21. A disadvantage of solid-dose medications is:
    a. longer shelf life before expiration.
    b. dosing is more accurate.
    c. patients are able to self-administer.
    d. they take longer to be absorbed.

22. Creams are:
    a. semisolid.
    b. solid.
    c. semiliquid.
    d. jellyfied.

Match the following drugs with their sources.

23. _____ morphine
24. _____ aspirin
25. _____ human growth hormone
26. _____ vincristine
27. _____ OxyContin
28. _____ Pepsin
29. _____ adrenaline
30. _____ digoxin

    a. synthesized epinephrine
    b. the stomach of a cow
    c. synthetic opium
    d. periwinkle
    e. pituitary gland
    f. opium poppy plant
    g. white willow bark
    h. foxglove

Fill in the blanks.

31. A drug is _____ if it is a naturally occurring substance that has been chemically altered.

32. _____ release carbon dioxide when they come into contact with liquid.

33. Collodions are alcoholic solutions that contain _____.

34. Oleaginous ointments are _____ used to soothe and cool the skin or mucous membranes.

35. Emulsions are comprised of _____ and _____.

PHARMACY CALCULATION PROBLEMS

Calculate the following.

1. Levetiracetam is usually initiated at 20 mg/kg/day in two divided doses for a pediatric patient. Determine the dose in milligrams for a boy who weighs 45 pounds.

2. Levetiracetam comes in a 100 mg/mL oral solution. How many milliliters will you need per dose for the patient in question #1?

3. If a patient is receiving ondansetron 4 mg IVP tid prn, what is the maximum daily dosage the patient will receive in milligrams?

4. If an acetaminophen 80 mg suppository is prescribed q6–8 hr prn, what is the maximum number of suppositories the patient can receive in a day?

5. What amount of active ingredient is contained in 60 gm of a 2.5% cream?

PTCB EXAM PRACTICE QUESTIONS

1. The best known example of a sublingual tablet formulation is:
   a. hydrochlorothiazide.
   b. nitroglycerin.
   c. digoxin.
   d. codeine.

2. Which would *not* be caused by particulate material in an intravenous injection?
   a. air emboli
   b. thrombus
   c. phlebitis
   d. necrosis

3. Emulsions are likely to be used in which route of administration?
   a. oral
   b. buccal
   c. topical
   d. sublingual

4. Which ophthalmic formulation will maintain the drug in contact with the eye the longest?
   a. solution
   b. gel
   c. suspension
   d. ointment

5. Which is the most common and uncomplicated route of administration?
   a. buccal
   b. intravenous
   c. oral
   d. topical

ACTIVITY 6-1: Case Study—Pain and Therapy

Instructions: Read the following scenario and then answer the critical thinking questions.

Mrs. Gupta, a mother of three children (all of whom are under 12 years of age), still has a fair amount of pain after her car accident nearly six months ago. She hurt her shoulder and has experienced radiating pain around the upper back, shoulder, and neck for months now. However, the doctors say that nothing major is wrong, and she does not need surgery.

Initially Mrs. Gupta was prescribed a strong painkiller, along with ibuprofen for the inflammation; then she was taken off the painkiller. However, her pain continued even weeks after the accident, and she was prescribed Vicodin one to two tablets two to three times daily as needed. Mrs. Gupta is in so much pain that if she does not take the Vicodin in time, she is unable to move for a while after ingesting the dose. Whenever she exerts herself, she finds that the pain intensifies, and she can barely make it to the next timed dose. If she takes the Vicodin on time, she is relaxed so much that the pain is just a memory.

In addition to the pain medication, her doctor is going to order physical therapy for Mrs. Gupta, in an attempt to help with mobility. The doctor has the nurse phone the therapy center and arrange for a recurring appointment for Mrs. Gupta to begin physical therapy.

1. What are some considerations regarding therapy scheduling for Mrs. Gupta?

   _____

   _____

   _____

2. Even though Mrs. Gupta blames all of her pain on the car accident, do you think the fact that she has three children at home contributes to her condition? Why or why not?

   _____

   _____

   _____

3. Can you think of other side effects that Mrs. Gupta might experience from the pain medicine when the physical therapy begins?

   _____

   _____

4. Mrs. Gupta is currently taking oral medications to treat her pain. What other route(s) of administration may be effective for treating pain? Why?

   _____

   _____

   _____

5. What concerns must be considered regarding Mrs. Gupta's current therapy plan?

   _____

   _____

   _____

ACTIVITY 6-2: Case Study—The Elderly and Medicine

Instructions: Read the following scenario and then answer the critical thinking questions.

Mrs. Wheaten is a lovely 87-year-old woman who reminds you of your grandmother. When she was in her 50s, she was diagnosed with bipolar depression; she has been coming to the retail pharmacy where you work for more than 22 years. Over the years, she has slowed down a bit and has had a few medical conditions arise. For example, she has high blood pressure that is hard to control, and sometimes has trouble breathing. She is also being treated with lithium for her bipolar condition. Other than that, she is much healthier than many people 10 years younger.

Today she presents at the pharmacy with a cough, stuffy nose, and slight headache. As with most people in the winter, Mrs. Wheaten has developed a cold with cough. She requests a box of pseudoephedrine, which is behind the counter. She also requests a recommendation from the pharmacist as to which cough medicine to take, how often, for how long, and how much. Mrs. Wheaten has an aspirin allergy and would like to stay away from drugs containing aspirin.

1. What does the pharmacist take into consideration about Mrs. Wheaten before recommending a drug selection and dose?

   _____

   _____

   _____

2. How do you handle her request for pseudoephedrine?

_____

_____

_____

3. Mrs. Wheaten would also like to know how much ibuprofen she can take to make her headache go away. How much should be given in this situation?

_____

_____

_____

ACTIVITY 6-3: Case Study—Long-Acting Option

Instructions: Read the following scenario and then answer the critical thinking questions.

Cedric is a 45-year-old male who has been battling depression for a very long time. At your pharmacy, his medication history is a catalogue of one depression medicine after another, with each one seeming to fail only to be replaced by a prescription for another. Because he usually takes his medicine two to three times a day, the number of tablets dispensed to Cedric over the last year alone totals about 1,000.

You feel sorry for this patient because he visits so much—approximately every two to three weeks—for a new medication. Sometimes his mood is pleasant and he can carry on a conversation, but during some visits he seems disorganized and lost, and talks to himself. Some of the pharmacy staff refer to him as "The Ghost of Mr. Cedric." You think at first that Cedric seems scattered at times because his medicine is changed so often.

During one of the conversations you had with Cedric, he told you that a friend comes by at seven in the morning and cooks him a nice breakfast, complete with a glass of milk. The rest of the day he either sleeps or gets busy. He says that his thoughts get so scattered as the day progresses that he becomes forgetful and cannot remember a thing.

Today Cedric has come to the pharmacy to pick up yet another new medicine for his depression: bupropion 75 mg twice a day. While at the intake window, you ask if he needs anything else and he says he sure doesn't think so, that he has enough medicine to supply an army.

1. Why do you think Cedric has an overstock of medication?

_____

_____

_____

2. Can you see any medication option for Cedric's situation today?

_____

_____

_____

3. What is the advantage of the option you selected over what he has been prescribed over the past year?

_____

_____

_____

ACTIVITY 6-4: Dosage Forms

Correct interpretation of standard pharmacy abbreviations found on prescriptions and medical orders is critical in your role as a pharmacy technician. Equally important is your ability to determine the appropriate route of administration for the dosage form given.

Activity:

The three scenarios that follow document each patient's current medical condition or history. After reading each scenario, use your knowledge of that patient's unique situation to determine which dosage form would be most beneficial to her or him.

Scenario 1

Briana, a 37-year-old woman, has just been hospitalized. She has a stomach virus and has been experiencing vomiting and diarrhea for three days. The doctor wants to give her ondansetron 4 mg tid prn for the nausea. He has also ordered IV fluids to help with her dehydration.

Scenario 2

Jacob, a 7-year-old boy, has been admitted to the hospital. His mother brought him in because he had a bad seizure an hour and a half ago. He was diagnosed with a seizure disorder the year before. Jacob seems coherent, and has no other medical issues. His physician would like to start him on a different medication, levetiracetam 200 mg bid.

Scenario 3

Aydin, a 3-year-old boy, has been complaining of a sore throat and is having trouble swallowing. He also has a mild fever. His mother called his pediatrician, who said to give him acetaminophen 80 mg every 4–6 hours until the doctor could see him the next morning.

Questions:

1. What is the best dosage form of ondansetron for Briana, based on her current medical condition?

    _____

    _____

    _____

    _____

2. What is the best dosage form of levetiracetam for Jacob?

    _____

    _____

    _____

    _____

3. Which dosage form would you choose to give to Aydin for his fever and sore throat?

    _____

    _____

    _____

    _____

4. Why do you think there are so many different kinds of dosage formulations?

_____

_____

_____

_____

5. What is the difference between transdermal and topical routes of administration?

_____

_____

_____

_____

6. What is the difference between sublingual and buccal routes of administration?

_____

_____

_____

_____

7. See how well you remember the abbreviations for the common routes of administration and dosage formulations by completing the following table.

	Route of Administration	Abbreviation
a.	Buccal	
b.	by mouth	
c.	External	
d.	Inhalation	
e.	Injection	
f.	Intradermal	
g.	Intramuscular	
h.	Intravenous	
i.	intravenous push	
j.	mouth/throat	
k.	Nasal	
l.	Ophthalmic	
m.	Oral	
n.	Otic	
o.	Rectally	
p.	Subcutaneous	
q.	Sublingual	
r.	Transdermal	

LAB 6-1: Identifying Chemical, Generic, and Brand Names of Drugs

Objectives:

Recognize and describe the differences between chemical, generic (nonproprietary), and brand/trade (proprietary) drug names.

Explain which types of names are commonly used and the purpose of the United States Adopted Names Council (USAN).

Pre-Lab Information:

- Review Chapter 6, "Dosage Formulations and Administration," in your textbook.
- Search on the Internet for the United States Adopted Names Council. One webpage you might try is http://www.ama-assn.org/ama/pub/physician-resources/medical-science/united-states-adopted-names-council.page. Research the USAN's main purpose, scope of practice, and approved drug-name stems.

Explanation:

When a drug company develops a new drug, it has to name it. Three different names are assigned to the drug. The chemical name, which is based on the chemical formula of the medication, is rarely used in pharmacy practice. For example, the full chemical name of Tylenol is *N*-acetyl-*p*-aminophenol. (You can see why it is used by only a handful of people, generally scientists or chemists.)

A generic name or nonproprietary name is also assigned to each drug. Generic drug names are not usually capitalized. If the medication is in the same class as another medication, it may have a similar suffix or stem. For example, most beta blockers have an "-olol" ending, like ateno*lol* or metopro*lol*. The drug manufacturer may enlist the help of the USAN to give a unique generic name to the new drug. USAN's primary goal is to create a name that will not look or sound like that of another drug already in existence.

The proprietary name (brand/trade name) is always capitalized, and symbols may indicate that the name is trademarked. This usually also indicates that the company has a patent on the medication. While under patent protection, the drug will be marketed exclusively under the brand name. A drug patent is good for 20 years, but after research, development, and animal and clinical trials, only a few years may actually be left on the patent. After the patent expires, other companies can manufacture the drug under its generic name.

Activity:

Part One

In each of the following questions there are three drug names. You must determine which are the chemical, generic, and trade names. In addition, you must search USAN's approved stems on the Internet, and determine the appropriate category for each drug based on its generic name. Finally, list the available dosage formulation(s) and routes of administration(s) for the medication.

> Hint:
> Look at the suffix. For example, for candesartan, look for "-sartan" on the USAN stems page; you will find that it is an angiotensin II receptor antagonist.

1. sodium hydrogen bis(2-propylpentanoate) _____

   divalproex sodium _____

   depakote _____

   Category: _____

   Dosage formulation(s): _____

   Route(s) of administration: _____

2. famciclovir _____

   famvir _____

   2-[2-(2-amino-9H-purin-9-yl)ethyl]-1,3-propanediol diacetate _____

   Category: _____

   Dosage formulation(s): _____

   Route(s) of administration: _____

3. adipex-p _____

   α α Dimethylphenethylamine hydrochloride _____

   phentermine hydrochloride USP _____

   Category: _____

   Dosage formulation(s): _____

   Route(s) of administration: _____

4. 3-[2-(dimethylamino)ethyl]-N-methyl-indole-5-methanesulfonamide succinate (1:1) _____

   imitrex _____

   sumatriptan succinate _____

   Category: _____

   Dosage formulation(s): _____

   Route(s) of administration: _____

5. celecoxib _____

   celebrex _____

   4-[5-(4-methylphenyl)-3-(trifluoromethyl)-1H-pyrazol-1-yl] benzenesulfonamide _____

   Category: _____

   Dosage formulation(s): _____

   Route(s) of administration: _____

Part Two

Review the following list of drug names, and note for each whether it is a brand (B) or generic (G) name. Then, determine the route of administration of each drug. Note that all drug names in the list appear in lower case so as not to give you any clues.

Drug	Brand or Generic?	Route of Administration?
1. caduet		
2. pulmicort respules		
3. miconazole		
4. tetrahydrozoline		
5. cortisporin		
6. insulin		
7. amoxicillin clavulanate		
8. atorvastatin		
9. janumet		
10. zolpidem		
11. enbrel		
12. medrol		
13. oxycodone		
14. spiriva		
15. duragesic		
16. flonase		
17. rhinocort aqua		
18. benzaclin		
19. restoril		
20. warfarin sodium		

Student Name: _____

Lab Partner: _____

Grade/Comments: _____

_____

_____

Student Comments: _____

_____

_____

_____

LAB 6-2: Identifying Dosage Forms

Objectives:

Recognize and distinguish the various types of pharmaceutical dosage forms.

Pre-Lab Information:

• Review Chapter 6, "Dosage Formulations and Routes of Administration," in your textbook.

Explanation:

Medications are available in various dosage forms; the term refers to how the medication is prepared for administration to the patient. Common dosage forms include tablets, solutions, suspensions, inhalants, creams, and ointments. A single medication may be available in multiple dosage forms to allow use for various disease states, patient age ranges, and desired results.

Activity:

Observe various medications, either set out by your instructor or shown as images. For each medication, identify the correct dosage form—being as specific as possible. For example, if it is a liquid medication, is it a solution, a suspension, an emulsion, etc. In addition, list at least one potential advantage and one possible disadvantage for the dosage formulation, based on information presented in the textbook.

1. Dosage Form: _____
   Advantage(s): _____
   Disadvantage(s): _____

2. Dosage Form: _____
   Advantage(s): _____
   Disadvantage(s): _____

3. Dosage Form: _____
   Advantage(s): _____
   Disadvantage(s): _____

4. Dosage Form: _____
   Advantage(s): _____
   Disadvantage(s): _____

5. Dosage Form: _____
   Advantage(s): _____
   Disadvantage(s): _____

Student Name: _____

Lab Partner: _____

Grade/Comments: _____

_____

Student Comments: _____

_____

LAB 6-3: Identifying Routes of Administration

Objectives:

Recognize and distinguish the various routes of administration.

Pre-Lab Information:

• Review Chapter 6, "Dosage Formulations and Routes of Administration," in your textbook.

Explanation:

Medications are delivered to a patient by a variety of routes of administration. The route of administration (ROA) is simply the method by which a medication is introduced into the body for absorption and distribution. The route of administration can vary from patient to patient and depends on the effect desired from the administered medication.

Activity:

Observe various medications, either set out by your instructor or shown as images. For each medication, identify the correct route of administration—being as specific as possible. For example, if it is a parenteral medication, is it to be administered IV, IM, etc. In addition, list at least one potential advantage and one possible disadvantage for the dosage formulation, based on information presented in the textbook.

1. Route of Administration: _____
   Advantage(s): _____
   Disadvantage(s): _____

2. Route of Administration: _____
   Advantage(s): _____
   Disadvantage(s): _____

3. Route of Administration: _____
   Advantage(s): _____
   Disadvantage(s): _____

4. Route of Administration: _____
   Advantage(s): _____
   Disadvantage(s): _____

5. Route of Administration: _____
   Advantage(s): _____
   Disadvantage(s): _____

Student Name: _____

Lab Partner: _____

Grade/Comments: _____

_____

_____

Student Comments: _____

_____

CHAPTER 7
Referencing and Drug Information Resources

After completing Chapter 7 from the textbook, you should be able to:	Related Activity in the Workbook/Lab Manual
1. Explain the need for referencing and drug information resources.	Review Questions, PTCB Exam Practice Questions, Activity 7-1, Lab 7-1, Lab 7-2, Lab 7-3, Lab 7-4
2. Outline and describe the proper steps for referencing drug information resources.	Review Questions, Activity 7-1, Lab 7-1, Lab 7-2, Lab 7-3, Lab 7-4
3. Explain how package insert monographs are used for referencing.	Review Questions, PTCB Exam Practice Questions, Lab 7-1
4. List and describe the most commonly used printed drug reference books in pharmacies.	Review Questions, PTCB Exam Practice Questions, Activity 7-1, Lab 7-2, Lab 7-3
5. List and describe the most commonly used electronic and web-based references in pharmacies.	Review Questions, Lab 7-4
6. Outline and describe the proper steps for evaluating the credibility of a website for use as a reference.	Review Questions, Activity 7-2, Lab 7-4
7. List and describe the most commonly used journals and magazines in pharmacies	Review Questions

INTRODUCTION

Pharmacy practice relies on accurate and timely information, and new, revised, and updated information occurs at a frequent pace within health care sciences. Physicians, nurses, pharmacists, pharmacy technicians, and other health care professionals must stay constantly informed on the latest drugs, therapeutic indications, dosing standards, and clinical evidence. Pharmacy professionals, in particular, must stay well informed as both patients and health care professionals, such as doctors and nurses, often turn to the pharmacist for answers to their medication-related questions. The pharmacist commonly handles these inquiries through the process of referencing. As a pharmacy technician, therefore, mastering the ability to reference drug information resources is critical. Although in many cases the information will be able to be communicated only by the pharmacist, a pharmacy technician can play a vital role in helping the pharmacist look up the needed information. In other cases, pharmacy technicians will rely on the ability to reference drug information resources for their roles in pharmacy practice.

REVIEW QUESTIONS

Match the following.

1. _____ referencing
2. _____ drug information resources
3. _____ off-label usage
4. _____ drug classification
5. _____ therapeutic indication
6. _____ index
7. _____ apps

a. any source providing credible, evidence-based, and evaluated drug information.

b. grouping drugs together based on similar chemical structures, mechanisms of action, or pharmacologic effects.

c. an alphabetical listing of names or subjects with page references for ease of use.

d. the specific disease or condition a drug is intended to treat.

e. using drug information resources to find evidence-based information.

f. applications, can refer to use on computers, smartphones, tablets, etc.

g. the practice, regulated by the FDA, of physicians prescribing approved medications for use other than their intended indication.

Choose the best answer.

8. Off-label usage is regulated by the _____.
   a. DEA
   b. FDA
   c. SBOP
   d. USP

9. _____ refers to a specific disease or condition a drug is intended to treat.
   a. Drug classification
   b. Drug indication
   c. Therapeutic classification
   d. Therapeutic indication

10. Which reference book contains average wholesale prices (AWP) for prescription drugs?
    a. *AHFS-DI*
    b. *Facts and Comparisons*
    c. *RED BOOK*
    d. *USP-NF*

11. The _____ contains detailed information on more than 1,000 of the most prescribed drugs, but it is designed primarily for use in physician offices.
    a. *AHFS-DI*
    b. *FDA Orange Book*
    c. *PDR*
    d. *USP-NF*

12. _____ is part of the U.S. National Library of Medicine.
    a. Medline
    b. MEDMARX
    c. Micromedex
    d. none of the above

13. The *Handbook on Injectable Drugs* contains all of the following information on parenteral drugs, except:
    a. compatibility.
    b. pricing.
    c. sizes.
    d. strengths.

14. Determining the appropriate reference source is the _____ step in referencing.
    a. first
    b. second
    c. third
    d. fourth

15. Skyscape is an example of a _____ reference source:
    a. book-based
    b. journal-based
    c. website-based
    d. all of the above

Identify which of the following reference sources contain drug monograph information.

16. _____ PDR
17. _____ Handbook on Injectable Drugs
18. _____ Remington
19. _____ Medline
20. _____ USP-NF
21. _____ Goodman & Gilman's
22. _____ AJHP
23. _____ Orange Book
24. _____ RED BOOK
25. _____ Facts and Comparisons

a. contains drug monograph information
b. does NOT contain drug monograph information

Fill in the blanks.

26. _____ is the largest registry of adverse drug events in the United States.
27. _____ is the Micromedex product that assists in the identification of unknown drugs by imprint code or slang term.
28. *Drug Topics*, *Pharmacy Times*, and *U.S. Pharmacist* are all published _____ times per year.
29. _____ is the most commonly used drug information reference used in community pharmacies.
30. AHFS Drug Information is primarily used in _____ pharmacies.

PHARMACY CALCULATION PROBLEMS

Calculate the following.

1. $1/8 + 1/4 =$

2. $3/5 - 1/10 =$

3. $4 \times 1/3 =$

4. $1/8 \div 2/3 =$

5. $5\ 3/7 \times 2\ 1/2$

PTCB EXAM PRACTICE QUESTIONS

1. On a package insert, the _____ section lists the types of patients who should not use the medication.
   a. contraindications
   b. clinical pharmacology
   c. indications and usage
   d. warnings

2. Which of the following reference sources does not contain drug monographs?
   a. *American Drug Index*
   b. *Facts and Comparisons*
   c. *Geriatric Dosage Handbook*
   d. *Remington*

3. The _____ requires package inserts as part of the labeling of a drug.
   a. CDC
   b. DEA
   c. FDA
   d. USP

4. _____ allows facilities to anonymously and voluntarily report adverse drug events.
   a. Medline
   b. Medscape
   c. MEDMARX
   d. Micromedex

5. The _____ is published by the FDA.
   a. *American Drug Index*
   b. *Orange Book*
   c. *RED BOOK*
   d. *USP-NF*

ACTIVITY 7-1: Selecting the Best Reference Source

Instructions: Describe a scenario in which each of the following sources would be the best choice as a reference source.

1. *Martindale*

   _____
   _____
   _____
   _____

2. *USP-NF*

   _____
   _____
   _____
   _____

3. *Handbook on Injectable Drugs*

   _____
   _____
   _____
   _____

4. *RED BOOK*

_____

_____

_____

_____

5. MEDMARX

_____

_____

_____

_____

_____

ACTIVITY 7-2: Case Study—Analyzing Credible Sources

Instructions: Read the following scenario and then answer the critical thinking questions.

Adriana is 34 years old and a regular patient at your pharmacy. She comes in on a Saturday minutes before the pharmacy is scheduled to close. She explains to the pharmacist that she has been experiencing mild to sharp pains in her lower abdomen for roughly 24 hours. Adriana wants to know which laxative the pharmacist recommends.

Although the pharmacist would typically provide a recommendation for a brand of laxative upon request, the pharmacist is curious why the patient is looking for a laxative if she is only experiencing abdominal pain. Constipation can certainly cause moderate to sharp pain in the lower abdomen, but it could be something else. After asking Adriana several questions, the pharmacist learns that she has been having regular bowel movements, but she is convinced that she must be constipated.

Adriana explains that she used the Symptom Checker on WebMD and that adult constipation was one of the top three possible conditions. She fails to mention that there were 56 other possible conditions listed, including appendicitis, irritable bowel syndrome, urinary tract infection, and more.

1. How should the pharmacist respond to Adriana? What recommendation(s) could be made?

_____

_____

_____

2. What possible outcome(s) might have occurred if the patient simply asked the pharmacist for a recommendation for laxatives, without providing any other information?

_____

_____

_____

3. Self-diagnosis and misguided health decisions are growing exponentially as a result of the Internet. How can pharmacy professionals aid in reducing this trend?

_____

_____

_____

LAB 7-1: Using a Package Insert for Referencing

Objective:

Demonstrate the ability to obtain pertinent drug information by using a package insert as a reference source.

Pre-Lab Information:

Review Chapter 7, "Referencing and Drug Information Resources," in your textbook.

Explanation:

Pharmacy professionals must stay well informed as both patients and health care professionals often turn to the pharmacist for answers to medication-related questions. Although the pharmacist handles these questions, pharmacy technicians can play a valuable role by aiding with the referencing and research process. This exercise will help you gain experience in referencing drug resources.

Activity:

Using a package insert from a prescription drug, locate and document the following information:

Drug Name (Brand/Generic): _____

1. Available dosage forms
   _____
   _____

2. Available strengths
   _____
   _____

3. Storage requirements
   _____
   _____

4. Common adult dosage
   _____
   _____

5. Indication(s)
   _____
   _____

6. Mechanism of action
   _____
   _____

7. Contraindication(s)

_____

_____

8. Precaution(s)

_____

_____

9. Warning(s)

_____

_____

10. Adverse reaction(s)

_____

_____

Student Name: _____

Lab Partner: _____

Grade/Comments: _____

_____

_____

Student Comments: _____

_____

_____

LAB 7-2: Using Drug Fact and Comparisons or AHFS-DI for Referencing

Objective:

Demonstrate the ability to obtain pertinent drug information by using either *Drug Facts and Comparisons* or *AHFS-DI* as a reference source.

Pre-Lab Information:

Review Chapter 7, "Referencing and Drug Information Resources," in your textbook.

Locate a copy of either *Drug Facts and Comparisons* or *AHFS-DI*.

Explanation:

Pharmacy professionals must stay well informed as both patients and health care professionals often turn to the pharmacist for answers to medication-related questions. Although the pharmacist handles these questions, pharmacy technicians can play a valuable role by aiding with the referencing and research process. This exercise will help you gain experience in referencing drug resources.

Activity:

Using *Drug Facts and Comparisons* or *AHFS-DI*, select one of the following prescription drugs, locate, and document the following information:

Choose one of the following medications: Ceclor, Levsin SL Mannitol I.V., Seroquel XR, or Zoloft.

Reference Source Used: _____

Drug Name (Brand/Generic): _____

1. Available dosage forms

   _____

   _____

2. Available strengths

   _____

   _____

3. Storage requirements

   _____

   _____

4. Common adult dosage

   _____

   _____

5. Indication(s)

   _____

   _____

6. Mechanism of action

_____

_____

7. Contraindication(s)

_____

_____

8. Precaution(s)

_____

_____

9. Warning(s)

_____

_____

10. Adverse reaction(s)

_____

_____

Student Name: _____

Lab Partner: _____

Grade/Comments: _____

_____

_____

Student Comments: _____

_____

_____

LAB 7-3: Selecting and Using a Drug Reference Source

Objective:

Demonstrate the ability to obtain pertinent drug information by using various drug reference sources.

Pre-Lab Information:

Review Chapter 7, "Referencing and Drug Information Resources," in your textbook.
Select an appropriate drug reference source.

Explanation:

Pharmacy professionals must stay well informed as both patients and health care professionals often turn to the pharmacist for answers to medication-related questions. Although the pharmacist handles these questions, pharmacy technicians can play a valuable role by aiding with the referencing and research process. This exercise will help you gain experience in referencing drug resources.

Activity:

Using a credible drug reference source, select one of the following prescription drugs, locate and document the following information:

Choose one of the following medications: alprazolam, Bacitracin, Factor IX Complex, ketoprofen, or Pepcid Injection.

Reference Source Used: _____

Drug Name (Brand/Generic): _____

1. Available dosage forms

   _____

   _____

2. Available strengths

   _____

   _____

3. Storage requirements

   _____

   _____

4. Common adult dosage

   _____

   _____

5. Indication(s)

   _____

   _____

6. Mechanism of action

_____

_____

7. Contraindication(s)

_____

_____

8. Precaution(s)

_____

_____

9. Warning(s)

_____

_____

10. Adverse reaction(s)

_____

_____

Student Name: _____

Lab Partner: _____

Grade/Comments: _____

_____

_____

Student Comments: _____

_____

_____

LAB 7-4: Analyzing the Credibility of a Website as a Reference

Objective:

Demonstrate the ability to obtain pertinent drug information from a credible website.

Pre-Lab Information:

Review Chapter 7, "Referencing and Drug Information Resources," in your textbook.

Explanation:

The Internet contains a vast amount of information on medical conditions and prescription drugs; however, all websites are not equal. With the ease of creating and publishing online content, medical information is being provided by both trustworthy and untrustworthy sources. This exercise will help you gain experience in researching medical information online and assessing the credibility of the content.

Activity:

Choose any disease state or medical condition that you are interested in researching. Using the Internet, search for information on the condition, assessing the credibility of the website and source. The website that you use does not have to be a credible source, for this lab activity.

Do NOT use WebMD or Wikipedia for this activity.

Selected Condition/Disease State: _____

Website address: _____

Step 1. Determine the website's authority and accuracy.

1. Who is the author of the content? What are their qualifications/credential/expertise?

   _____

   _____

2. Is the information provided reliable?

   _____

   _____

Step 2. Analyze the website's purpose and content.

3. What is the purpose of the website?

   _____

   _____

4. Does the website provide clinical, educational, or factual information?

   _____

   _____

5. Is the website balanced, objective and informational, or is it subjective and biased?

   _____

   _____

6. Is the website owned or sponsored by a commercial interest?

_____

_____

Step 3. Review the currentness of the website.

7. When was the website last revised/updated? How current is the information provided?

_____

_____

Step 4. Consider the website's design, organization, and ease of use.

8. Is the website clearly organized and easy to navigate and read?

_____

_____

9. Does the website have an appropriate search capability?

_____

_____

10. Does the website provide a help section for instructions on use?

_____

_____

Your assessment:

Is this website a credible and trustworthy source that could be used as a reference source? Explain.

_____

_____

_____

_____

_____

_____

Student Name: _____

Lab Partner: _____

Grade/Comments: _____

_____

_____

Student Comments: _____

_____

_____

Chapter 8
Retail Pharmacy

After completing Chapter 8 from the textbook, you should be able to:	Related Activity in the Workbook/Lab Manual
1. Explain the ambulatory pharmacy practice setting.	Review Questions, Activity 8-2
2. Describe the two main types of retail pharmacies.	Review Questions, Activity 8-2
3. List the various staff positions in retail pharmacies.	Review Questions, Activity 8-2, Activity 8-5
4. Describe the typical work environment of a retail pharmacy.	Review Questions, Activity 8-2, Lab 8-6
5. Discuss the two agencies that regulate retail pharmacy practice.	Review Questions, PTCB Exam Practice Questions
6. List the legal requirements of a prescription medication order.	Review Questions, PTCB Exam Practice Questions, Activity 8-4, Lab 8-1
7. Describe the different ways prescriptions arrive at a retail pharmacy.	Review Questions, Activity 8-1, Lab 8-4, Lab 8-5
8. List the steps required for a prescription to be filled.	Review Questions, PTCB Exam Practice Questions, Activity 8-1, Activity 8-2, Lab 8-4, Lab 8-5
9. Discuss the various job duties of technicians in retail pharmacies.	Review Questions, Activity 8-1, Activity 8-2, Activity 8-4, Activity 8-5, Lab 8-1, Lab 8-2, Lab 8-3, Lab 8-4, Lab 8-5, Lab 8-6
10. Discuss the importance of confidentiality for personal health information.	Review Questions, PTCB Exam Practice Questions, Activity 8-3

INTRODUCTION

The two main types of pharmacy practice are ambulatory and institutional. An institutional pharmacy is located on the site of the patients' residence; pharmacies within hospitals, nursing homes, hospices, and long-term care facilities are examples. Most other pharmacies fall into the category of ambulatory. Examples of ambulatory settings, which are usually called *community-based* or *retail pharmacies*, are privately owned, chain, and franchise pharmacies, as well as clinics. Retail pharmacy is the largest category of pharmacy in the United States. These types of pharmacies serve the community in which they are located.

The staff at a retail pharmacy includes the pharmacist in charge (PIC), pharmacy manager, staff pharmacists, pharmacy technicians, and, in many cases, pharmacy clerks. It is a fast-paced work environment where pharmacy professionals interact with patients face to face. Pharmacy technicians have numerous job responsibilities, from taking care of inventory orders, rotations, returns, and billing to counting, measuring, filling, and labeling. In the retail environment, you may also help patients find over-the-counter (OTC) medications or lead them to the pharmacist for counseling, to name only a few of your daily tasks. In ambulatory pharmacy, every day is another opportunity to serve the community.

REVIEW QUESTIONS

Match each of the following.

1. _____ chain pharmacy
2. _____ franchise pharmacy
3. _____ neighborhood pharmacy
4. _____ outpatient pharmacy

a. owned by an individual, with several different owner-operated locations

b. privately owned, relatively small in size, pharmacy

c. corporately owned, more than four pharmacies

d. affiliated with a health care system, hospital, clinic, or ambulatory care facility

Fill in the blanks.

5. The process of transmitting a prescription electronically to the appropriate insurance carrier for approval is called _____.

6. The code DAW, when written by the prescriber, means _____.

7. An electronic record stored in the pharmacy computer system detailing the patient's personal and billing information, prescription records, and medical conditions is known as a/an _____.

8. When the patient resides where the medication is kept, the pharmacy there is described as a/an _____ pharmacy.

9. The agency that registers and regulates pharmacies, pharmacists, and pharmacy technicians, as well as the practice of pharmacy, is known as the _____.

10. The _____ conducts inspections to ensure compliance with its guidelines and also approves reimbursement for Medicare and Medicaid.

True or False?

11. Retail pharmacy practice allows for a more hands-on approach.

    T   F

12. The term "Pharm.D." is used to designate a Director of Pharmacy.

    T   F

13. Pregnancy tests can be obtained only with a prescription.

    T   F

14. Any OTC product may be kept behind the counter if the pharmacist chooses.

    T   F

Choose the best answer.

15. Which of the following is not an approved prescriber?
    a. DDS
    b. PA
    c. DVM
    d. RN

16. Which of the following is a valid DEA number for Dr. Rebecca Carey?
    a. AC5932764
    b. BC8162753
    c. BC3791250
    d. AC79131591

17. A C-III prescription may be refilled:
    a. six times.
    b. zero times.
    c. for six months from the date it was written.
    d. for one year from the date it was first filled.

18. Which of the following is not required on a prescription?
    a. route of administration
    b. patient's age
    c. strength of drug
    d. prescriber's signature

19. The prescriber wrote Mr. Mallory's prescription for Synthroid® on 12/14/2008 with prn refills. Mr. Mallory had the prescription filled for the first time on 03/09/2009. He may continue receiving monthly refills until:
    a. 12/14/2009.
    b. 12/14/2008.
    c. 03/09/2010.
    d. 03/09/2009.

20. The second group of numbers in an NDC code signifies:
    a. package size.
    b. manufacturer.
    c. drug, strength, and form.
    d. cost (AWP).

21. Once a medication has left the pharmacy counter, it may:
    a. not be returned for resale.
    b. not be returned for a refund.
    c. not be returned for resale or refund.
    d. be refunded and/or resold if the pharmacist allows.

22. Most pharmacies and insurance providers require a prescription to be _ used before it may be refilled.
    a. 50%
    b. 90%
    c. 75%
    d. 100%

23. Most states restrict controlled medications with refills:
    a. to a maximum of one transfer.
    b. to zero transfers; controlled substances may not be refilled.
    c. so that all refills written by the prescriber may be transferred.
    d. to a maximum of three refills that are transferred.

24. It is not a technician's responsibility to:
    a. verify the information in a patient's profile.
    b. counsel a patient on the use of a medication.
    c. double-count a controlled medication for accuracy.
    d. contact an insurance provider on behalf of a patient.

25. When Mrs. Rigby asked to have her Lunesta® prescription transferred from across town, the technician should:
    a. explain to her that controlled medications cannot be transferred.
    b. inform her that the sending pharmacy has to call.
    c. check her profile to see if the prescription had been transferred before and if there are any refills remaining.
    d. apprise her that it may take up to 24 hours to complete the transfer.

PHARMACY CALCULATION PROBLEMS

Calculate the following.

1. The directions for a prescription cough medicine states: Take 5 mL po q4h prn. If the patient takes the maximum daily amount, how long will a 120 mL bottle last?

2. If the sig on the prescription states "2 tabs po q hs," how many tablets will you need to dispense in order to last for 28 days?

3. If a patient is taking tetracycline 500 mg caps po bid, how many capsules are needed for a 30-day supply?

4. Jill is compounding a prescription that requires $\frac{3}{4}$ oz. of hydrocortisone 1% cream, $\frac{1}{4}$ oz. nystatin cream, and $\frac{1}{4}$ oz. of clotrimazole 1% cream. How many ounces will be in the finished product?

5. The directions for a prescription antibiotic state: Give 5 mL tid. Disp: 150 mL. What is the correct days supply for this prescription?

PTCB EXAM PRACTICE QUESTIONS

1. Which organization oversees the practice of community pharmacies in the United States?
   a. FDA
   b. DEA
   c. SBOP
   d. APHA

2. In the following number, NDC 51285-601-05, the first set (51285) represents which of the following?
   a. drug name
   b. manufacturer
   c. dosage form
   d. capsule size

3. How many times can you refill a prescription for Viagra®?
   a. As many times as indicated by the prescriber.
   b. As many times as indicated by the prescriber within one year from the date the prescription was written.
   c. Six times within six months.
   d. None.

4. Which law provides for protection of patient confidentiality?
   a. HIPAA
   b. TJC
   c. OSHA
   d. CSA

5. A technician receives a prescription for a controlled substance. The prescription is from out of state and the technician is unfamiliar with the physician and the customer. The DEA number for the physician is AG8642123. Based on the physician's DEA number, is this a fraudulent prescription?

ACTIVITY 8-1: Prescription Translation Worksheet

Review each of the following five prescriptions, then translate the information contained in each one.

Rx #1

Towne Center Family Medicine
40 Towne Center Drive
Pleasantville, Texas 77248-0124
Phone 281-555-0134 Fax 281-555-0125

James L. Brook, MD BB1234563   Rebecca Smith, MD AS1234563   Walter Roberts, MD AR1234563
Sharon Ortiz, NP   Beth Matthews, NP   Terri King, NP

Name_ *Melvin Brooks* _____ Age_____

Address_____ Date_ *Nov 21* _____

R_x

       Isordil 10 mg

           #60

        Tpo bid

Refill _____ times

_____
                Signature

A generically equivalent drug product may be dispensed unless the practitioner hand writes the words 'Brand Necessary' or 'Brand Medically Necessary' on the face of the prescription.

6HUR133050

1. Patient name: _____
2. Prescriber: _____
3. Drug name and strength: _____
4. Is generic substitution permitted? _____
5. Quantity to dispense: _____
6. Directions/ SIG: _____
7. Refills authorized: _____

Rx #2

Towne Center Family Medicine
40 Towne Center Drive
Pleasantville, Texas 77248-0124
Phone 281-555-0134 Fax 281-555-0125

James L. Brook, MD BB1234563   Rebecca Smith, MD AS1234563   Walter Roberts, MD AR1234563
Sharon Ortiz, NP   Beth Matthews, NP   Terri King, NP

Name_____*Beth Andrews*_____ Age_____

Address_____ Date__*03/12*_____

Rx

          Allegra 60mg

                  #60

          T po Bid

Refill____*2*____times

                            Signature

A generically equivalent drug product may be dispensed unless the practitioner hand writes the words
'Brand Necessary' or 'Brand Medically Necessary' on the face of the prescription.

                                                  6HUR133050

---

1. Patient name: _____
2. Prescriber: _____
3. Drug name and strength: _____
4. Is generic substitution permitted? _____
5. Quantity to dispense: _____
6. Directions/ SIG: _____
7. Refills authorized: _____

Rx #3

Towne Center Family Medicine
40 Towne Center Drive
Pleasantville, Texas 77248-0124
Phone 281-555-0134 Fax 281-555-0125

James L. Brook, MD BB1234563   Rebecca Smith, MD AS1234563   Walter Roberts, MD AR1234563
Sharon Ortiz, NP   Beth Matthews, NP   Terri King, NP

Name _Stephanie Ruiz_____ Age_____

Address_____ Date _March 12_____

℞

Azelex 308

#1

U UD

Refill ___3___ times

_____
Signature _Becky Smith_

A generically equivalent drug product may be dispensed unless the practitioner hand writes the words
'Brand Necessary' or 'Brand Medically Necessary' on the face of the prescription.

6HUR133050

1. Patient name: _____
2. Prescriber: _____
3. Drug name and strength: _____
4. Is generic substitution permitted? _____
5. Quantity to dispense: _____
6. Directions/ SIG: _____
7. Refills authorized: _____

Rx #4

Towne Center Family Medicine
40 Towne Center Drive
Pleasantville, Texas 77248-0124
Phone 281-555-0134 Fax 281-555-0125

James L. Brook, MD BB1234563   Rebecca Smith, MD AS1234563   Walter Roberts, MD AR1234563
Sharon Ortiz, NP   Beth Matthews, NP   Terri King, NP

Name _Algooter Prince_____ Age _____

Address _____ Date _4/20_____

Rx

Leset 80mg
#30

T + D

Refill __5___ times

Terri King
Signature

A generically equivalent drug product may be dispensed unless the practitioner hand writes the words
'Brand Necessary' or 'Brand Medically Necessary' on the face of the prescription.

6HUR133050

---

1. Patient name: _____
2. Prescriber: _____
3. Drug name and strength: _____
4. Is generic substitution permitted? _____
5. Quantity to dispense: _____
6. Directions/ SIG: _____
7. Refills authorized: _____

Rx #5

Towne Center Family Medicine
40 Towne Center Drive
Pleasantville, Texas 77248-0124
Phone 281-555-0134 Fax 281-555-0125

James L. Brook, MD BB1234563   Rebecca Smith, MD AS1234563   Walter Roberts, MD AR1234563
Sharon Ortiz, NP   Beth Matthews, NP   Terri King, NP

Name _Elesabeth Beastese_____ Age_____

Address_____ Date _3/20_____

℞

Damler 25 mg

#90

TP TID

Refill _____ times

_Terri King_____
Signature

A generically equivalent drug product may be dispensed unless the practitioner hand writes the words
'Brand Necessary' or 'Brand Medically Necessary' on the face of the prescription.

6HUR133050

1. Patient name: _____
2. Prescriber: _____
3. Drug name and strength: _____
4. Is generic substitution permitted? _____
5. Quantity to dispense: _____
6. Directions/ SIG: _____
7. Refills authorized: _____

ACTIVITY 8-2: Role Play—Retail Pharmacy Scenarios

Using the information provided, act out the scenario described, then reflect about the exercise through the use of the discussion questions.

Scenario 1

Cast:

- Customer
- Pharmacy Technician
- Pharmacist

Scene:

A customer approaches the pharmacy technician. The customer begins to describe experiencing symptoms of fever, body aches, and chills. The customer then asks the technician what over-the-counter product to purchase in order for the customer to feel better. The technician suggested to the customer to speak with the pharmacist. The customer agreed to the technician's suggestion. The pharmacist listened to the customer describing the symptoms being experienced. The pharmacist then recommended an over-the counter product to the customer.

Discussion Questions:

1. Was the pharmacy technician effective in his or her communication with the customer?

   _____

   _____

   _____

2. Did the pharmacy technician stay within his or her scope of practice while interacting with the customer?

   _____

   _____

   _____

3. At what point did the pharmacist become involved in assisting the customer? Was this appropriate?

   _____

   _____

   _____

Scenario 2

Cast:

- Pharmacy Technician
- Patient

Scene:

The patient brings in a prescription to be filled. The pharmacy technician explains that the current wait time is 30 to 45 minutes, which then outrages the patient. The technician apologizes for the wait time and the patient is still upset about the given time frame.

Discussion Questions:

1. Was the pharmacy technician professional in his or her communication with the patient?
   _____
   _____
   _____

2. How well did the pharmacy technician handle the upset patient?
   _____
   _____
   _____

3. Would you have handled the situation differently? Why? If so, what would you have done?
   _____
   _____
   _____

Scenario 3

Cast:

- Pharmacy Technician
- Patient

Scene:

The patient brings in a prescription to be filled, and the pharmacy technician explains that the current wait time is 30 minutes. The patient explains that he or she is going to run a quick errand and will then return. Upon returning, the pharmacy technician explains to the patient that the prescription will not be available until the following day at 10:30 a.m., after the pharmacy's morning delivery, because the pharmacy is out of the medication. The patient is unhappy that he or she was not informed of this when the prescription was first dropped off to be filled.

Discussion Questions:

1. What mistakes, if any, did the pharmacy technician make?
   _____
   _____
   _____

2. How did the pharmacy technician resolve the situation with the patient?
   _____
   _____
   _____

3. Would you have handled the situation differently? Why? If so, what would you have done?

_____

_____

_____

ACTIVITY 8-3: Case Study — Privacy/HIPAA

Instructions: Read the following scenario and then answer the critical thinking questions.

A remodel of the work space at the retail pharmacy in which you work has finally begun. Many people were involved in the design planning, including various construction personnel. However, no one from the pharmacy itself was included on the planning committee. Weeks pass, and it appears that the newly remodeled pharmacy will allow a more efficient use of space.

The remodel is completed on a Friday, and everyone returns to work on Monday excited to see the new space. Almost immediately, everyone notices that the redesigned space lacks an adequate area for patient counseling. HIPAA mandates that every pharmacy have a patient counseling area.

The pharmacy does not close down while this space is added, but instead remains open for business, and pharmacy personnel are asked to "work around" the inconvenience. You are told that the counseling area will be in place after two more weeks of construction. In the meantime, it seems almost impossible to find a private space to counsel patients.

1. What are some creative ways in which the pharmacy could assure patient privacy during counseling until construction is complete?

_____

_____

_____

_____

2. What effect might this inconvenience have on the pharmacy workload, in terms of time?

_____

_____

_____

3. Describe what a HIPAA-compliant counseling area, which protects patient privacy, might look like or include.

_____

_____

_____

_____

Research: Research more information about HIPAA-compliant counseling areas for pharmacy. Does any of the information you find surprise you? How does the information you discover compare with the reality of the pharmacy you personally use?

ACTIVITY 8-4: Case Study—Biases

Instructions: Read the following scenario and then answer the critical thinking questions.

A gangly, unkempt, middle-aged man with a slightly offensive odor presents a prescription at your pharmacy for hydrocodone bitartrate 5 mg/acetaminophen 500 mg #120 to be taken twice daily as needed for pain. He attempts to rush you through the process, talking excessively and stating that he should be getting more than what was prescribed. His actions make you suspicious, in that he appears nervous, is constantly looking around, and becomes increasingly agitated with each question you ask, such as his address and phone number. It appears that the amount of tablets may have been altered, but you are not quite certain, as this provider's writing is not very legible.

The man becomes more and more uncooperative as you try to gain the information you need to process the prescription, but finally you have everything you need. You have been trained to notice things that may raise questions as to the validity of prescriptions and feel that this may be one such situation. You bring this to the attention of the pharmacist in charge, who in turn calls to verify the prescription. It turns out that the prescription is legitimate and the patient has some mental health issues.

1. What were some factors in this scene that made the technician suspect that this might be a fraudulent prescription?

   _____

   _____

   _____

   _____

2. Can you identify any communication barriers present with this type of patient?

   _____

   _____

   _____

   _____

3. Do you think that the way the patient was dressed or acted contributed to the assessment that his might be a fraudulent prescription?

   _____

   _____

   _____

   _____

ACTIVITY 8-5: Case Study—Patient Requests Recommendations

Instructions: Read the following scenario and then answer the critical thinking questions.

Mrs. Hornbuckle, with her 4-year-old daughter in tow, approaches the pharmacy counter and requests some assistance in locating the Children's Tylenol Liquid. You are the only person available, and state that it is located on aisle 6 toward the back of the store; you then offer to show her to the area. Mrs. Hornbuckle accepts your offer and the three of you head to aisle 6.

You point out the Children's Tylenol Liquid section, but before you can walk away, Mrs. Hornbuckle begins asking questions about the wide array of Tylenol liquid preparations. She states that her daughter has a really bad cough and wants to know which one works best, the grape- or the cherry-flavored. Meanwhile, she is picking up boxes and reading the information on the back.

You explain that a pharmacist could answer any questions she may have about the medicines. With a frustrated sigh, she says, "Forget it," and starts to walk out in a huff, obviously upset that you were not able to answer the questions yourself.

1. Why might Mrs. Hornbuckle have felt that you could (and should) have answered her questions about medications?

_____

_____

_____

_____

2. Do you think pharmacy technicians should identify themselves as such, or would it matter to the general public, who may not know the difference between pharmacy technicians and pharmacists?

_____

_____

_____

_____

3. How would you explain to a patient/customer, in an understanding way, your limited authority as a pharmacy technician?

_____

_____

_____

_____

LAB 8-1: Checking a Prescription for Completeness

Objective:

To interpret some sample prescriptions, identify their key components, and then determine if the prescriptions contain all of the necessary information required for processing.

Pre-Lab Information:

Review Tables 5-4, 5-5, 5-6, and 5-7 from Chapter 5 of your textbook to re-familiarize yourself with various medical terms and abbreviations.

Explanation:

Many times a legitimate prescription lacks some of the information required for processing. This exercise will help you review the key components of a prescription, practice translating prescriptions, as well as for you to identify any imperative missing information required for processing.

Activity:

Four prescriptions have been dropped off at the pharmacy to be filled. The first step is to put the data from the prescriptions into the computer. Translate the prescription, note all key points that must be printed on the labels, and determine if the prescriptions contain all the information needed for processing.

Name _Jill Johnson_____ Age_____

Address___79 Holiday Rd_____ Date _06/08/15_____

Rx

Metoprolol tablets

#60

Sig: 1 po bid

Refill____5____times

L. MacCoy
_____
Signature

A generically equivalent drug product may be dispensed unless the practitioner hand writes the words
'Brand Necessary' or 'Brand Medically Necessary' on the face of the prescription.

6HUR133050

1. Does the information seem correct on the prescription for Jill Johnson? How would you translate the instructions for the prescription label? Is there any imperative missing information from this prescription?

_____

_____

_____

Dr. Fillmore McGraw
100 Hollywood Blvd.
Los Angeles, CA 00000
(800) 123-4567

Name _Britanny Spires_____ Age_____

Address _6002 Hillside Place_____ Date _07/02/15_____

R

Xanax 0.25 mg tablet

Sig: 1 po tid prn anxiety

Refill ____0____ times

Fillmore McGraw
Signature

A generically equivalent drug product may be dispensed unless the practitioner hand writes the words
'Brand Necessary' or 'Brand Medically Necessary' on the face of the prescription.

6HUR133050

2. Does the information seem correct on the prescription for Britanny Spires? How would you translate the instructions for the prescription label? Is there any imperative missing information from this prescription?

_____

_____

_____

Name Sandy Deitz   Age _____

Address 123 Laramy Ct   Date 05/14/15

Rx

Sig: Promethazine 25 mg

1 q4-6hrs prn nausea

Refill _____ 0 _____ times

Elsie Kumar, MD
Signature

A generically equivalent drug product may be dispensed unless the practitioner hand writes the words 'Brand Necessary' or 'Brand Medically Necessary' on the face of the prescription.

6HUR133050

3. Does the information seem correct on the prescription for Sandy Deitz? How would you translate the instructions for the prescription label? Is there any imperative missing information from this prescription?

_____

_____

_____

Timothy Stiles, DDS
65 Main St.
Davenport, IA 00000
(563) 111-2222

Name _Jeremy Jacobsen_____ Age _____

Address _455 Brady Street_____ Date _7/25/15_____

R℞

Amoxicillin 500 mg

Sig: 1 po TID X 10 days

Refill ____O____ times

_____
Signature

A generically equivalent drug product may be dispensed unless the practitioner hand writes the words
'Brand Necessary' or 'Brand Medically Necessary' on the face of the prescription.   6HUR133050

---

4. Does the information seem correct on the prescription for Jeremy Jacobsen? How would you translate the instructions for the prescription label? How many capsules will be needed to fill this prescription? Is there any imperative missing information from this prescription?

   _____

   _____

   _____

Student Name: _____

Lab Partner: _____

Grade/Comments: _____

_____

Student Comments: _____

_____

_____

LAB 8-2: Counting Oral Medication in a Community Pharmacy Setting

Objective:

To demonstrate the ability to count oral medications manually as well as gain experience with cleaning procedures in the pharmacy.

Pre-Lab Information:

- Review Chapter 8, "Retail Pharmacy," in the textbook.
- Gather the following supplies:
- Pill counting tray and spatula
- Large bag of M&Ms®, Skittles®, or other small-sized hard candy
- Prescription vials, plastic sandwich bags, or other containers for the "tablets"
- Isopropyl alcohol (70%)

Explanation:

This exercise will give you the opportunity to practice counting "tablets" manually. In the pharmacy, tablets are generally counted in increments of five, while using a pill counting tray and spatula on a clean, clutter-free counter. It requires ongoing practice for you to feel confident and efficient in counting tablets by fives. Until you gain experience, please remember to count tablets twice before giving them to the "pharmacist."

Option: You can complete this lab utilizing automated counting and dispensing equipment to gain experience in using this equipment.

Activity:

Part 1

For this first exercise, you will count 15 tablets.

1. Prepare a clean, clutter-free work surface, and then place a clean pill counting tray and spatula in front of you.
2. Pour a substantial amount of your "tablets" into the counting tray. Then open the lid of the pour compartment.
3. Begin counting the "tablets" in increments of five while using the counting spatula. Slide each group of five "tablets" into the pour compartment of your tray. Count by fives until you reach 15 tablets. Then close the lid of the pour compartment.
4. Return any unused "tablets" that remain in your counting tray to their original container or bag.
5. Select an appropriate-sized prescription vial and place it on the counter next to the counting tray.
6. Pour or "re-dispense" the "tablets" you counted into the vial.
7. Now pour the "tablets" you counted back into your counting tray and count them again to make sure you have 15.
8. Repeat step 6. Then place the appropriate-sized lid on the prescription vial.

Part 2

For this next exercise, you will use the materials from the previous activity to prepare the following "prescriptions" for "dispensing."

1. Ibuprofen [M&Ms] 800 mg

   Sig: 1 tab tid × 10 days

   Count the correct number of "tablets" required to fill this prescription.

2. M&Mcycline 320 mg tabs

   Sig: 1 tab qid × 5 days

   Count the correct number of "tablets" required to fill this prescription.

3. M&Mnisone 20 mg tabs

   Sig: 1 tab qid × 2 days; 1 tab tid × 2 days; then 1 tab daily × 2 days

   Count the correct number of "tablets" required to fill this prescription.

Feel free to continue counting until all of the "tablets" are "re-dispensed."

Part 3

To complete this lab activity, please clean your materials and work area using a disinfectant solution of water and 70% isopropyl alcohol. Spray the solution on the counting tray and spatula, then wipe them both with a paper towel and return them to the shelf or appropriate storage location. Then, spray the counter with the solution and wipe the counter down.

Student Name: _____

Lab Partner: _____

Grade/Comments: _____

_____

_____

Student Comments: _____

_____

_____

LAB 8-3: Processing a New Patient

Objective:

Demonstrate the ability to follow the procedure for processing a new patient.

Pre-Lab Information:

Review Chapter 8 in your textbook.

Explanation:

As a pharmacy technician working in a retail pharmacy, you will need to create a new patient profile for each new customer. The patient profile is an electronic record stored in the pharmacy computer system that details the patient's personal and billing information, prescription records, and medical conditions.

Activity:

In this exercise, you will work with a partner to create a mock patient profile and insurance card. You will then trade information and each create a new patient profile in the computer.

Materials Needed

- Pharmacy computer station
- Patient profile information
- Insurance information

Procedure

1. Complete a new patient profile form using the blank form that follows. The information you enter should be fictitious; do not use your own personal information.
2. Create an insurance card by using the template provided. Again, use fictitious information.
3. Trade information with your lab partner and add your partner's information to the pharmacy computer system as though your partner were a new patient.

4. Review the information entered for accuracy.

PATIENT PROFILE

Patient Name

_____   _____   _____

          Last   **First**   **Middle Initial**

- -

_____

        Street or PO Box

_____   _____   _____

       City   State   Zip

- -

Phone   Date of Birth   Social Security No.
( ) _____ _____   □ Male □ Female   ___ ___ ___
           Month   Day   Year

□ Yes, I would like medication dispensed in a child-resistant container.
□ No, I do not want medication dispensed in a child-resistant container.
Medication Insurance   Card Holder Name _____
□ Yes   □ No   □ Card Holder   □ Child   □ Disabled Dependent
                       □ Spouse   □ Dependent Parent   □ Full Time Student

MEDICAL HISTORY

HEALTH		ALLERGIES AND DRUGS REACTIONS
□ Angina	□ Epilepsy	□ No known drug allergies or reactions
□ Anemia	□ Glaucoma	□ Aspirin
□ Arthritis	□ Heart Condition	□ Cephalosporins
□ Asthma	□ Kidney Disease	□ Codeine
□ Blood Clotting Disorders	□ Liver Disease	□ Erythromycin
□ High Blood Pressure	□ Lung Disease	□ Penicillin
□ Breast Feeding	□ Parkinson's Disease	□ Sulfa Drugs
□ Cancer	□ Pregnancy	□ Tetracyclines
□ Diabetes	□ Ulcers	□ Xanthines

Other Conditions _____   Other Allergies/Reactions _____
_____
_____

Prescription Medication Being Taken   OTC Medication Currently Being Taken
_____   _____
_____   _____
_____   _____

Would You Like Generic Medication Where Possible? □ Yes □ No

Comments _____

Health information changes periodically. Please notify the pharmacy of any new medications, allergies, drug reactions, or health conditions.
_____ Signature _____ Date □ I do not wish to provide this information.

United Health Care
1-800-555-3456

Subscriber No.   Group No.

_____   _____

Name _____

Patient Code_____

Rx 10/25/50   Effective 01/09

Discussion Questions:

1. Did you enter the patient's information accurately on the first attempt? If not, what mistake(s) did you make?

   _____

   _____

2. Why is the information on the patient profile form so important?

   _____

   _____

   _____

   _____

3. What are the most common patient codes, and what do they represent?

   _____

   _____

Student Name: _____

Lab Partner: _____

Grade/Comments: _____

_____

_____

Student Comments: _____

_____

_____

LAB 8-4: Processing a New Prescription

Objective:

Demonstrate ability to follow the procedure for processing a new prescription.

Pre-Lab Information:

Review the steps listed in Procedure 8-2, "Entering a Prescription," in Chapter 8 of your textbook.

Explanation:

As a pharmacy technician working in a retail pharmacy, you will need to process new prescriptions for your customers. This process has many steps, including receiving the order either in person, or by phone, fax, or e-mail, depending on the regulations of your particular state. Next you must review the order for legality and correctness, and then translate the order. This all happens before the prescription may be entered into the computer system.

Activity:

In this exercise, you will enter the mock prescription that follows into the computer system and print a label.

Materials Needed

- Pharmacy computer station
- Prescription
- Printer
- Prescription labels

Procedure

1. Enter the prescription that follows into the pharmacy computer system.
2. Review the information as entered for accuracy.
3. Print a prescription label.

Towne Center Family Medicine
40 Towne Center Drive
Pleasantville, Texas 77248-0124
Phone 281-555-0134 Fax 281-555-0125

James L. Brook, MD BB1234563   Rebecca Smith, MD AS1234563   Walter Roberts, MD AR1234563
Sharon Ortiz, NP   Beth Matthews, NP   Terri King, NP

Name___Taylor Payne_____   Age_____

Address_____   Date___April 21_____

R℞

Amoxil 500mg
#20
T POBFD X 10D

Refill_____times

_____ _Becky Smith_
                                Signature

A generically equivalent drug product may be dispensed unless the practitioner hand writes the words
'Brand Necessary' or 'Brand Medically Necessary' on the face of the prescription.

6HUR133050

Discussion Questions:

1. Whom did you list as the prescriber?

   _____

2. What is the proper days supply for this prescription?

   _____

3. If the patient approved generic substitution, what drug name should be printed on the label?

   _____

Optional Activity:

For additional practice, process the prescriptions provided in Activity 8-1, "Prescription Translation Worksheet."

Student Name: _____

Lab Partner: _____

Grade/Comments: _____

_____

_____

Student Comments: _____

_____

_____

LAB 8-5: Processing a Refill Request

Objective:

Demonstrate ability to follow the procedure for processing a refill request.

Pre-Lab Information:

Review Chapter 8 in your textbook.

Review the steps listed in Procedure 8-4, "Requesting a Refill Authorization," in Chapter 8 of your textbook.

Explanation:

As a pharmacy technician working in a retail pharmacy, you will need to process prescription refills. This involves documenting patient refill orders, verifying prescription refills, processing orders with refills available, and contacting prescribers to seek approval for prescriptions for which additional refills are needed.

Activity:

Review the two prescription refill requests that follow and list the specific steps necessary to perform each one.

Rx #1

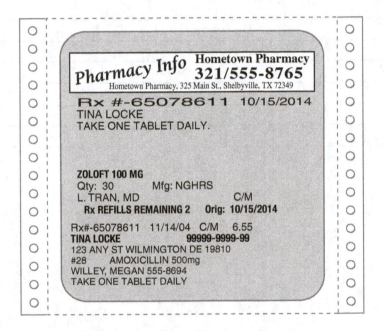

List the steps for processing this prescription refill:

_____

_____

_____

_____

_____

Rx #2

```
Date – April 5
For – Patient, Jim Roberts
Message – Needs a refill for his blood pressure medication
```

After looking up the patient's profile, you determine that he has no remaining refills for his blood pressure medication.

List the steps for processing this prescription refill:

_____
_____
_____
_____
_____
_____

Student Name: _____

Lab Partner: _____

Grade/Comments: _____
_____
_____

Student Comments: _____
_____
_____

LAB 8-6: Cash Register Maintenance

Objective:

Demonstrate skill in replacing cash register tapes and ribbons.

Pre-Lab Information:

- Familiarize yourself with the cash register used in your lab and instructions on how to replace cash register tape and ink ribbons.

Explanation:

As a pharmacy technician working in a retail pharmacy, you will need to be able to operate the cash register, including changing cash register tape and ink ribbons.

Materials Needed

- Cash register
- Cash register tape
- Cash register ink ribbons

Activity:

Replace the cash register tape according to the instructions specific to your cash register.

1. List the steps for changing cash register tape.

_____

_____

_____

_____

_____

Replace the cash register ink ribbon according to the instructions specific to your cash register.

2. List the steps for changing cash register ink ribbon.

_____

_____

_____

_____

_____

_____

Student Name: _____

Lab Partner: _____

Grade/Comments: _____

_____

_____

Student Comments: _____

_____

_____

CHAPTER 9
Health-System Pharmacy

After completing Chapter 9 from the textbook, you should be able to:	Related Activity in the Workbook/Lab Manual
1. Describe the health-system pharmacy practice setting.	Review Questions, PTCB Exam Practice Questions, Activity 9-1, Activity 9-3, Activity 9-5
2. Describe the advantages of a unit-dose system.	Review Questions, PTCB Exam Practice Questions, Activity 9-4
3. List the necessary components of a medication order.	Review Questions, Activity 9-2, Lab 9-1, Lab 9-2, Lab 9-3
4. Compare the duties of a technician with those of a pharmacist in accepting a medication order in a health-system setting.	Review Questions, Activity 9-2, Activity 9-3, Activity 9-5
5. Compare centralized and decentralized unit-dose systems.	Review Questions, Activity 9-4
6. Compare the duties of a technician with those of a pharmacist in filling a medication order in a health-system setting.	Review Questions, Activity 9-2, Activity 9-3, Activity 9-5, Lab 9-1, Lab 9-2, Lab 9-3
7. Define the tasks pharmacy technicians perform in health-system settings.	Review Questions, Activity 9-1, Activity 9-2, Activity 9-3, Activity 9-5, Lab 9-1, Lab 9-2, Lab 9-3

INTRODUCTION

A health-system pharmacy, also called an *institutional pharmacy*, is designed to serve patients who live onsite. Examples of facilities that might include an institutional pharmacy are long-term care facilities, nursing homes, hospitals, correctional facilities, and hospices. Regardless of the type of facility, the on-site pharmacy is responsible for all patients' medications; pharmacy staff must ensure that drug therapies are appropriate, effective, and safe. The health-system pharmacist also identifies, resolves, and prevents medication-related problems. As a pharmacy technician working in this setting, you must understand the policies and procedures of your institution, as well as state and federal laws. In addition to filling pre-scriptions and medication orders, you might also work with several distribution systems, repackage bulk medications for floors and patient care areas, use unit-dose and automatic dispensing systems, and handle sterile products.

REVIEW QUESTIONS

Match each of the following.

1. _____ blister packs
2. _____ decentralized pharmacy system
3. _____ centralized pharmacy system
4. _____ emergency medication orders
5. _____ floor stock
6. _____ POE system
7. _____ unit dose
8. _____ STAT order
9. _____ standing order
10. _____ patient prescription stock system
11. _____ PRN order

a. a specific order required to respond to a medical emergency
b. medication order that takes priority over other orders and requests
c. orders are reviewed, prepared, verified, and delivered to the patient
d. allows prescribers to enter orders directly into the pharmacy computer system
e. scheduled order to be administered throughout the day
f. consists of central, inpatient, outpatient, and satellite pharmacies
g. unit-dose packages
h. all pharmacy-related services are performed in one location
i. order used only as necessary or needed
j. medication order is filled for no more than a 24-hour period
k. medications stored on the same floor where patients' rooms are, for patient distribution

Choose the best answer.

12. A licensed individual who is trained to examine patients, diagnose illnesses, and prescribe/administer medication is a:
    a. doctor of medicine (MD).
    b. doctor of osteopathy (DO).
    c. licensed nursing assistant (LNA).
    d. licensed practical nurse (LPN).

13. An individual who is licensed to provide basic care, such as administering medication under the supervision of an RN, is a:
    a. doctor of medicine (MD).
    b. doctor of osteopathy (DO).
    c. licensed nursing assistant (LNA).
    d. licensed practical nurse (LPN).

14. An individual who is registered to assist physicians with specific procedures, administer medication, and provide patient care is a:
    a. licensed practical nurse (LPN).
    b. licensed nursing assistant (LNA).
    c. registered nurse (RN).
    d. nurse practitioner (NP).

15. An individual who is certified to assist RNs and LPNs in providing patient care, but is not permitted to administer medication, is a:
    a. licensed practical nurse (LPN).
    b. licensed nursing assistant (LNA).
    c. registered nurse (RN).
    d. nurse practitioner (NP).

16. An individual who is licensed to work closely with a physician in providing patient care, typically under the supervision of a physician, is a:
    a. licensed practical nurse (LPN).
    b. licensed nursing assistant (LNA).
    c. registered nurse (RN).
    d. nurse practitioner (NP).

17. A licensed individual, who is trained to coordinate patient care under the supervision of a medical or osteopathic doctor, is a:
    a. licensed practical nurse (LPN).
    b. licensed nursing assistant (LNA).
    c. physician's assistant (PA).
    d. nurse practitioner (NP).

18. A pharmacy that provides services to onsite patients 24 hours a day, 365 days each year, is called a:
    a. mail-order pharmacy.
    b. health-system pharmacy.
    c. community pharmacy.
    d. all of the above.

19. The American Hospital Association (AHA) categorizes hospitals as community-based, federal government, psychiatric, long-term care, or institutional hospital units. Which represent 85% of the total number of registered hospitals?
    a. community-based
    b. federal government
    c. long-term care
    d. psychiatric

Match the following organizations/agencies/regulations to their area of influence.

20. _____ HIPAA
21. _____ OBRA
22. _____ CMS
23. _____ SCHIP
24. _____ DPH
25. _____ CLIA

a. laboratories
b. children
c. privacy
d. counseling
e. regulates hospitals
f. Medicare/Medicaid

PHARMACY CALCULATION PROBLEMS

Calculate the following.

1. A hospitalized patient needs a 24-hour supply of sucralfate 1 gm tablets. How many tablets will be dispensed if the patient is administered it as a qid dose?

2. A patient on the infectious disease floor takes 10 mL of levofloxacin syrup bid. If the product is only available as a 5 mL unit-dose oral syringe, how many syringes will the technician prepare for a 24-hour supply?

3. A technician is checking floor stock on one of the nursing units. She notices that the floor has five acetaminophen 325 mg tablets left, but their par level is 20. How many tablets should the technician restock?

4. While checking a crash cart tray that was recently used for a code, Bill finds that there are two epinephrine syringes left in the tray. When the tray is fully stocked, it contains 12 epinephrine syringes. How many syringes should be restocked in the tray?

5. Karen is repackaging cyanocobalamin 1,000 mcg tablets into unit dosages on February 16, 2014. The manufacturer's expiration date for the product is December 2015. What expiration date should Karen assign to the repackaged medication?

PTCB EXAM PRACTICE QUESTIONS

1. Which of the following health care practitioners is not considered a prescriber?
   a. medical doctor (MD)
   b. physician assistant (PA)
   c. nurse practitioner (NP)
   d. certified nursing assistant (CNA)

2. A unit dose is a:
   a. package that contains all non-controlled medications for a given day.
   b. package that contains all medications for a given day.
   c. controlled substance.
   d. package that contains the amount of given day medication for one dose.

3. Which of the following allows a patient to receive medications on an as-needed basis?
   a. STAT order
   b. standing order
   c. parenteral
   d. PRN order

4. Nurses track medication administration on a/an:
   a. PCU.
   b. PRN.
   c. STAT.
   d. MAR.

5. In the health-system setting, needles and other items that can cut or puncture the skin should be thrown away in:
   a. MSDS.
   b. designated sharps containers.
   c. red garbage bags.
   d. regular garbage cans.

ACTIVITY 9-1: Role Play—Health-System Pharmacy Scenarios

Using the information provided, act out the scenario described, then reflect about the exercise through the use of the discussion questions.

Scenario 1

Cast:

• Pharmacy Technician
• Pharmacist
• Nurse

Scene:

The pharmacy technician is on the phone with a nurse who is complaining that the PRN floor stock medication is running low and that it should be refilled. While the technician is on the phone, the pharmacist brings a STAT order to the technician to fill for the emergency room.

Discussion Questions:

1. How did the pharmacy technician prioritize his or her work? Was this correct?

   _____

   _____

2. Did the pharmacy technician remain calm and professional or become flustered?

   _____

   _____

3. What, if anything, would you have done differently?

   _____

   _____

Scenario 2

Cast:

- Pharmacy Technician
- Pharmacist

Scene:

While preparing three IV bags, the pharmacy technician forgets to have the pharmacist check the measured volumes of medication before it is added to the IV bags. The technician knows that the medication is very expensive and is very nervous about alerting the staff pharmacist about the mishap.

Discussion Questions:

1. What could have caused the pharmacy technician's error?

   _____

   _____

2. How did the pharmacist and pharmacy technician resolve the matter? Was this appropriate?

   _____

   _____

3. How else could this situation have been resolved?

   _____

   _____

Cast:

- Pharmacy Technician 1
- Pharmacy Technician 2

Scene:

Pharmacy Technician 1 is training Pharmacy Technician 2 on how to establish expiration dates when repackaging medication into blister packs. They are working with ibuprofen 600 mg, which (according to the manufacturer) will expire in 18 months.

Discussion Questions:

1. Did the two pharmacy technicians establish a proper expiration date for the repackaged medication?

   _____

   _____

2. Was Pharmacy Technician 1 effective in teaching Pharmacy Technician 2?

   _____

   _____

3. Would you have handled the situation differently? Why? If so, what would you have done?

   _____

   _____

ACTIVITY 9-2: Medication Order Translation Worksheet

Review and translate each of the medication orders provided below.

Medication Order #1

<table>
<tr><td colspan="2">PHYSICIAN'S ORDER WORKSHEET</td><td>45671001   311A
Eckels, Ruby G.
04-10-1943

Dr. C. Thomsen</td></tr>
</table>

NOTE: *Person initiating entry should write legibly, date the form using (Mo/Day/Yr.), enter time, sign, and indicate their title.*

USE BALL POINT PEN (PRESS FIRMLY)

Date	Time	Treatment
10/18	4:30	Dilaudid 0.5 mg IV inject q 3h prn pain

(2)

	Distribution:	
PHYSICIAN'S ORDER WORKSHEET	(Original) Medical Record Copy (Plies 3, 2, & 1) Pharmacy	**T-5**

1. Patient name: _____
2. Prescriber: _____
3. Drug name and strength: _____
4. Directions/SIG: _____

CHAPTER 9 *Health-System Pharmacy*   **143**

Medication Order #2

PHYSICIAN'S ORDER WORKSHEET

NOTE: *Person initiating entry should write legibly, date the form using (Mo/Day/Yr.), enter time, sign, and indicate their title.*

USE BALL POINT PEN (PRESS FIRMLY)

132445855   210
Sanchez, Roberto L.
10-01-1940

Dr. L. Hubbard

Date	Time	Treatment
7/14	10:30	Vevaquin 500 mg IV infusion over 6hr
		②

PHYSICIAN'S ORDER WORKSHEET

Distribution:
(Original) Medical Record Copy
(Plies 3, 2, & 1) Pharmacy

T-5

1. Patient name: _____
2. Prescriber: _____
3. Drug name and strength: _____
4. Directions/SIG: _____

Medication Order #3

PHYSICIAN'S ORDER WORKSHEET

NOTE: *Person initiating entry should write legibly, date the form using (Mo/Day/Yr.), enter time, sign, and indicate their title.*

USE BALL POINT PEN (PRESS FIRMLY)

82347665   835 A
George, Sarah M.
02-17-1961

Dr. L. Montgomery

Date	Time	Treatment
4/10	13:00	Ibuprofen 600 mg po q 6hr
		②

 PHYSICIAN'S ORDER WORKSHEET   Distribution:
(Original) Medical Record Copy
(Plies 3, 2, & 1) Pharmacy   **T-5**

1. Patient name: _____
2. Prescriber: _____
3. Drug name and strength: _____
4. Directions/SIG: _____

Medication Order #4

PHYSICIAN'S ORDER WORKSHEET

NOTE: *Person initiating entry should write legibly, date the form using (Mo/Day/Yr.), enter time, sign, and indicate their title.*

USE BALL POINT PEN (PRESS FIRMLY)

782467199   1410 B
Smith, Cody M.
11-18-1975

Dr. L. Halberdier

Date	Time	Treatment
8/14	13:15	Ranitidine 150 mg Infuse over 24 hr
		②

	PHYSICIAN'S ORDER WORKSHEET	Distribution: (Original) Medical Record Copy (Plies 3, 2, & 1) Pharmacy	T-5

1. Patient name: _____
2. Prescriber: _____
3. Drug name and strength: _____
4. Directions/SIG: _____

ACTIVITY 9-3: Case Study—Health Care Professional Demands Medication

Instructions: Read the following scenario and then answer the critical thinking questions.

You are one of two pharmacy technicians working the graveyard shift at a local community hospital of 230 beds. The single pharmacist working the same evening is currently out of the pharmacy, consulting on a dosing recommendation for a powerful IV antibiotic, which must be administered to an inpatient soon. A nurse practitioner calls in to the pharmacy and frantically tells you that a loading dose of 1,500 mg IV vancomycin is needed, to be started right away on another patient. The nurse practitioner reinforces the urgent request by saying, "Have it ready when I get there in less than 2 minutes," and hangs up abruptly. Clearly, the NP is on the way to the pharmacy.

You decide to head into the IV room to start preparing the sterile solution while the other pharmacy technician attempts to contact the pharmacist, who is still out of the pharmacy.

1. What would you do if the nurse practitioner appeared at the pharmacy, demanding the IV vancomycin, while the pharmacist was still unavailable?

   _____

   _____

   _____

2. Can you think of any situation in which a pharmacy technician would be allowed to hand over the medication before a pharmacist checks it?

   _____

   _____

   _____

3. Is it a good idea to begin making the IV vancomycin to save time?

   _____

   _____

   _____

4. Can you think of another way to accomplish this task other than the solution given?

   _____

   _____

   _____

© 2014 Pearson Education, Inc.

CHAPTER 9 *Health-System Pharmacy* **147**

ACTIVITY 9-4: Case Study—Unit Dosing

Instructions: Read the following scenario and then answer the critical thinking questions.

Pharmacy technicians have always packaged the unit-dose medications in the nursing home where you work. In recent weeks, it seems the procedures have not been followed according to policy. In light of this information, you have been placed in charge of the unit-dosing processes for all ward stock areas. Three other pharmacy technicians also help out in this area, all working different shifts.

Numerous unit-dose medications are available for patients on the wards. You inspect the wards and notice that there are also large bottles of such items as Maalox®, Benadryl® liquid, Tylenol®, and docusate sodium. It seems that almost every patient receives these medications, and a nursing staff explains that it is easier just to have these large bottles available. Besides, these are all OTC medications anyway. Your understanding of the Joint Commission on the Accreditation of Healthcare Organizations recommendations is that all medications on ward stock are to be unit dosed, if unit doses are available from the manufacturer or when repackaging by the pharmacy into unit doses is feasible. You must decide whether to unit dose these bulk items you find in the ward stock areas.

1. What factors would you use to determine when unit dosing is feasible? Give examples.

   _____

   _____

   _____

2. Which of the medications mentioned in the scenario would you unit dose? What other types of bulk medications would normally be used in a ward stock situation?

   _____

   _____

   _____

3. How would you communicate any updates to the process to the other pharmacy technicians who work with unit dosing? How would you convey the importance of your decisions?

   _____

   _____

   _____

4. What regulations from what agencies can you find that relate to the unit dosing of medications?

   _____

   _____

   _____

ACTIVITY 9-5: Case Study—Outside Request for Dosing Information on Patient

Instructions: Read the following scenario and then answer the critical thinking questions.

All nine certified pharmacy technicians at the 120-bed community hospital where you work have received ongoing education through the facility monthly for the past three years. This CE has placed special emphasis on cyber-security and HIPAA.

An outside call comes in one evening while you are working and the person at the other end of the line begins asking a simple question. The caller goes on to explain that her father was recently a patient at the hospital and his outside doctor needs to know what dose of digoxin was prescribed while the father was a patient. The caller states that she knows it was 0.25 mg every day, but wants to verify it now. Your train of thought leads to your recent training and you inform this person that you are unable to answer that question; instead, you refer her to another source.

The person on the phone now informs you that she called the previous day and whoever answered then gave her the information that the digoxin dose was 0.25 mg per day. You ask the caller if she knows who she spoke to, and she names one of the certified pharmacy technicians who was answering phones that day.

1. Should this concern you? If so, for what reason?

_____

_____

_____

2. Can you give the information requested to the outside person on the phone? Why or why not?

_____

_____

_____

3. To what source did you refer this outside relative for answers to her question?

_____

_____

_____

4. What regulation(s) or guideline(s), in both the cyber-security and HIPAA arenas, do you know of that would govern why you would or would not divulge this information?

_____

_____

_____

LAB 9-1: Locating Basic Lab Values

Objective:

Become familiar with common lab values that the health-system pharmacist may use to monitor patients.

Pre-Lab Information:

- Review Chapter 9, "Health-System Pharmacy," in your textbook.
- Visit the following website as an introduction to normal human lab values: http://www.globalrph.com /labs.htm

Explanation:

It is important for you to have a basic understanding of the laboratory values used in the health-system and other pharmacy settings. This exercise will help you gain experience by looking up the most common "labs."

Activity:

Go to the website http://www.globalrph.com/labs.htm. Look up the information included in the following tables. Add the normal lab values for each item.

CBC		
Hemoglobin (g/dL)	Male Normal _____ g/dL	Female Normal _____ g/dL
Hematocrit (%)	Male Normal _____ %	Female Normal _____ %
Platelet Count	Normal Range _____	
White Blood Count (WBC)	Normal Range _____	

Metabolic Panel	Normal Range
Sodium	
Potassium	
Calcium (ionized)	
Chloride	
Glucose	
Blood Urea Nitrogen (BUN)	
Creatinine	
Albumin	
Alkaline phosphatase (ALP)	
Aspartate aminotransferase (AST)	
Alanine aminotransferase (ALT)	

Lipid Panel	Normal Range
Total cholesterol	
HDL cholesterol	
LDL cholesterol	
Triglycerides	

Student Name: _____

Lab Partner: _____

Grade/Comments: _____

_____

_____

Student Comments: _____

_____

_____

LAB 9-2: Filling a Medication Order

Objective:

To follow the proper procedure for filling a medication order.

Pre-Lab Information:

Review Chapter 9, "Health-System Pharmacy," in your textbook.

Explanation:

The medication order form is a multipurpose tool for communication among various members of the health care team who are working within a health system. In addition to the listed prescribed medications, this form can be used by the physician for ordering lab values, dietary considerations, X-rays, or other medical procedures. It is imperative that all pharmacy personnel be able to properly distinguish and interpret medication orders.

Hospitals may use a physical, hard-copy medication order form. Alternatives to a hard-copy medication order form are: a physician order entry system (POE) or a computerized physician order entry system (CPOE). The CPOE is a computerized system in which orders are entered electronically into the hospital's networked system.

Activity:

Review each of the following medication orders. Please enter each of them into the pharmacy computer system to generate the appropriate labels. Then fill the medications, and label the prescriptions for the pharmacist to review.

If you do not have access to a pharmacy computer system, you may use the blank label that appears at the end of this lab.

PHYSICIAN'S ORDER WORKSHEET

NOTE: *Person initiating entry should write legibly, date the form using (Mo/Day/Yr.), enter time, sign, and indicate their title.*

USE BALL POINT PEN (PRESS FIRMLY)

```
63450091          105
Randall, Kristen F.
09-28-63

Dr. R. Manini
```

Date	Time	Treatment
3/30	10:5?	Restoril 15mg po qhs prn sleep
		②

PHYSICIAN'S ORDER WORKSHEET

Distribution:
(Original) Medical Record Copy
(Plies 3, 2, & 1) Pharmacy

T-5

Medication Order # 2

PHYSICIAN'S ORDER WORKSHEET

NOTE: *Person initiating entry should write legibly, date the form using (Mo/Day/Yr.), enter time, sign, and indicate their title.*

USE BALL POINT PEN (PRESS FIRMLY)

```
51298556          620 B
Nguyen, Kim T.
05-05-1971

Dr. K. Tran
```

Date	Time	Treatment
9/8	8:30	Vicodin 5/500 PO PRN PAIN
		②

PHYSICIAN'S ORDER WORKSHEET

Distribution:
(Original) Medical Record Copy
(Plies 3, 2, & 1) Pharmacy

T-5

Medication Order #3

PHYSICIAN'S ORDER WORKSHEET

NOTE: *Person initiating entry should write legibly, date the form using (Mo/Day/Yr.), enter time, sign, and indicate their title.*

USE BALL POINT PEN (PRESS FIRMLY)

93471287   515B
Goodman, Ronald B.
06-15-1958

Dr. K. Patel

Date	Time	Treatment
4/10	11:20	Diflucan 200 mg IV over 4 hrs
		②

| | PHYSICIAN'S ORDER WORKSHEET | Distribution: (Original) Medical Record Copy (Plies 3, 2, & 1) Pharmacy | **T-5** |

Use the following label template to perform this lab if you do not have access to a computer.

Hometown Pharmacy, 325 Main St., Shelbyville, TX 72349, phone 321-555-8765

Prescription #:

Patient:

Prescriber:

Prescription:

Quantity:

Directions:

SIG:

Date Filled:

Refills Remaining:

Discussion Questions:

1. What was the most challenging aspect of this lab for you? Why?

   _____

   _____

   _____

2. Did you enter and fill each prescription accurately and correctly? If not, what mistakes did you make? How will you avoid making such errors in the future?

   _____

   _____

   _____

Student Name: _____

Lab Partner: _____

Grade/Comments: _____

_____

_____

Student Comments: _____

_____

_____

LAB 9-3: Processing a New Medication Order

Objective:

To follow the proper procedures for processing a new medication order.

Pre-Lab Information:

Review Chapter 9, "Health-System Pharmacy," in your textbook.

Explanation:

As a pharmacy technician in a health-system setting, you will need to know the correct procedures for entering a new medication order into the computer system.

Activity:

Materials Needed

- Pharmacy computer station
- Prescription
- Printer
- Prescription labels

Procedure

1. Enter the prescription provided below to you into the pharmacy computer system.
2. Review the information entered for accuracy.
3. Print a prescription label.

If you do not have access to a pharmacy computer system, you can use the blank label that appears at the end of Lab 9-2.

PHYSICIAN'S ORDER WORKSHEET

NOTE: *Person initiating entry should write legibly, date the form using (Mo/Day/Yr.), enter time, sign, and indicate their title.*

USE BALL POINT PEN (PRESS FIRMLY)

10875532   1218 A
Luke, Monica S.
01-15-1955

Dr. W. Huey

Date	Time	Treatment
12/10	6:15	Furosemide 10 mg q d
		②

PHYSICIAN'S ORDER WORKSHEET

Distribution:
(Original) Medical Record Copy
(Plies 3, 2, & 1) Pharmacy

T-5

Discussion Questions:

1. Whom did you list as the prescriber?

   _____

2. Is this prescription to be administered by mouth or intravenously?

   _____

3. What is the brand name of the medication prescribed?

   _____

Optional Activity:

For additional practice, process the prescriptions provided in Activity 9-2, "Medication Order Translation Worksheet."

Student Name: _____

Lab Partner: _____

Grade/Comments: _____

_____

_____

Student Comments: _____

_____

_____

LAB 9-4: Tech-Check-Tech (T-C-T)

Objective:

To become familiar with the process and procedures of Tech-Check-Tech in the acute care inpatient setting.

Pre-Lab Information:

- Review Chapter 9, "Health-System Pharmacy" in your textbook.
- Visit the following website as an introduction to Tech-Check-Tech:http://www.ashp.org/s_ashp/docs /files/TCTTrainingPacket.pdf

Explanation:

As more states have adopted into law the Tech-Check-Tech procedures and processes for the acute care inpatient setting, it is important for you, as a technician, to understand the basic concepts.

Activity:

Review each of the following three orders for three separate "patients" in order to fill their unit-dose cassettes. Then elect a "pharmacist-in-charge," a "lead-technician," and a "trainee" as the three will be a part of the activity. Have the "trainee" fill the three orders as accurately as the "trainee" can. Then have the "lead-technician" check the "trainee's" cassettes. Please have the "pharmacist-in-charge" audit the three cassettes. Finally have the "lead-technician" generate and submit a report for the "pharmacist-in-charge" to review.

Medication Order #1

PHYSICIAN'S ORDER WORKSHEET

NOTE: *Person initiating entry should write legibly, date the form using (Mo/Day/Yr.), enter time, sign, and indicate their title.*

USE BALL POINT PEN (PRESS FIRMLY)

401

Jane Dustin

Four (geriatrics)

Dr. Knoes

Date	Time	Treatment
13		clopidogrel 75 mg, 1t, qd
		metoprolol 100mg 1t, bid,
		APAP 500mg 1-2t, q4-6 h, prn
		②

 PHYSICIAN'S ORDER WORKSHEET

Distribution:
(Original) Medical Record Copy
(Plies 3, 2, & 1) Pharmacy

T-5

Medication Order #2

PHYSICIAN'S ORDER WORKSHEET

NOTE: *Person initiating entry should write legibly, date the form using (Mo/Day/Yr.), enter time, sign, and indicate their title.*

USE BALL POINT PEN (PRESS FIRMLY)

Date	Time	Treatment
		glyburide 2.5 mg, 1t. qd
		atenolol 50 mg, 1t, bid
		①

PHYSICIAN'S ORDER WORKSHEET

Distribution:
(Original) Medical Record Copy
(Plies 3, 2, & 1) Pharmacy

T-5

Medication Order #3

PHYSICIAN'S ORDER WORKSHEET

NOTE: *Person initiating entry should write legibly, date the form using (Mo/Day/Yr.), enter time, sign, and indicate their title.*

USE BALL POINT PEN (PRESS FIRMLY)

515

Cathy Cakes

Five (pediatrics)

Dr. Knoes

Date	Time	Treatment
		amoxil 250mg, 1t, tid
		fluconazole 100mg, 1t, qd
		APAP 500mg 1-2t, q4-6 h, prn
		③

‖‖‖ **PHYSICIAN'S ORDER WORKSHEET** | Distribution: (Original) Medical Record Copy (Plies 3, 2, & 1) Pharmacy | **T-5**

Student Name: _____

Lab Partner: _____

Grade/Comments: _____

_____

_____

Student Comments: _____

_____

_____

LAB 9-5: Unit-Dosing and Repackaging

Objective:

To become familiar with the process and procedures of unit-dosing and repackaging in inpatient settings.

Pre-Lab Information:

• Review Chapter 9, "Health-System Pharmacy" in your textbook.

Explanation:

As nursing homes and long-term care facilities, as well as closed-door pharmacies, often fill for their patients a unit-dose supply of medications, the technician is relied upon to repackage the orders for each patient.

Activity:

Review each of the following orders for the two "patients." Fill each of the orders using a 30-day blister card. This will be for a cold-seal tray. Make sure to notate the expiration date and lot number of each medication.

Patient #1: James Kicks

PHYSICIAN'S ORDER WORKSHEET

James Kicks

NOTE: *Person initiating entry should write legibly, date the form using (Mo/Day/Yr.), enter time, sign, and indicate their title.*

USE BALL POINT PEN (PRESS FIRMLY)

Date	Time	Treatment
		Truvada \t, qd
		Isentress \t, bid
		Multivitamin \t, qd

	PHYSICIAN'S ORDER WORKSHEET	Distribution: (Original) Medical Record Copy (Plies 3, 2, & 1) Pharmacy	T-5

Patient #2: Karen Sweets

PHYSICIAN'S ORDER WORKSHEET

Karen Sweets

NOTE: *Person initiating entry should write legibly, date the form using (Mo/Day/Yr.), enter time, sign, and indicate their title.*

USE BALL POINT PEN (PRESS FIRMLY)

Date	Time	Treatment
		warfarin 2.5 mg tt, qd, M,W,F, Sun
		warfarin 5 mg tt, qd, Tues, Thur. Sat
		②

  PHYSICIAN'S ORDER WORKSHEET | Distribution:
(Original) Medical Record Copy
(Plies 3, 2, & 1) Pharmacy | **T-5**

Student Name: _____

Lab Partner: _____

Grade/Comments: _____

_____

_____

Student Comments: _____

_____

_____

CHAPTER 10
Technology in the Pharmacy

After completing Chapter 10 from the textbook, you should be able to:	Related Activity in the Workbook/Lab Manual
1. List the hardware and software components used in pharmacy computers and summarize their purpose.	Review Questions, PTCB Exam Practice Questions, Activity 10-6
2. Describe and discuss the use of automation and robotics in community pharmacies.	Review Questions, PTCB Exam Practice Questions, Activity 10-5, Lab 10-1
3. Describe and discuss the use of automation and robotics in health-system pharmacies.	Review Questions, Activity 10-1, Activity 10-5, Lab 10-2
4. Define and explain telepharmacy practice.	Review Questions
5. Summarize the impact of patient confidentiality regulations on the use of technology in the pharmacy.	Review Questions

INTRODUCTION

Over the past few decades, technology has revolutionized the practice of pharmacy. Today, virtually every pharmacy uses computers, automated systems, and other technology platforms for its operations and management of pharmaceutical care. Technology is used in both community and health-system pharmacies. As a pharmacy technician, it is important for you to have a basic understanding of the different technologies that are available and being used in pharmacies. These include basic tools, such as computers, printers, modems, and scanners, as well as more advanced tools, such as automatic counters, dispensing systems, bar coding, and even robots. Although you will certainly learn a lot on the job, if you enter the workplace computer literate and familiar with some basic concepts, you will be comfortable managing technological changes as they arise.

REVIEW QUESTIONS

Match the following.

1. _____ hardware   a. connects computers via phone lines or cable
2. _____ hard drive   b. lists of information ordered in specific ways
3. _____ database   c. hardware that allows information to be entered
4. _____ CPU   d. primary software/program of a computer system
5. _____ applications   e. uses advanced telecommunications technology
6. _____ input devices   f. brain of the computer system
7. _____ keyboard   g. permanent memory for essential operations
8. _____ modem   h. mechanical and electrical components of a computer
9. _____ software   i. primary input device of a computer
10. _____ ROM   j. temporary memory used for inputting
11. _____ RAM   k. software/programs that perform specific functions
12. _____ operating system   l. main storage device
13. _____ EHRs   m. programs and applications that control computers
14. _____ telepharmacy   n. electronic accessible patient records

True or False?

15. Electronic counters are a threat to pharmacy technician jobs.

    T   F

16. The FDA mandates that all prescription medications contain a bar code.

    T   F

17. A faxed prescription is considered a legal document in most states.

    T   F

18. Patient profiling is a violation of federal discrimination laws.

    T   F

19. Pharmacists and technicians may now research a patient's EHR.

    T   F

Fill in the blank.

20. Using telecommunications technology, pharmacists can provide care to patients in medically under-served areas at a distance. This is called _____.

PHARMACY CALCULATION PROBLEMS

Calculate the following.

1. A patient's medical order reads: "cefazolin 1,000 mg IVPB q8hr 3 days." How many grams of cefazolin will the patient receive in total?

2. A patient is going to receive 1,500 mg of vancomycin IVPB daily in three divided doses. How many milligrams will the patient receive in each dose?

3. A technician runs a report and finds that an automated dispensing unit in the ER has only two vials of ondansetron left. The maximum par level for that medication is 20 vials. That item also has a minimum par set of five vials. How many vials should the technician restock?

4. A patient needs 25 mg hydroxyzine IV push. The vial contains 50 mg in each mL. How many milliliters will the patient need?

5. A patient is receiving 100 mL of NACl IV every hour. How long will a 1,000 mL IV bag last?

PTCB EXAM PRACTICE QUESTIONS

1. What part of a computer is responsible for interpreting commands and running software applications?
   a. JAZ
   b. RAM
   c. CPU
   d. ROM

2. E-prescribing greatly reduces:
   a. illegible physician handwriting.
   b. forgeries.
   c. medication errors.
   d. all of the above.

3. Which of the following examples of pharmacy technology has not been associated with improved patient safety?
   a. computerized patient profiles
   b. automated dispensing systems
   c. central processing unit
   d. prescription filling robot

4. What information is contained in the bar code mandated by the FDA?
   a. NDC code
   b. DEA number
   c. Social Security number
   d. AWP

5. Which of the following is considered a hardware output device?
   a. keyboard
   b. mouse
   c. printer
   d. scanner

ACTIVITY 10-1: Case Study—Bar Coding

Instructions: Read the following scenario and then answer the critical thinking questions.

The University Teaching Hospital is buzzing about its recently purchased new technology, which will help dispense medications for patients. The new equipment that everyone is excited about will bring many conveniences to the facility, including the ability to perform electronic prescribing, which feeds into an automated medication delivery system throughout the hospital system. The system is comprised of numerous 200-draw-type units on each ward, in an area that is easily accessible to health care providers and requires bar coding for medication verification.

From the point of electronic entry, once the pharmacist verifies the medication, the drug can then be withdrawn from a cabinet by health care personnel where the patient is located. For example, nurses are able to view and withdraw medications from a current, active medication profile.

On one particular patient's profile, a prescription for aspirin 81 mg has been entered. The patient's nurse is attempting to pull the medication from one such cabinet after it has been verified by the pharmacist. The nurse electronically logs in and looks for the aspirin. It is there, but for some reason is not available for withdrawal. A message pops up on the screen, stating "medication not found"—yet it is right there on the screen. The nurse calls in to the pharmacy and asks for help.

1. Using what you know and can research about bar-coding technology, why might this message appear?

   _____

   _____

   _____

   _____

2. What is a possible reason why the automated medication delivery system is unable to "read" the aspirin prescribed, even after verification and after it appears on the patient profile?

   _____

   _____

   _____

   _____

3. What must be done to make the medication available to the health care personnel from the automated medication delivery unit?

   _____

   _____

   _____

   _____

ACTIVITY 10-2: Case Study—New Software, Not-So-New Help

Instructions: Read the following scenario and then answer the critical thinking questions.

For years your pharmacy has utilized MBC Data software for processing all its prescriptions. This system has worked flawlessly for the pharmacy as long as the data entered is correct. When the correct NDC number is entered, the prescription is just a few seconds away from being completed and a label printed, complete with auxiliary labels. Billing processes can sometimes be difficult, but overall the software gets the job done.

This is the only system most of your pharmacy staff has ever worked on, and the news that a new software application system is being installed takes them by surprise. In addition to seamless prescription processing and online billing, this new system is supposed to integrate with inventory and has the ability to create numerous valuable reports for management. Despite the apparent advantages, most, but not all, of the staff are upset with this change and actively demonstrate their resistance through actions and words. Regardless, the new system will be in place within two weeks, going live on a Monday.

The training consists of one week in a computer lab where company trainers walk your staff through various prescription scenarios. The company presents you with two user manuals. Three trainers state that they will be present when the system goes live on Monday.

Monday arrives. One trainer makes it in, but is kept busy by the data systems department, so the trainer is deemed unavailable for staff questions. As predicted, there are many problems, as the staff is too unfamiliar with this new system that must get information in certain places in order to work properly. Pandemonium breaks out, and the staff becomes extremely frustrated as the day moves on due to the lack of assistance with the new system. Rejections of the new software are adding up.

1. What are some resources you could locate in a scenario such as this?

   _____

   _____

   _____

   _____

2. How would you go about calming down your fellow workers so that everyone can concentrate?

   _____

   _____

   _____

   _____

3. What person in the pharmacy should be taking the lead here?

   _____

   _____

   _____

   _____

ACTIVITY 10-3: Case Study—New Equipment Considerations

Instructions: Read the following scenario and then answer the critical thinking questions.

As a new manager in your pharmacy, you have recently taken on more responsibilities such as: scheduler, coordinator, trainer, counselor, and committee participant. One of the committees to which you have been assigned is the pharmacy equipment committee. This committee meets annually to evaluate the equipment/supply needs of the pharmacy.

Some of the equipment in your pharmacy is outdated to where new models could be very useful. In addition to your existing responsibilities, you have now been assigned the task of researching any new equipment that would be beneficial to your pharmacy. Excitedly, you begin your searching.

1. What are some ways that you can learn about new or updated equipment that is available?

    _____

    _____

    _____

    _____

2. Which types of existing equipment would most likely be outdated after one year?

    _____

    _____

    _____

    _____

3. Who can you contact to discuss new models of pharmacy equipment and their pricing?

    _____

    _____

    _____

    _____

ACTIVITY 10-4: Case Study—Online Billing

Instructions: Read the following scenario and then answer the critical thinking questions.

Third-party billing is a complicated part of pharmacy. It is not the same for every transaction. Different providers require different methods of data entry.

Both pharmacy technicians in the billing department of your facility are very efficient at what they do. It is said that if anyone can get a bill paid, it is these two pharmacy technicians. Other pharmacy technicians rotate through this billing realm periodically, but these two are the primary billers. No one person knows everything about billing except these two.

During the course of the summer, one of the pharmacy billing technicians goes on maternity leave for at least 12 weeks, leaving the one other expert biller alone. Coincidentally, within weeks the other billing person expert breaks her leg and is placed on medical leave for at least three months. Suddenly, the billing is piling up. Other pharmacy technicians are filling in, but they cannot keep pace with the workload, and there is much information that has not been disseminated.

You look around their work areas and the entire pharmacy, hoping to find something that will give you a clue as to how to perform the billing duties—but you find nothing. What do you do?

1. As you looked around the pharmacy, what did you hope to find to help?

    _____

    _____

    _____

    _____

2. What would have been a good resource for this, and who should have provided it?

_____

_____

_____

3. What role do you think the third-party insurers have as far as providing information? What could they provide?

_____

_____

_____

ACTIVITY 10-5: Exploring Technology in the Institutional Pharmacy

In a busy institutional pharmacy, it is vital that medications reach the patients as quickly and safely as possible. Modern conveniences such as phones, fax machines, and computerized physician order entry (CPOE) systems are now commonplace, and have increased the daily number of orders a pharmacy can fill. However, newer technology that has slowly been making its way into the pharmacy not only helps the staff process more orders quickly but also decreases the drug dispensing errors that are far too common. Three different types of technology commonly used in pharmacy practice are the automated dispensing unit, bar-coding technology, and the pneumatic tube system. These three pieces of technology serve different but complementary functions. You may discover that this technology is not really all that new. You may have seen it in places outside the pharmacy in a different shape or form.

The Automated Dispensing Unit

Automated dispensing units have become very popular in recent years. In the past, most medications for hospital patients had to come directly from the pharmacy. This entailed sending an order to the pharmacy, having the pharmacy input the order into the computer, and then filling the order. After the orders were filled a pharmacy technician would deliver the medications to the unit on rounds. This process multiplied hundreds of times over during a day, produced huge workloads, and slow turnaround times.

An automated dispensing unit consists of a cabinet containing locked drawers and cabinets, each filled with the medications needed. This advanced computerized "vending machine" is linked to the main computer, which maintains all the patient profiles. When a nurse needs to dispense a medication, she simply enters her user name and password, accesses the patient's profile, and selects the medication that the patient needs. Then, a drawer or cabinet unlocks, and the nurse can retrieve the medication. The patient will simultaneously be billed for this medication. These automated dispensing units can be found in every major unit in the hospital, such as the OR, ER, and medical units. Each one is customized to carry a large percentage of the medications that the specific unit uses most frequently. When an item gets low or runs out, a report is generated (either automatically or manually), and a pharmacy technician is cued to restock the unit.

This system greatly decreases the amount of time it takes for a patient to receive a medication, resulting in greater customer satisfaction. With fewer phone calls and medication requests, the pharmacy can operate with much higher efficiency, and the pharmacy staff is able to concentrate more on other tasks. Automated dispensing units also decrease the risk of dispensing errors and reduce waste. This is accomplished by stocking the units with unit-dose medications. Unit-dose medications are individually packaged, either by the manufacturer or by the pharmacy. Each dose has all the necessary drug information on each package, such as drug, strength, lot number, expiration date, and manufacturer. Each unit dose also contains a bar code, which will indicate the same information when scanned. The nurse does not open a unit-dose medication until it is to be given to the patient, so there is little wasted medication. In addition, many institutions require the nurse to scan the bar code on the unit-dose medication along with the bar code on the patient's wristband. This practice increases safety by assuring that the right patient is receiving the right medication.

Despite the many advantages of automated dispensing systems, because of the nature of technology, sometimes things do not always work as they should. Pharmacy technicians need to be familiar with this technology, so that they will be better able to respond to unusual situations. For example: Have you ever lost a bag of chips in a vending machine because it was stuck to the coil? You only brought exact change with you, so you left it there, dangling from the coil. Then, the next person who wanted those same chips received two bags, because your bag finally fell down. Similarly, some automated units have small, removable cartridges that can hold 20 or more pills between the coils, like a smaller version of the chip vending machine. Occasionally, one pill will get hung up and will not dispense.

Overall, though, these automated dispensing units are convenient, efficient, and improve patient safety. As a pharmacy technician working at a hospital, you will most likely become familiar with this type of technology and learn how to maintain such units.

Matching Game

Even technology breaks down sometimes. Now that you have read about automated dispensing units, see if you can troubleshoot some common issues listed in Column A by matching them with the (often) simple solutions in Column B. To make this more fun, some of the solutions apply to more than one problem—and some problems have more than one solution!

Problem	Solution
1. _____ Biometric (fingerprint) scanner does not work.	a. Place the extra tablet back into the dispenser.
2. _____ One of the medication drawers will not open.	b. Reboot the system.
3. _____ A nurse requested one tablet for a patient, but the dispenser issued two.	c. Hold your finger up to your mouth and lightly breathe on it.
4. _____ While restocking, a technician found that a morphine syringe was stuck in the dispenser.	d. Try inserting a long, thin object, like a ruler or a chopstick, in the crack.
5. _____ The keypad and/or the touch screen is not responding.	e. Clean it off with an alcohol swab, then try again.
	f. Unscrew the dispenser from the unit.

Bar-Coding Technology:

Bar-coding technology has been around for decades. You can find bar codes on almost any product you buy, from food to clothing. Only recently, however, were laws passed requiring bar-code technology to be used in pharmacies. Requiring bar-code scans significantly reduces the possibility of drug errors. In all types of pharmacies, bar codes are found on all medication stock bottles and unit-dose packages. In an institutional pharmacy, every unit dose must have a bar code. If the manufacturer does not make unit-dose forms of a certain drug, the pharmacy does its own repackaging. This includes all dose forms, including oral liquids. Each unit dose, whether manufactured or repackaged by the pharmacy, has to contain a bar code indicating the drug name, strength, lot number, expiration date, and manufacturer. When a technician fills an order for a medication, a handheld scanner can be used to scan the medication's bar code and the bar code on the patient's order. This assures that the technician has chosen the correct medication for that order. Earlier, it was mentioned that many hospitals also require the nurse to scan both the patient's ID band and the medication to be given, to guarantee that the right patient is receiving the right medication.

Bar coding does have some minor flaws. When a medication is repackaged in the pharmacy, the technician needs to make sure to enter all the information into the repackaging/unit-dose computer correctly. If any manual overrides are performed, it greatly increases the risk of having a bar code with incorrect information. With bar coding, the exact product must be chosen. If your usual generic brand of ibuprofen 400 mg tablets is on backorder and the procurement technician ordered a different manufacturer's brand of ibuprofen 400 mg, the bar code will not match the new brand. This is because each manufacturer uses a specific NDC (National Drug Code) number for its product. Another product from another manufacturer has its own NDC number. When this occurs, the existing medication order must be modified or changed, using the new drug or NDC number. Once this is done, the product and new label can be rescanned and will match.

Using a bar-coding system takes a little extra time, but for the most part, implementation of bar coding is positive as well as mandatory. It significantly reduces errors in the pharmacy and on the nursing units. Because of the accuracy of bar coding, mistakes can be caught before they ever leave the pharmacy.

Pneumatic Tube Stations

Whether you realize it or not, you have been exposed to pneumatic tube systems for most of your life. When you use a bank drive-through, most have tube stations installed to assist in sending your transactions. It increases the number of customers they can help during busy times. Many larger hospitals have incorporated complex pneumatic tube systems that can deliver all sorts of things throughout the entire hospital. Most areas have a station from which they can receive and send medication orders, medications, X-rays, supplies, and so on. Each station has an identifying code or "address," so to speak. If you want to send something to the emergency room, you just load the item in the tube, place the tube on its launching pad, and enter in the code for the ER. These tubes or pods are heavy duty, and can withstand a heavy load, such as a 1-L bag of fluid or several piggybacks. Pneumatic tube stations are a convenient way to get something from one end of the building to the other without having to deliver it in person.

Most pharmacy items can be sent via pneumatic tube. However, most institutions have policies and procedures regarding proper use of the tube system and products that should not be tubed. Foam padding is sometimes used to help cushion fragile items during transport. Most institutions require that any sort of liquid IV bag be placed in a zip-lock plastic bag before it is placed into a tube for transport. If for any reason the IV bag breaks, the zip-lock bag will contain the spill inside. A spill that occurs within the pneumatic tube system is expensive to clean up, and the system is difficult to repair. A system that is down for repairs will also contribute to longer wait times for medication.

Policies vary from institution to institution, but most have a list of drugs/products that should not be tubed. Medications with a protein base, such as insulin vials or total parenteral nutrition (TPN) solutions, should not be tubed. These items are sensitive to shaking, which causes the proteins within the medications to break down. Chemotherapy medications should not be tubed, because of their toxic nature. Items that could easily be broken, like glass evacuated bottles, may also be on the "do not tube" list. Other items that may be excluded from the tube system include: expensive medications, medications that are in limited supply, infected blood samples, carbonated items, and combustible items.

Pneumatic tube stations are just one of many modern conveniences that help improve patient care in hospitals. Many items can be tubed to different locations in much less time than it would take to deliver them by foot. With the implementation of automated dispensing units and bar-code technology, fewer medication errors occur, and patients receive their medications in a timely manner, thus increasing customer satisfaction. These newer technologies have greatly improved work flow in the pharmacy and contributed significantly to better patient care. Technology will continue to play a major role in the pharmacy in years to come.

Critical Thinking Questions:

1. A 200-bed private hospital is considering implementing either automated dispensing units for all of the major areas in the hospital, or a pneumatic tube system. The hospital's budget is small, so it can only afford to install either the dispensing units or the tube system. If you were on the budget committee representing the pharmacy, which system would you choose? Explain your choice.

   _____

   _____

   _____

   _____

2. Do you feel that bar coding should be mandatory for all pharmacies? Explain your answer.

   _____

   _____

   _____

   _____

3. Can you think of any reasons why you should not tube a drug that is in limited supply? How about a syringe that is worth $12,000?

   _____

   _____

   _____

   _____

4. A nurse requested two oxycodone 5 mg tablets for John Jones, but the automated dispensing unit only dispensed one tablet. How do you think this error might affect the inventory count of this medication? How do you think it might affect Mr. Jones's billing account? Without having any experience with these units, can you think of any ways to resolve these issues?

   _____

   _____

   _____

   _____

Web Activity:

Go to the following websites to research different automated dispensing units and hospital-grade pneumatic tube systems. Navigate around each site to see the different types of units that are available for hospital use.

www.omnicell.com

www.pyxis.com

www.swisslog.com

www.pevco.com

ACTIVITY 10-6: Identifying the Parts of a Computer

You learned about technology used in pharmacies in Chapter 10 of the textbook. Without returning to the textbook, see how much you remember by listing some examples of each of the following technology categories.

1. What is hardware?

   Definition: _____

   _____

2. Name three examples of input devices.

   1. _____

   2. _____

   3. _____

3. Name three examples of processing components.

   1. _____

   2. _____

   3. _____

4. Name two examples of output devices.

   1. _____

   2. _____

5. What is software?

   Definition: _____

   _____

6. Name three examples of automation or robotics used in pharmacies.

   1. _____

   2. _____

   3. _____

LAB 10-1: Technology in Community Pharmacies

Objective:
Become familiar with two technological devices that are commonly used in the community pharmacy setting.

Pre-Lab Information:
Review Chapter 10, "Technology in the Pharmacy" in your textbook.

Explanation:
Automation in the community pharmacy setting allows and enables accuracy and speed for prescription processing. Counting machines and bar-coding equipment are commonly used by the pharmacy technician.

Activity:
Select five medications from the pharmacy inventory to fill for a "prescription." Use the counting machine to count out the following number of capsules or tablets:

1. 20 capsules or tablets
2. 30 capsules or tablets
3. 60 capsules or tablets
4. 14 capsules or tablets
5. 90 capsules or tablets

Be sure to account for accuracy of the quantities that the machine has counted out.

With those same prescriptions which have been counted, using the scanning device, scan the medications into the computer to ensure accuracy and patient safety.

Student Name: _____

Lab Partner: _____

Grade/Comments: _____

_____

_____

Student Comments: _____

_____

_____

LAB 10-2: Technology in Health-System Pharmacies

Objective:

Become familiar with automation in a health-system pharmacy setting.

Pre-Lab Information:

Review Chapter 10, "Technology in the Pharmacy" in your textbook.

Explanation:

Automation in the health-system pharmacy setting allows and enables accuracy and speed with processing. The automated medication delivery system has been an innovative and secure piece of technology for technicians to use at a health-system pharmacy.

Activities:

Review the following website and read through all of the products that are related to "Pyxis" technology. Answer the questions as they pertain to the related products. http://www.carefusion.com/medical-products/medication-management/medication-technologies/pyxis-medstation-system.aspx

1. What four critical areas do the analytical solutions focus on for the Med Analytics Service for Pyxis MedStation system?

   _____

   _____

2. What are the three areas of the CUBIE system that will help health-system pharmacies reduce the risk of medication errors, drug diversion, and activities that are time consuming and non-valued?

   _____

   _____

   _____

3. What kind of technology does the Pyxis PARx system use as a solution to maintain the chain of custody for medications?

   _____

   Talk with your instructor about arranging a field trip to a local area health-system pharmacy.

Student Name: _____

Lab Partner: _____

Grade/Comments: _____

_____

_____

Student Comments: _____

_____

CHAPTER 11
Inventory Management

After completing Chapter 11 from the textbook, you should be able to:	Related Activity in the Workbook/Lab Manual
1. List and describe the various purchasing systems used in pharmacies.	Review Questions, PTCB Exam Practice Questions Lab 11-1
2. List and describe the various methods of purchasing available in pharmacies.	Review Questions, PTCB Exam Practice Questions
3. Define and describe prescription formularies.	Review Questions, PTCB Exam Practice Questions *Activity 12-2, Lab 12-3
4. Describe and perform the steps necessary for placing orders.	Review Questions, PTCB Exam Practice Questions, Lab 11-1
5. Describe and perform the steps necessary for receiving orders.	Review Questions, PTCB Exam Practice Questions, Activity 11-1, Lab 11-3
6. List the atypical products to consider with inventory management.	Review Questions, PTCB Exam Practice Questions, Lab 11-1
7. List the reasons for back-ordered products and outline appropriate methods to communicate changes in product availability.	Review Questions, PTCB Exam Practice Questions, Activity 11-2, Lab 11-3, Lab 11-4
8. Classify the reasons for product returns and describe the process of making returns.	Review Questions, PTCB Exam Practice Questions, Activity 11-1, Lab 11-2
9. List and explain the three classifications of drug recalls.	Review Questions, PTCB Exam Practice Questions, Lab 11-2
10. Describe the process of handling expired drugs.	Review Questions, PTCB Exam Practice Questions

11. Identify the problems with having excessive inventory.	Reveiw Questions, PTCB Exam Practice Questions, Lab 11-1
12. Describe the issue of drug theft and diversion.	Review Questions, PTCB Exam Practice Questions, Activity 11-1

INTRODUCTION

One of the most common duties you will perform as a pharmacy technician is inventory management.

A pharmacy cannot dispense prescriptions if the proper medications are not in stock. A pharmacy obtains its inventory through a purchasing system, either as a member of a group purchasing system (GPO) or independently. The inventory is often based on an organization's formulary or the formularies approved by insurance carriers. A pharmacy's inventory must be closely and regularly monitored to ensure that adequate stock is available, to remove expired drugs, and to comply with any product recalls.

Although the management of inventory varies by facility, as a pharmacy technician, you will be available to assist the pharmacist by handling these responsibilities and allowing the pharmacist to focus on more clinical aspects of pharmaceutical care provision.

REVIEW QUESTIONS

Fill in the blanks.

1. A _____ is a collective purchasing system in which a pharmacy joins a GPO, which contracts with pharmaceutical manufacturers on behalf of its members.

2. A purchasing system in which the pharmacy is responsible for establishing contracts directly with each pharmaceutical manufacturer is a/an _____.

3. A procedure for obtaining medications, devices, and products for an organization is known as a/an _____.

4. The process through which a drug manufacturer or the FDA requires that specific drugs be returned to the manufacturer because of a specific concern is known as a/an _____.

5. A _____ enables the pharmacy to purchase a large number of products, from various manufacturers, from a single source.

Choose the best answer.

6. Formularies are used by:
   a. institutional pharmacies.
   b. insurance companies.
   c. ambulatory pharmacies.
   d. all of the above.

7. Inventory should be checked for "outdates":
   a. weekly.
   b. monthly.
   c. yearly.
   d. whenever there is time.

8. OTC products may be recalled by the:
   a. FDA.
   b. DEA.
   c. AFT.
   d. FTC.

9. The P&T Committee is composed of:
   a. physicians.
   b. pharmacists.
   c. nurses.
   d. all of the above.

10. Evaluating the costs of medications will vary greatly depending on:
    a. its NDC number.
    b. the wholesaler.
    c. if the drug is a brand or a generic.
    d. contracted prices between the manufacturer and the pharmacy.

Match the following.

11. _____ Class I Recall   **a.** someone has or could die from using a drug
12. _____ Class II Recall   **b.** a drug has been mislabeled or is noncompliant
13. _____ Class III Recall   **c.** a drug could cause harm, but is not deadly

PHARMACY CALCULATION PROBLEMS

Calculate the following.

1. The pharmacy's automated order system indicates that there are 240 hydrochlorothiazide 25 mg tablets left in inventory. If the system is programmed to reorder when the order point falls below 200, how many bottles of 100 tablets will the system order?

2. The pharmacy's automated order system indicates that there are seven vials of Humulin R insulin left. How many vials will the system order if the reorder point falls below 10?

3. A small, independent pharmacy has a manual ordering system with maximum/minimum levels (in bottles) written on the shelf under the drug. If the maximum/minimum levels for nabumetone 500 mg are 4/2, and there is one bottle on the shelf, how many bottles should be reordered?

4. A customer is picking up three prescriptions and owes a co-pay of $7.50 on each one. If she hands the pharmacy clerk $30, how much change should the customer receive?

5. A pharmacy is running a special on cold medicines: buy two and get the third for 50% off. If a customer purchases three cold medicines that are all regularly $5.99 each, how much is the total cost to the customer?

PTCB EXAM PRACTICE QUESTIONS

1. A listing of the goods or items that a business will use in its normal operation is called a/an:
   a. purchasing.
   b. inventory.
   c. open formulary.
   d. closed formulary.

2. The goal of inventory management is:
   a. to ensure that drugs are available when they are needed.
   b. to maintain MSDS.
   c. to develop closed formularies.
   d. to increase use of wholesalers.

3. What do we call the minimum and maximum stock levels that are used to determine when to reorder a drug and how much to order?
   a. reorder points
   b. automatic ordering
   c. POS
   d. turnovers

4. Medications that are dropped on the floor should be:
   a. re-dispensed to the patient.
   b. swept up right away and packaged.
   c. put back into the original container.
   d. taken home by the technician for store credit or proper disposal.

5. Counterfeit medications should be reported to:
   a. the FDA.
   b. supervisors.
   c. appropriate authorities.
   d. all of the above

ACTIVITY 11-1: Case Study—DEA Forms and Shipment Do Not Match

Instructions: Read the following scenario and then answer the critical thinking questions.

In your pharmacy, controlled medications are ordered by the vault technician. The process specifies that the vault technician fills out the DEA 222 forms and has the head pharmacist sign them. Upon arrival, two people check in the freight, matching up the shipment to the order. For many months, the two who have checked in the freight each time are the exact same pharmacist and pharmacy technician. This is acceptable because they are not the same persons who do the ordering.

One day, the pharmacy technician who checks in orders is absent and you are asked to help receive a shipment. You have the forms, and you and the pharmacist begin opening the totes. You work without incident until you get to the third tote and notice that the red locking tie is not sealed. You point it out to the pharmacist, who brushes it off, stating that it probably got caught on something. The pharmacist is also rushing you along because he has prescriptions to check. Continuing to match up the medications to the order form, you realize that you are short one #30-count bottle of Oxycontin® 10 mg. A recount brings about the same results.

You expect the pharmacist to be concerned, but he is not. He just keeps pushing you to "get on with it" and says that he will figure it out later. You are very uncomfortable with this direction; however, this is your head pharmacist giving the order.

1. What is the right thing to do here?

   _____

   _____

   _____

   _____

2. What are some possible explanations for the one missing bottle?

   _____

   _____

   _____

   _____

3. Can and should the ordering/checking-in process be altered to better prevent such situations?

_____

_____

_____

4. Is there any reason why you should not do what the pharmacist directs you to do here?

_____

_____

_____

_____

ACTIVITY 11-2: Case Study—Out-of-Stock Item

Instructions: Read the following scenario and then answer the critical thinking questions.

It is late on a Saturday evening and the rural southwestern hospital where you work is the only medical facility open to the public. A middle-aged female comes into the emergency room after she has reported a sexual assault to the authorities. The physician on duty prescribes a post-exposure prophylaxis (PEP) regimen for the patient. PEP is a course of antiretroviral medications (ARVs) which are taken within 72 hours after the possible and potential exposure to human immunodeficiency virus (HIV). The regimen includes: one zidovudine 300 mg/ lamivudine 150 mg tablet and one tablet of tenofovir 300 mg. These medications, when taken within 72 hours after the potential exposure to HIV, may help keep the patient from converting to an HIV+ status.

For some reason, either through poor supply or high demand, you discover that your pharmacy is completely out of tenofovir. You are left with the task of obtaining tenofovir as soon as possible for this patient. There are only two independent pharmacies in the rural town where the hospital is located, and neither will be open on Sunday, leaving you unable to obtain a supply for at least two days. The nearest town is a two-and-a-half-hour drive away. What do you do?

1. What options do you have for obtaining the medication quickly?

_____

_____

_____

2. Where do you think you can find this medication in the time allowed?

_____

_____

_____

3. Detail how you would go about obtaining this medication, from time of contact to time of possession. How long does it actually take?

_____

_____

_____

LAB 11-1: Maintaining a Manual Inventory Using Par Levels

Objective:

Practice ordering medications manually using a mock par-level system.

Pre-Lab Information:

Review Chapter 11, "Inventory Management," in the textbook for an overview of the different types of inventory systems.

Explanation:

Some smaller institutional and retail pharmacies do not have the volume or financial means to implement an automated inventory system. When a point of sale (POS) or other automated inventory system is un-available, inventory may be maintained through a par-level system. Generally, maximum and minimum par levels are noted on the shelf below each medication, indicating how many bottles, packages, and so forth should be kept on hand.

For example, sertraline 100 mg tablets are ordered in bottles of 100. The maximum/minimum par levels are set to 3/1, indicating that the pharmacy should have three full bottles as maximum inventory, but no less than one full bottle. When the minimum falls below one full bottle (only a partial bottle left), the pharmacy should reorder enough to bring the quantity back up to the maximum par level (three bottles). If inventory is somewhere between one and three bottles, no stock is reordered, as it is in the acceptable par-level range. Depending on the company's reorder policies, this technique could vary (perhaps the facility keeps only a minimum or an ideal par level).

Activity:

In this activity, you will be given information regarding the par levels of certain medications along with the current level of inventory. Based on these quantities, determine whether a product should be reordered and, if so, how many bottles/packages should be reordered.

> ✓ **Tip:** If an item is in the range of the maximum/minimum par level, you do not need to reorder. If an item falls below the recommended minimum par level, you should reorder enough to bring the inventory back up to the maximum level of full bottles/packages.

1. Fluticasone 0.05% nasal spray (each)

   Max/min: 5/2
   On hand: 3
   How many nasal sprays should be reordered? _____

2. Furosemide 40 mg tablets (bottle)

   Max/min: 3/1
   On hand: partial bottle
   How many bottles should be reordered? _____

3. Hydralazine 25 mg tablets (bottle)

   Max/min: 2/1
   On hand: 1 bottle
   How many bottles should be reordered? _____

4. Enoxaparin 30 mg syringes (box)

   Max/min: 4/2

   On hand: 1 box

   How many boxes should be reordered? _____

5. Nifedipine 10 mg capsules (bottle)

   Max/min: 4/1

   On hand: 1 bottle

   How many bottles should be reordered? _____

6. Albuterol 17 g inhalers (each)

   Max/min: 12/4

   On hand: 2 inhalers

   How many inhalers should be reordered? _____

7. Nystatin ointment, 15 g tube (each)

   Max/min: 3/1

   On hand: 2 tubes

   How many tubes should be reordered? _____

8. Clonidine 0.2 mg transdermal patches (box)

   Max/min: 5/2

   On hand: 2 boxes

   How many boxes should be reordered? _____

9. Valacyclovir 500 mg tablets (bottle)

   Max/min: 2/1

   On hand: partial bottle

   How many bottles should be reordered? _____

10. Metoprolol 100 mg tablets (bottle)

    Max/min: 3/2

    On hand: 1 full bottle and a partial bottle

    How many bottles should be reordered? _____

Student Name: _____

Lab Partner: _____

Grade/Comments: _____

_____

_____

Student Comments: _____

_____

_____

LAB 11-2: Drug Recalls

Objective:

To become familiar with the drug recall process.

Pre-Lab Information:

Review the FDA website: http://www.recalls.gov/medicine.html

Explanation:

As a pharmacy technician, you may be involved with a drug recall and will have to be put to the task of "pulling" a drug from the shelves in order to discontinue the dispensing of that drug. This exercise is designed to help you become familiar with the FDA's definitions and processes that are used when a drug is recalled.

Activity:

Review the following website and read through "FDA 101: Product Recalls—From First Alerts to Effectiveness Check": http://www.fda.gov/ForConsumers/ConsumerUpdates/ucm049070.htm

You could also watch the video "FDA 101: Product Recalls (Consumer Update)" too.

Review the following website and answer the questions: http://www.fda.gov/oc/po/firmrecalls/recall_defin.html

1. Define a Class I recall.

   _____

   _____

   _____

2. Define a Class II recall.

   _____

   _____

   _____

3. Define a Class III recall.

   _____

   _____

   _____

4. Describe the First Alert process and strategy.

   _____

   _____

   _____

5. List three FDA-regulated products which are subjected to recall.

_____

_____

_____

6. What is the most recently posted drug recall on the FDA website?

_____

Student Name: _____

Lab Partner: _____

Grade/Comments: _____

_____

_____

Student Comments: _____

_____

_____

LAB 11-3: Stocking an Order

Objective:

To become familiar with stocking medications in the pharmacy after a shipment has been delivered.

Pre-Lab Information:

Review Chapter 11, "Inventory Management" in your textbook.

Explanation:

The community pharmacy setting has a very valuable inventory and overhead. A primary responsibility for the technician is to stock the inventory after the shipment has been delivered and the inventory has been accounted for.

Activity:

In the mock pharmacy laboratory, the instructor will fill up a tote with 10 to 15 of different mock medications for you to stock the pharmacy with. The lab is arranged in a route of administration format. While stocking the medications, you realize that this is a great opportunity for you to become familiar with brand and generic medication names, as well as their varying strengths and dosage forms.

From the medications that you stocked in your lab, list the medication name, the strength, and the dosage form of each medication.

1. _____

_____

2. _____

_____

3. _____

_____

4. _____

_____

5. _____

_____

6. _____

_____

7. _____

_____

8. _____

_____

9. _____

_____

10. _____

_____

11. _____

_____

12. _____

_____

13. _____

_____

14. _____

_____

15. _____

_____

Student Name: _____

Lab Partner: _____

Grade/Comments: _____

_____

_____

Student Comments: _____

_____

_____

LAB 11-4: Communicating Changes in Product Availability

Objective:

To become comfortable and familiar with effective communication as it applies to a technician notifying patients about a recent change in product availability.

Pre-Lab Information:

Review Chapter 11, "Inventory Management" in your textbook.

Explanation:

As more drug shortages are becoming problematic for patients and providers alike, pharmacy technicians will need to effectively communicate drug changes to patients and providers in the proper manner.

Activity:

Select a team of four, which will include a "pharmacist," a "technician," a "patient," and a "nurse." Decide upon which participant will take on each of the roles in these activities/scenarios.

Scenario 1:

The technician comes to work and has just learned that the medication amikacin sulfate is not available due to a nationwide shortage. A nurse calls to the pharmacy and is requesting that the medication be ordered for a pediatric patient. What should the technician do and say to appease the nurse and more importantly, the patient?

_____

_____

_____

Scenario 2:

Role Play

One of the more difficult geriatric patients walks into the pharmacy. The patient is carrying an order for a generic medication that he or she is currently taking as maintenance therapy. The original version of the medication has been taken by the patient on a consistent basis. A recent change in availability from the original generic manufacturer, due to a formulation processing error, has left the technician to fill the order with a different version of the generic medication prescribed to the patient. The tablets are different in both shape and color. The pharmacist, after his or her final check, has given the technician permission to apprise the patient of this change.

Choose a partner and role play this scenario. Be sure to consider what the technician should say to the patient, what the patient might say about this recent change to his or her medication, and if the pharmacist is needed to intervene. After five minutes, switch roles and act out the scenario again. What worked best in each role play? What was less effective? How might you apply what you learned in a similar "real life" situation?

_____

_____

_____

Student Name: _____

Lab Partner: _____

Grade/Comments: _____

_____

_____

Student Comments: _____

_____

_____

CHAPTER 12
Insurance and Third-Party Billing

After completing Chapter 12 from the textbook, you should be able to:	Related Activity in the Workbook/Lab Manual
1. Define and describe drug utilization reviews (evaluations).	Review Questions, PTCB Exam Practice Questions
2. List and describe the various types of insurance.	Review Questions, PTCB Exam Practice Questions
3. Describe and differentiate Medicare and Medicaid.	Review Questions, PTCB Exam Practice Questions, Activity 12-2, Lab 12-3
4. Recognize and define terms commonly used in insurance billing.	Review Questions, PTCB Exam Practice Questions, Lab 12-1
5. Describe and perform the steps required in collecting data for insurance purposes.	Review Questions, PTCB Exam Practice Questions, Lab 12-1
6. Describe and perform the steps necessary to transmit a prescription for insurance.	Review Questions, PTCB Exam Practice Questions, Activity 12-1, Activity 12-3, Lab 12-1, Lab 12-3
7. List and explain common insurance billing errors and their solutions.	Review Questions, PTCB Exam Practice Questions, Lab 12-2
8. Define fraud as it pertains to insurance billing.	Review Questions, PTCB Exam Practice Questions

INTRODUCTION

To operate effectively, the pharmacy must be reimbursed by insurance carriers in a timely fashion. Insurance billing requires a comprehensive knowledge of billing terms, codes, and policies, such as DAW codes, authorized days supply, and formularies. As a pharmacy technician, you can help prevent many insurance claim rejections by ensuring that all information is correctly entered into the pharmacy's computer system before a claim is submitted.

Although the process of insurance and third-party billing can vary by facility, as a pharmacy technician, you will be available to assist the pharmacist by handling these responsibilities and allowing the pharmacist to focus on more clinical aspects of pharmaceutical care provision.

REVIEW QUESTIONS

Fill in the blanks.

1. A request for reimbursement, from a health care provider to an insurance provider, for products or services rendered is known as a/an _____.

2. The portion of the cost of a service or product that a patient pays out of pocket each time the service or product is provided is called the _____.

3. _____ is the notation used by prescribers to instruct the pharmacy to use the exact drug written (usually a brand-name drug).

4. _____ is the number of days a dispensed quantity of medication will last.

5. A set amount that a client pays up front before insurance coverage applies is known as the _____.

6. A federally funded, state-administered insurance program for low-income and disadvantaged persons is _____.

7. The federally funded and administered health insurance program is called _____.

8. A company hired by the insurer to process claims is a/an _____.

9. HIPAA formed the Healthcare Fraud and Abuse Control Program to catch and prosecute any _____.

10. DUR stands for _____.

PHARMACY CALCULATION PROBLEMS

Calculate the following.

1. A physician orders amoxicillin 250 mg tid ×10 d. Calculate the quantity to be dispensed and the days supply for this order.

2. The oncologist orders ondansetron 0.15 mg/kg 30 minutes prior to the first dose of chemotherapy for a patient who weighs 150 lbs. for a 15 minute infusion. After the chemotherapy treatment, two subsequent doses of ondansetron 0.15 mg/kg are going to be administered four and eight hours after the first dose of ondansetron. How much ondansetron will be administered for each dose and what is the total volume for the three doses?

3. The oncologist has ordered for the same patient in question two gemcitabine as a part of the patient's chemotherapy regimen. The order is for 1,000 mg/m^2 over 30 minutes on Days 1 and 8 of each 21-day cycle. Factoring in the patient's weight from question two, the patient's height is 5′7″. What is the BSA for this patient and what is the volume for each dose?

4. A physician orders 8 oz. of Hycodan cough syrup, with directions of 1 tsp q 4–6h. What is the correct day's supply to be entered for insurance purposes?

5. What quantity should be dispensed for a 90-day supply of capsules to be taken qod?

PTCB EXAM PRACTICE QUESTIONS

1. What do we call the portion of the price of the medication that the patient is required to pay?
   a. co-insurance
   b. co-pay
   c. maximum allowable cost
   d. usual and customary price

2. The process of transmitting a prescription electronically to the proper insurance company or third-party biller for approval and billing is called:
   a. notification.
   b. adjudication.
   c. settlement.
   d. accreditation.

3. A form of insurance for employees who are injured while at work is called:
   a. Medicaid.
   b. Worker's Reimbursement.
   c. Worker's Compensation.
   d. Worker's Reparation.

4. HIPAA stands for:
   a. Health Insurance Probability and Accountability Act.
   b. Health Insurance Portability and Accountability Acts.
   c. Health Insurance Portability and Accountability Act.
   d. Health Institution Portability and Accountable Act.

5. A pharmacy system should provide support for the following activities performed in the pharmacy except for:
   a. inpatient order entry, management, and dispensing.
   b. manufacturing and compounding.
   c. management and dispensing.
   d. All of the above are acceptable activities.

ACTIVITY 12-1: Case Study—Delayed Patient Refill Date

Instructions: Read the following scenario and then answer the critical thinking questions.

Mrs. Walker is a regular customer at your retail pharmacy; today she comes in a little upset. She explains that she requested a refill of her monthly prescription for phenytoin 100 mg earlier in the day and was told that it was "too early" to get a refill. She states she was also told that her medicine could not be refilled for another 12 days, although she has no medicine left. Knowing that the customer/patient cannot go without a dose, you look up her prescription and find that indeed it appears she is not due to get a refill for 12 days.

You ask Mrs. Walker if you could call her after you have had some time to research this and find out what happened. She agrees.

Upon further research, you discover that what happened in this case was that Mrs. Walker did receive her medication on the 12th of last month, but her insurance did not accept the transaction until the 24th of that month. To the brand-new pharmacy technician who processed her prescription that day, this information made it seem that the 24th was the day she actually received it. The same pharmacy technician was the person Mrs. Walker saw earlier, who told her the refill request was too early. You diplomatically explain to Mrs. Walker, in terms she will understand, what has occurred and assure her that you have refilled her medicine.

1. How did you explain to Mrs. Walker, in lay terms, what happened?

   _____

   _____

   _____

   _____

2. Do you have a conversation with the pharmacy technician who processed the prescription? If so, what do you say?

   _____

   _____

   _____

   _____

3. Is there any way you can evaluate the process and prevent this from happening again, either with this or other future prescriptions? How?

   _____

   _____

   _____

   _____

4. Do you think the insurance company has some accountability here?

   _____

   _____

   _____

   _____

ACTIVITY 12-2: Drug Formularies

As you learned in Chapters 11 and 12 in the textbook, a *drug formulary* is a listing of drugs. HMOs, hospitals, insurance companies, and other health care systems use formularies to keep track of what drugs have been approved for use. Some systems have an *open formulary* that allows the purchase of any drug a doctor prescribes. Other systems have *closed formularies* and require a physician to obtain prior approval to prescribe a drug that is not on the formulary. A quick way to get a feeling for formularies is to investigate drugs covered by Medicare Part D.

Activity:

1. Go to the Medicare website (www.medicare.gov) and follow the Formulary Finder link.
2. Choose your state.
3. Add the following drugs to your list:

- Lipitor
- Nexium
- Prevacid
- Ambien
- Glucotrol
- Ventolin
- Singulair

Questions

1. How many health plans in your state have the drugs you selected on their formularies?

2. Now select one of the health plans whose formulary includes the drugs on your list. List the formulary status of each drug.

Lipitor _____

Nexium _____

Prevacid _____

Ambien _____

Glucotrol _____

Ventolin _____

Singulair _____

3. Which tier covers non-preferred brand-name drugs?
   _____

4. Do any of the drugs on your list require prior authorization?
   _____

5. Do any of the drugs on your list have quantity limits?
   _____

6. Do you think drug formularies are a good idea? What are some benefits of using drug formularies (a) to the health plan and (b) to the patient?

   a. _____
   _____
   _____

   b. _____
   _____
   _____

ACTIVITY 12-3: Case Study: Refill Too Soon

One area of third-party billing, which can be confusing for both the patient and the pharmacy technician alike, is when there is an error message of "Too early to refill." The primary reason for this error message is when the patient has not taken at least 75% of his or her medication before the next refill can be processed. Other reasons for this error message are:

A: The patient is going on a vacation or traveling outside of the United States and they are requesting another refill on the medication(s).

B: The patient has lost or has had stolen a portion or all of their medication.

C: The day supply of the medication may not have been entered correctly by the pharmacy team.

In any of these cases, it is important for the technician to recognize the error message as well as be able to relate the error message and the reason behind the message to the patient in a clear, effective and professional manner. Vacation supplies overrides from the pharmacy benefit management company are a benefit to a patient. A lost or stolen override also from the pharmacy benefit management company may be provided to a patient, provided that the medication is not a Schedule II medication.

Activity:

Calculate the following prescriptions' days supply as it relates to the corresponding requested refill dates. Given that the patient will need to take 75% of the medication. Each prescription has two refills remaining for the patient to submit.

1: metoprolol 100 mg po bid. Original fill date is 10/1/12. Requested refill date is 10/25/12. Can the patient refill this medication?

_____

2: albuterol inhaler two puff q 4–6 hrs prn. Original fill date is 11/15/12. Requested refill date is 12/9/12. Can the patient refill this medication?

_____

3: A patient comes in for his refill of his maintenance medication escitalopram 5 mg. He states that he is going on a vacation and he will not have a sufficient amount of the medication. He will be out of the country before he can refill the medication again. Can the patient refill this medication?

_____

LAB 12-1: Insurance Billing

Objective:

Practice looking at insurance information and calculating prices in different insurance situations.

Pre-Lab Information:

Read Chapter 12, "Insurance and Third-Party Billing," in your textbook.

Explanation:

As a pharmacy technician, in the community pharmacy setting, you will be involved with third-party billing on a daily basis. It is important for you to understand where to find the information required to process pharmacy claims accurately. It is equally important for you to understand the impact of billing on the pharmacy business. These exercises are designed to help you experience working with this type of information.

Activity:

Review the following three scenarios and answer the associated questions.

Scenario 1

Some insurance companies have contracts with participating pharmacies that include a monthly capitation fee for each patient. This means that the pharmacy gets paid the same amount every month for each patient member of that plan, regardless of the number or cost of prescriptions filled for that patient.

For example, the pharmacy may have two patients with the same HMO for which the monthly capitation fee is $100. That means the pharmacy will receive $100 for each patient. The patients will each have a $5.00 co-pay amount for each prescription filled.

Mr. Smith has three monthly prescriptions that cost $23, $36, and $32. Mrs. Lee has two prescriptions costing $13 and $128. In questions A–H below, calculate the patient's cost as well as the pharmacy's total profit or loss for the two patients.

  A. Mr. Smith's monthly prescription cost: $_____

  B. Mr. Smith's capitation fee + co-pays: $_____

  C. Mrs. Lee's monthly prescription cost: $_____

  D. Mrs. Lee's capitation fee + co-pays: $_____

  E. Pharmacy profit or loss from Mr. Smith's prescriptions: $_____

  F. Pharmacy profit or loss from Mrs. Lee's prescriptions: $_____

  G. Combined profit or loss from both patients: $_____

  H. Did the pharmacy have a profit or a loss? _____

Scenario 2

Mr. Thomas's insurance company reimburses the pharmacy using the formula AWP minus 10% plus a $5.00 dispensing fee. Mr. Thomas is paying a $10.00 co-pay for each of his prescription. The actual acquisition cost of his medicine is $95 for 100 tablets, and the AWP is $125 for 100 tablets.

In questions A–F below, calculate how much the pharmacy will receive from the insurance company for a 30-day supply if Mr. Thomas takes one tablet bid. Calculate the pharmacy's gross profit for each prescription.

A. Acquisition cost for 60 tablets: $_____

B. AWP for 60 tablets: $_____

C. Insurance reimbursement for 60 tablets: $_____

D. (AWP – 10%): $_____

E. Plus $5.00 dispensing fee = _____ = insurance reimbursement

F. Plus patient's co-pay = $_____

G. Less acquisition cost (from above) = gross profit: $_____

Scenario 3

Consider the following insurance card. Fill in the information for the patient on the attached patient profile. Then, fill in the blanks labeled A–J in the chart.

ACME HMO   Group. 00001681
                                               Member#: 00004568
                                               Effective: 01/01/2014

Member: Mary T. Smith
PCP: James S. Thomas, MD
Phone#: 321-123-3231   Co-Pays
Network: Mountain Medical Group   RX: Generic $10, Brand $30

Patient Profile

Patient	Address	Phone	D.O.B.	Allergies	Insurance	Plan/Group #	ID #	Co-Pay
Smith, Mary T	11334 Park NY, NY	444-3457	02/01/43	Sulfa	A.	B.	C.	D.

Rx #	Date	Drug	Directions	Quantity	AWP	Prescriber	Charge to Patient
60456	03/15/14	furosemide 40 mg	1 tab PO q.a.m.	30	$1.75	Thomas	E.
60457	03/15/14	Plavix 20 mg	1 tab PO q.a.m.	30	$124.74	Thomas	F.
60458	03/15/14	lisinopril 10 mg	1 tab PO bid	60	$6.45	Thomas	G.
60458	03/15/14	Lantus insulin	10 Units S.CUT. QHS	10 mL	$86.76	Thomas	H.
				TOTAL COST	J	TOTAL	I.

Student Name: _____

Lab Partner: _____

Grade/Comments: _____

_____

_____

Student Comments: _____

_____

_____

LAB 12-2: Troubleshooting Insurance

Objective:
Recognizing error messages and finding solutions during the troubleshooting process.

Pre-Lab Information:
Read Chapter 12, "Insurance and Third Party Billing," in your textbook.

Explanation:
Many times in the community pharmacy setting, pharmacy claims that process via the online adjudication method may produce an error message that a pharmacy technician will have to troubleshoot.

Activity:
Select a team of three, which will include a "pharmacist," a "technician," and a "patient." Decide upon which team member will take on each of the roles in this activity/scenario.

Scenario 1:

A transgender male to female patient brings in new prescriptions for the hormone therapy drugs of estrogen, estradiol, and conjugated estrogens. The patient is listed as a male in the patient profile. The error message that populates for both medications is that the "drug is not covered." The medications are approved on the insurance company's formulary.

What are the options you can choose to do and steps to take with troubleshooting the claims in order for them to be paid for by the insurance company?

1: _____

_____

_____

2: _____

_____

_____

3: _____

_____

_____

4: _____

_____

_____

Scenario 2:

A patient requests refills on all of their maintenance medications, which were filled for a 30-day supply less than two weeks ago. The insurance company rejects the claims as "Refills Too Soon." The patient explains that they are leaving in a few days for a four-week international business trip, which means they will run out of their medications while out of the country.

What are the options you can choose to do and steps to take with troubleshooting these claims in order for them to be paid for by the insurance company?

1: _____

_____

_____

2: _____

_____

_____

3: _____

_____

_____

4: _____

_____

_____

Student Name: _____

Lab Partner: _____

Grade/Comments: _____

_____

_____

Student Comments: _____

_____

_____

LAB 12-3: Drug Formularies

Objective:

To become familiar with types of formularies.

Pre-Lab Information:

Read Chapter 12, "Insurance and Third Party Billing," in your textbook.

Explanation:

Formularies exist to help ensure and maintain patient safety as well as control costs of medication therapy management. The technician is heavily relied upon to be aware of and understand which medications are approved and not approved on a third-party plan benefit.

Activity:

Research the following two websites and notate three medications from each site that are approved formulary drugs.https://www.healthnet.com/portal/member/content.do?mainResourceFile=/content/general/unprotected/html/ca/pharmacy/rec_drug_list.html

1: _____
2: _____
3: _____

https://www.uhcmedicaresolutions.com/health-plans/medicare-advantage-plans/resources-plan-material/drug-list.html#4

1: _____
2: _____
3: _____

Student Name: _____

Lab Partner: _____

Grade/Comments: _____

_____

_____

Student Comments: _____

_____

_____

CHAPTER 13
Over-the-Counter (OTC) Products

After completing Chapter 13 from the textbook, you should be able to:	Related Activity in the Workbook/Lab Manual
1. Define and describe the FDA categories and regulations pertaining to OTC products.	Review Questions, PTCB Exam Practice Questions, Activity 13-3
2. Outline the process for prescription drugs to become approved for OTC classification.	Review Questions, PTCB Exam Practice Questions, Activity 13-3
3. List and describe common OTC analgesics and antipyretics.	Review Questions, PTCB Exam Practice Questions, Activity 13-1, Lab 13-1
4. List and describe common OTC respiratory agents.	Review Questions, PTCB Exam Practice Questions, Activity 13-1, Lab 13-1, Lab 13-2, Lab 13-3
5. List and describe common gastrointestinal system agents.	Review Questions, PTCB Exam Practice Questions, Activity 13-1, Lab 13-1, Lab 13-2, Lab 13-3
6. List and describe common OTC integumentary system agents.	Review Questions, PTCB Exam Practice Questions, Activity 13-1, Lab 13-1, Lab 13-2, Lab 13-3
7. List and describe common OTC central nervous system agents.	Review Questions, PTCB Exam Practice Questions, Activity 13-1, Lab 13-1, Lab 13-2, Lab 13-3
8. List and describe common OTC ophthalmic, otic, and oral agents.	Review Questions, PTCB Exam Practice Questions, Activity 13-1, Lab 13-1, Lab 13-2, Lab 13-3

9. List and describe common OTC contraceptive products.	Review Questions, PTCB Exam Practice Questions, Activity 13-1, Lab 13-1, Lab 13-2, Lab 13-3
10. List and describe common smoking cessation products.	Review Questions, PTCB Exam Practice Questions, Activity 13-1, Lab 13-1, Lab 13-2, Lab 13-3
11. List and describe common behind-the-counter (BTC) products.	Review Questions, PTCB Exam Practice Questions, Activity 13-1, Lab 13-1, Lab 13-2, Lab 13-3
12. List and describe common herbal and alternative treatments.	Review Questions, PTCB Exam Practice Questions, Activity 13-1, Lab 13-1, Lab 13-2, Lab 13-3
13. List and describe common vitamins and supplements.	Review Questions, PTCB Exam Practice Questions, Activity 13-1, Lab 13-1, Lab 13-2, Lab 13-3
14. List and describe common OTC medical devices and diagnostic agents.	Review Questions, PTCB Exam Practice Questions, Activity 13-1, Lab 13-1, Lab 13-2, Lab 13-3
15. List and describe common OTC fertility and pregnancy tests.	Review Questions, PTCB Exam Practice Questions
16. Describe the use of nebulizers.	Review Questions, PTCB Exam Practice Questions
17. List and describe common OTC test screening kits.	Review Questions, PTCB Exam Practice Questions
18. List and describe common OTC medical supplies.	Review Questions, PTCB Exam Practice Questions, Lab 13-3
19. Define and describe the pharmacy technician's role with OTC products, devices, and supplies.	Review Questions, PTCB Exam Practice Questions, Activity 13-3, Lab 13-3

INTRODUCTION

Pharmacy technicians who understand how over-the-counter (OTC) products effect prescription medications, or know how to educate patients on the use of medical devices, help to alleviate patient concerns and build avenues of trust. Although providing patients with the best possible route of care is important, the pharmacy technician must also remember what information is within their lawful scope of practice. It cannot be said enough; it is unlawful for pharmacy technicians to provide medical advice or medication information; whether it is prescription or OTC. If a technician has a patient who request information concerning OTC medications they should refer the patient to the pharmacist. Above all other things, concern for the patient's safety must be the pharmacy technician's main priority. A technician who not only understands this but also mimics it in their career will not only have a long career in pharmacy, but gain the respect of other health care professional.

REVIEW QUESTIONS

Fill in the blanks.

1. The drug manufacturer must first seek approval from the _____ and in order to do that they must prove the drug has potential benefit to the general public as well as a limited risk of safety.

2. In 1951 the _____ to the Food, Drug and Cosmetic Act of _____, created two distinct classes of drugs; prescription and nonprescription.

3. There are more than _____ nonprescription products on the U.S. market.

4. It takes a minimum of _____ and quite often longer, for the FDA to approve a drug switch to OTC status.

5. If at any time the FDA finds a nonprescription drug to be unsafe or without benefit to the average consumer, they may remove the drug from _____.

6. Ibuprofen and naproxen sodium belong to the _____ class of analgesics.

7. Antitussives are used to suppress _____ coughs.

8. The three most common dosage forms for OTC smoking cessation products are _____, _____ and _____.

9. Vitamin _____ and Vitamin _____ can have a negative effect on Coumadin.

10. Antacids, which are often used to treat heartburn, _____ stomach acid.

11. A(n) _____ is a machine used to vaporize medication into the air, in order to open up airways.

12. Antiemetics are used to treat _____ and _____.

13. A cough that is caused by a buildup of phlegm or mucus would be treated with a(n) _____.

14. "Lice season" typically peaks between the months of _____ and _____.

15. The FDA only permits sunscreens with an SPF of _____ or higher to be labeled as having the ability to aid in the prevention of skin cancer.

PHARMACY CALCULATION PROBLEMS

Calculate the following.

1. The volume of OTC cough syrup that the customer is purchasing is 120 mL. The directions for adults and children who are 12 years and older are; 2 teaspoons every 4 hours. How many days will this cough syrup last the patient?

2. A customer is asking you for two boxes of pseudoephedrine that he would like to purchase for personal use. Each tablet is 30 mg of pseudoephedrine. How many grams of pseudoephedrine are in each 24 count box? What is the total amount of pseudoephedrine for both boxes?

3. A patient brings in a prescription for nitroglycerin 1/150 g. How many milligrams does that equate to?

4. A customer brings in a prescription for guaifenesin AC 10 mg–200 mg/5 mL. The directions are; 2tsp po q4h not to exceed 60 mL per day for 5 days. What is the total volume needed to fill the order?

5. A customer is asking you about the multivitamins that are on sale this week. The retail price for a 60 count bottle is 14.99 with a 20% discount. How much will the discount be for the customer if he purchases three bottles?

PTCB EXAM PRACTICE QUESTIONS

1. A patient asks you if he or she can take low dose aspirin while on warfarin therapy. Your response is:
   a. no that is a fatal interaction.
   b. that should be fine to do.
   c. let me have the pharmacist speak with you.
   d. the pharmacist is busy right now.

2. Which of the following medications does not contain acetaminophen:
   a. percodan.
   b. Excedrin.
   c. hydrocodone/APAP.
   d. fioricet.

3. The most recently approved class of OTC product to combat acid reflux is:
   a. H2 antagonists.
   b. antacids.
   c. PPIs.
   d. acid reducers.

4. NSAID stands for:
   a. Nonsteroidal anti-irritation drug.
   b. Nonsteroidal anti-inflammation drug.
   c. Non-sedating anti-inflammatory drug.
   d. Nonsteroidal anti-inflammatory drug.

5. Claritin is to loratadine as Allegra is to:
   a. fluticasone.
   b. fexofenadine.
   c. fluoxetine.
   d. furosemide.

ACTIVITY 13-1: Classifying OTC Products

Instructions: Match the various classifications of OTC products from the lists below.

Set 1:

1. cetirizine _____
2. calcium carbonate _____
3. naproxen sodium _____
4. dextromethorphan _____
5. omeprazole _____

A. NSAID
B. PPI
C. Antitussive
D. Antihistamine
E. Antacid

Set 2:

1. aspirin _____
2. loratadine _____
3. pseudoephedrine _____
4. ibuprofen _____
5. simethacone _____

A. Antihistamine
B. Salicylate
C. Decongestant
D. Antiflatulent
E. NSAID

ACTIVITY 13-2: Case Study—Cold Season

Instructions: Read the following scenario and then answer the critical thinking questions.

A customer comes into the pharmacy and does not look well to you. The customer approaches the counter and states to you that she is feeling chilly and that she has also been coughing and producing mucous as well as being unable to successfully sleep throughout the night. The cough, cold, and flu season has arrived to her, and she is looking for recommendations from the pharmacy team for relief of her symptoms. After briefing the pharmacist about what the customer explained to you about her symptoms, you then apprise the pharmacist that the customer would like to speak with him or her about any OTC products which could be used to suppress the patient's symptoms.

The pharmacist recommends two OTC products to use for her fever and for her coughing. The customer pays for her products and thanks you and the pharmacist for being so helpful.

1. Was there any further information that you could have asked the customer prior to speaking with the pharmacist about her symptoms?

   _____

   _____

   _____

2. What OTC products can you think of that the pharmacist recommended to the patient?

   _____

   _____

   _____

3. Did you do anything outside of your scope of practice during this scenario?

   _____

   _____

   _____

ACTIVITY 13-3: Case Study—Rx to OTC Transition

Instructions: Visit the following website to view the listing of medications which have transitioned from a legend medication to an OTC product. List at least six OTC medications that have been approved for over the counter use in the past four years.http://www.fda.gov/AboutFDA/CentersOffices/OfficeofMedicalProductsandTobacco/CDER/ucm106378.htm

1: _____

2: _____

3: _____

4: _____

5: _____

6: _____

Part 2:

In your own words, describe the process for a prescription drug to become approved by the Food and Drug Administration for OTC classification. What questions about the drug must the FDA answer before it approves it for OTC use? Do you think additional questions are necessary to protect the safety of the public? Why or why not?

_____

_____

_____

_____

_____

_____

_____

_____

_____

_____

Research: Use the Internet to find examples where the FDA removed nonprescription status from an OTC drug. For each example, explain what events led up to this change.

LAB 13-1: Assisting Patients with OTC Products

Objective:

Exhibiting good customer service skills as well as memory recall.

Pre-Lab Information:

Review Chapter 13, "Over-the-Counter (OTC) Products," in the textbook.

Explanation:

There are numerous OTC products for customers to choose for various ailments. These products are at times readily available after a manufacturer has promoted it through successful marketing strategies. However, even with today's fast-paced environment of advertising techniques and mediums a product may not be as available as the media and manufacturer intended.

Any pseudoephedrine-containing product is now a BTC product. The sales of these products are facilitated and monitored by the pharmacy team.

Activity:

In this activity select a team of two, which will include a "technician" and a "patient." Decide upon which team member will take on each of the roles in this activity/scenarios.

Scenario 1

A customer comes in to purchase the latest product for his acid reflux symptoms. He approaches the counter and asks you if you currently have the product in stock as it has been advertised for the past week. Your shipment from the wholesaler had come in yesterday, and it did not include the product the customer is requesting. What should you do to help the customer?

_____

_____

_____

_____

Scenario 2

A customer comes in looking disheveled to both you and the pharmacy team. As she approaches the counter she asks you for four boxes of plain pseudoephedrine. You then tell the customer that only two boxes can be sold to her. She becomes frustrated and irritated by what you have just told her about the limitation. She then states that she will take two boxes and be on her way. As you leave the counter to retrieve the boxes, she becomes agitated and slams her hand on the counter. What should you do to help the customer?

_____

_____

_____

_____

Student Name: _____

Lab Partner: _____

Grade/Comments: _____

_____

Student Comments: _____

_____

_____

LAB 13-2: Classifying OTC Products

Objective:

Differentiating and classifying OTC products

Pre-Lab Information:

Review Chapter 13, "Over-the-Counter (OTC) Products," in the textbook.

Explanation:

Many OTC products have specific aisles or areas that they are housed in for ease of the consumer and for the pharmacy team to locate.

Activity:

In your mock pharmacy lab, the instructor will have a tote filled with various OTC products. Separate and count the different products and list them in the inventory.

	Class of product	Medication Name	Quantity
1:			
2:			
3:			
4:			
5:			
6:			
7:			
8:			
9:			
10:			
11:			
12:			
13:			
14:			
15:			

Student Name: _____

Lab Partner: _____

Grade/Comments: _____

_____

_____

Student Comments: _____

_____

_____

LAB 13-3: Helping a Patient Select a Blood Glucose Monitor

Objective:
To become familiar with blood glucose monitors.

Pre-Lab Information:
Review Chapter 13, "Over-the-Counter (OTC) Products," in the textbook.

Explanation:
Pharmacy technicians are often the first point of contact and advocate for patients who need a blood glucose monitor.

Activity:
Research the following websites to become familiar with three different types of blood glucose monitors. List the names of the monitors and what is different or unique about each monitor.

1: http://www.onetouch.com/onetouch-diabetes-testing-supplies

A: _____

B: _____

C: _____

2: https://www.myfreestyle.com/products.html

A: _____

B: _____

C: _____

3: https://www.accu-chek.com/us/

A: _____

B: _____

C: _____

Student Name: _____

Lab Partner: _____

Grade/Comments: _____

_____

_____

Student Comments: _____

_____

_____

CHAPTER 14
Introduction to Compounding

After completing Chapter 14 from the textbook, you should be able to:	Related Activity in the Workbook/Lab Manual
1. Explain the purpose and reason for compounding prescriptions.	Review Questions
2. Discuss the basic procedures involved in compounding.	Review Questions, PTCB Exam Practice Questions, Lab 14-1, Lab 14-2, Lab 14-3, Lab 14-4, Lab 14-5, Lab 14-6, Lab 14-7, Lab 14-8
3. List and describe the equipment, supplies, and facilities required for compounding.	Review Questions, PTCB Exam Practice Questions, Activity 14-2, Activity 14-3, Activity 14-4, Lab 14-1, Lab 14-2, Lab 14-3, Lab 14-4, Lab 14-5, Lab 14-6, Lab 14-7, Lab 14-8
4. List the major dosage forms used in compounding.	Review Questions, PTCB Exam Practice Questions, Activity 14-2, Lab 14-3, Lab 14-4, Lab 14-5, Lab 14-6, Lab 14-7, Lab 14-8
5. Discuss the considerations involved in flavoring a compounded prescription.	Review Questions, PTCB Exam Practice Questions, Activity 14-2, Activity 14-3, Activity 14-4

INTRODUCTION

Pharmaceutical *compounding* is the practice of extemporaneously preparing medications to meet the unique need of an individual patient according to the specific order of a physician or prescriber. Compounded medications may be either sterile or nonsterile and include suspensions, capsules, suppositories, topically applied medications, intravenous admixtures, and parenteral nutrition solutions.

Extemporaneous compounding is a special service provided by a number of community-based pharmacies. To assist the pharmacist in compounding medications, you will require additional training, skills, and practice. However, this unique area of pharmacy practice offers a number of advanced professional opportunities for those who pursue these skills.

REVIEW QUESTIONS

Match the following.

1. _____ comminuting
2. _____ compounding
3. _____ emulsion
4. _____ excipient
5. _____ geometric dilution
6. _____ suspension
7. _____ trituration

a. contains insoluble particles uniformly dispersed throughout the vehicle
b. another word for trituration
c. contains two immiscible liquids
d. any substance added to a prescription to make it a suitable consistency or to form the drug
e. reducing particle size of a substance by grinding
f. starts with smallest ingredient amount and doubles the portion by adding other ingredients
g. extemporaneously preparing medications to meet the unique need of an individual patient

Choose the best answer.

8. Which of the following is not a compounding resource?
   a. *United States Pharmacopoeia*
   b. Merck book of brand and generic drugs
   c. *Veterinary Drug Handbook*
   d. *Remington's Pharmaceutical Sciences*

9. Which of the following compounding steps should be completed before the others?
   a. Collecting all of the necessary ingredients.
   b. Writing up a compounding worksheet.
   c. Weighing each ingredient.
   d. Obtaining the formula from the pharmacist.

10. Which of the following is more appropriate for melting bases?
    a. a magnetic stirring plate
    b. a heat gun
    c. a hotplate
    d. an electronic mortar and pestle

11. When using geometric dilution, one should start with the:
    a. ingredient needed in the smallest amount.
    b. ingredient needed in the largest amount.
    c. equal amounts of each ingredient.
    d. the liquid or binding base.

12. Assuming that only the following dosage forms were suitable, which is the desirable choice for animal patients?
    a. cream
    b. ointment
    c. transdermal gel
    d. injection

Match the following.

13. _____ capsule
14. _____ emulsion
15. _____ stick
16. _____ troche

a. topical application of anesthetics or antivirals
b. dissipates into the skin when applied
c. liquid preparation that contains insoluble particles
d. oral dosage form, used for more than 100 years

17. _____ cream   e. oral form that disintegrates over time

18. _____ suspension   f. liquid/semisolid form that can be taken orally or applied topically

19. _____ paste   g. stiff, viscous ointment

20. _____ ointment   h. semisolid preparation that stays on top of skin

True or False?

21. Otic preparations may be used in the eye.

    T   F

22. The most common form of compounded transdermal gel therapy is a two-phase vehicle made from pluronic lecithin organogel.

    T   F

23. Using the proper coloring and flavoring in medications is important for patient compliance.

    T   F

24. One of the five basic flavoring techniques is physiological.

    T   F

25. Aseptic, or sterile, technique should be used in all extemporaneous compounding procedures.

    T   F

PHARMACY CALCULATION PROBLEMS

Calculate the following.

1. Tom is compounding a prescription that calls for 15 g betamethasone 0.05% cream, 15 g diphenhydramine cream, then qs ad 60 g with aquaphilic ointment. How much aquaphilic ointment will he need to add to this compound?

2. A prescription was brought to the pharmacy for a product that is not commercially available. It calls for clindamycin 4,500 mg qs ad 120 mL with lubricating lotion. If the clindamycin is available in 300 mg capsules, how many capsules should be opened for use in this compound?

3. How many sucralfate 1 g tablets will you need for an oral suspension that calls for 20 g sucralfate as the active ingredient?

4. A pharmacy received a faxed order from a veterinarian for celecoxib 25 mg chicken dog treats, #100. If the celecoxib comes in 100 mg capsules, how many capsules should be mixed in the chicken base to make 100 treats?

5. A special compound requires equal parts zinc oxide 20% ointment, nystatin ointment, and hydrocortisone 0.5% ointment. If the prescription calls for 60 g, how many grams of each ointment will be needed?

PTCB EXAM PRACTICE QUESTIONS

1. A two-phase system consisting of a finely divided solid dispersed in a liquid is a/an:
   a. suspension.
   b. emulsion.
   c. solution.
   d. trituration.

2. What is the on-demand preparation of a drug product according to a physician's prescription?
   a. IVPB
   b. extemporaneous compounding
   c. trituration
   d. spatulation

3. The fine grinding of a powder is called:
   a. extemporaneous compounding.
   b. suspension.
   c. emulsion.
   d. trituration.

4. Clear liquids in which the drug is completely dissolved are called:
   a. sublimations.
   b. suspensions.
   c. solutions.
   d. emulsions.

5. A system containing two immiscible liquids with one dispersed in the other is called a/an:
   a. emulsion.
   b. suspension.
   c. syrup.
   d. solution.

ACTIVITY 14-1: Case Study—Compounded Laser Gel

Instructions: Read the following scenario and then answer the critical thinking questions.

Note: Based partly on an actual event.

A 22-year-old college student decides she would like to use laser treatment to remove the hair from her legs. She hears that the benefits of laser treatment include a much longer time for hair to grow back. The negative, however, is that it can be a painful procedure. She finds a local "medical spa" that performs this procedure. The spa provides her with two tubes of anesthetic gel to apply just before her procedure; the gel was compounded in an outside compounding pharmacy. She is also told to wrap her legs in cellophane for better absorption. She is told that it is a numbing gel, but receives no counseling or patient information sheet about the product.

She applies the gel and cellophane wrap in anticipation of her appointment. As she is driving down the road, she begins to feel dizzy and pulls over. When she is found, she is unconscious and convulsing; she then goes into a coma.

The numbing product she received was called Laser Gel 10-10 and consisted of 10% lidocaine and 10% tetracaine with phenylephrine. After much media attention, several other cases are discovered in which people have gone into comas after using the anesthetic gel.

The spa's lawyer said the spa owners never knew that a prescription was needed for the gel, and they thought it was a safe and approved product. So did the 22-year-old college student.

1. In this case, from the information you have, what key elements are absent from the staff persons' knowledge about the gel?

_____

_____

_____

_____

2. Should the patient have questioned the product, or do you feel the responsibility lies with the medical spa?

_____

_____

_____

_____

3. What disciplinary measures, if any, do you think should be levied against the medical spa in this case? Against the compounding pharmacy?

_____

_____

_____

_____

ACTIVITY 14-2: Case Study—Veterinary

Instructions: Read the following scenario and then answer the critical thinking questions.

The veterinary compounding pharmacy where you work consists of three pharmacist/pharmacy technician teams. Pharmacists assist with dosing for the patients while the pharmacy technicians prepare the formulations and perform the administrative tasks. It is an optimum arrangement in which both staff members can practice their skill-sets. This pharmacy also encourages and provides yearly training to update skill-sets and learn new information. It does this through seminars, videos, and the purchase of materials such as reference books.

Calculations must be done for accurate and proper dosing as various drug forms may have to be created for better acceptance from the animal patients. Compounding for animals is a specialty area and can sometimes require some creativity. For example, when a dog will not swallow his or her prescribed medication, a flavoring agent might be added to help make it more palatable for the animal. Your team has been assigned a few cases today, each of which requires you to call upon your creativity:

- An elephant has recently had major eye surgery and has not eaten for days afterward. Elephants are notorious for not accepting oral medications. The elephant has been prescribed a sterile ophthalmic solution that must be compounded to acquire the correct dose. After consulting with the pharmacist, you now have a "recipe" or SOP to compound. However, you are told that elephants dislike having their eyes manipulated and will do anything to prevent access.

- A horse with equine Cushing's syndrome is prescribed pergolide mesylate and you are told that the horse can accept oral medications.

- A cat with leukemia has been prescribed chlorambucil. Although the cat can take medications orally, the owner has tried numerous times and has also failed to administer them successfully to the cat.

1. Can you think of a way to access the elephant's eye in order to administer the medication without touching any of the animal's eye area?

_____

_____

_____

_____

2. What oral drug forms could be used to compound the pergolide medication for administration to the horse?

_____

_____

_____

_____

3. Can you think of anything to do to the cat's medication to help the cat accept it?

_____

_____

_____

_____

ACTIVITY 14-3: Case Study—Childproof Containers

Instructions: Read the following scenario and then answer the critical thinking questions.

Mrs. Gaynor has been on estrogen therapy for a short time now and is beginning to feel much better. Her premenopausal hot flashes and night sweats have subsided. She receives an 8 oz. jar of a custom-compounded estrogen cream made specifically for her. She uses it daily and keeps the jar under a sink in the bathroom.

While her prepubescent grandson is visiting, he becomes curious and applies some of the cream. He thinks it must be something special because of the claims made on the jar about feeling much better. The grandson continues to do this, without anyone's knowledge, as he visits on a weekly basis. Meanwhile, Mrs. Gaynor is receiving more frequent refills through the compounding pharmacy.

Soon the grandson develops gynecomastia (the development of abnormally large mammary glands that can sometimes secrete milk). A doctor's visit confirms that the grandson has been exposed to large amounts of estrogen and enlists the family's help in finding the source.

1. What steps could the compounding pharmacy take to help prevent this situation?

_____

_____

_____

_____

2. What steps could the grandmother take to help prevent easy access by the grandson?

_____

_____

_____

_____

3. From the information provided, what signs or "flags" were present to indicate that there might be a problem?

_____

_____

_____

_____

ACTIVITY 14-4: Case Study—Medication Flavoring

Instructions: Read the following scenario and then answer the critical thinking questions.

An adult parent comes into the pharmacy with an already reconstituted prescription for amoxicillin suspension for her four-year-old daughter. After an unsuccessful attempt to administer the medication to her daughter earlier in the day, and prior to her coming back now, she first called the pharmacy to see if there was any option for the pharmacist to make the medication taste better in order for the daughter to take another dose.

You explain to the parent that there are three flavoring agents available to make the medication palatable for the patient.

1. What steps could the pharmacist or pharmacy technician have taken prior to the parent coming in a second time? What should the technician do the next time a prescription for a suspension that is prescribed for a child is going to be filled?

_____

_____

_____

2. What steps could the parent have taken to prevent a second trip to the pharmacy?

_____

_____

_____

3. What are the flavoring agents that the technician could suggest to make suspensions more palatable?

_____

_____

_____

_____

LAB 14-1: Measuring Liquids Accurately

Objective:

Gain experience in measuring liquids using graduated cylinders.

Pre-Lab Information:

- Review Chapter 14 in the textbook and visit http://pharmlabs.unc.edu/
- Gather the following materials:
  - 20, 50, and 100 mL graduated cylinders
  - chilled grape juice
  - chilled cranberry juice
  - chilled apple juice
  - paper cups to contain the liquid "medication"

Explanation:

This exercise gives you the opportunity to experience measuring liquids. You must be careful when pouring liquid medications, and it takes practice to accurately find the meniscus.

Activity:

Using the materials listed previously, prepare the following "prescriptions" for "dispensing":

1. apple juice 30 mL

    cranberry juice 20 mL

    grape juice 50 mL

    Sig: Mix together and enjoy UD

2. grape juice 55 mL

    apple juice 35 mL

    cranberry juice 80 mL

    Sig: Mix together and enjoy UD

Student Name: _____

Lab Partner: _____

Grade/Comments: _____

_____

_____

Student Comments: _____

_____

_____

LAB 14-2: Using the Prescription Balance

Objective:

Review use of the prescription balance, including taring the balance and using weights.

Pre-Lab Information:

- Review Chapter 14 in your textbook.
- Gather the following materials:
  - prescription torsion balance
  - prescription weights
  - weighing papers or boats
  - spatula
  - powder to weigh (could be flour, cake mix, or other kitchen ingredient)

Explanation:

Extemporaneous compounding has become increasingly important. Accurate use of the prescription balance is a vitally important aspect of compounding. The following exercise will help you develop a basic understanding of the process.

Activity:

Using the materials listed previously, weigh out 6.5 g of the powder.

Steps

1. Place the balance on a clean, flat surface away from moving air (windows, doors, etc.).
2. Check the balance pans for any residue left from previous use.
3. Move the calibration dial to zero.
4. Place a weighing boat or paper in the center of each pan.
5. Unlock the arrest knob and check that the balance is level.
6. If the pointer is not in the center, carefully rotate the leveling screws to bring the pointer to a level position. Lock the arrest knob.
7. Move the calibration dial to the 0.5 g mark.
8. Using tweezers, add a 5 g and 1 g weight to the boat or paper on the *right side* of the balance.
9. With the arrest knob still in the locked position, add a small amount of powder to the weighing boat on the *left side* of the balance.
10. Unlock the arrest knob and observe the balance pointer to see if the amount of powder added was too much or too little.
11. If the pointer rests to the left of the index center, you have added too much powder. If the pointer is to the right of the center, you have added too little powder.
12. Lock the arrest knob before adding or removing powder. When the pointer is near equilibrium, it will move back and forth within the index. At this point, you may leave the knob unlocked and add very small amounts of powder by placing a small amount of powder on the spatula and gently tapping the spatula.
13. Lock the arrest knob and remove the weighing boat or paper with the powder on it.

Questions

1. Why do you think it is necessary to use weigh boats or paper?

   _____

   _____

   _____

2. Why do you need to adjust the balance after a weigh boat has been placed on each pan?

   _____

   _____

   _____

3. Why is it a good idea to lock the pans in place before adding or removing weight from either pan?

   _____

   _____

   _____

Student Name: _____

Lab Partner: _____

Grade/Comments: _____

_____

_____

Student Comments: _____

_____

_____

LAB 14-3: Compounding Exercise—Capsules

Objective:

To give you experience in filling capsules using the punch method.

Pre-Lab Information:

- Review Chapter 14 in your textbook.
- Gather the following materials:
  - prescription torsion balance
  - prescription weights
  - weighing papers or boats
  - spatula
  - powder to weigh (could be flour, cake mix, or other kitchen ingredient)
  - gelatin capsules, size 0
  - ointment slab
  - powder paper or wax paper
  - nonsterile gloves

Explanation:

As a pharmacy technician, you should be familiar with the punch-filling of capsules to deliver custom-compounded medications to patients. This exercise is designed to give you practical experience with filling capsules.

Activity:

Using the materials outlined previously, follow these steps:

1. Using the steps from Lab 14-2, place the powder on the ointment slab that has been covered with powder paper or wax paper.
2. Using a spatula, form a smooth block that is about half the length of the capsule body.
3. Wearing gloves to prevent hand contact, separate five capsules and place them in an empty weighing boat.
4. Begin "punching" the capsules by taking the body of a capsule and holding it in an upright position. Punch the open end repeatedly into the powder until the capsule is full.
5. Replace the capsule cap and weigh each capsule, using an empty capsule on the other pan of the balance. Each capsule should weigh 500 mg; each must be between 90% and 110% of 500 mg.
6. Clean the capsules with a soft tissue and place them in an appropriate container.

Student Name: _____

Lab Partner: _____

Grade/Comments: _____

_____

_____

Student Comments: _____

_____

_____

LAB 14-4: Compounding Exercise—Solution

0.5% API Solution *

Suggested Formula for 2 oz

Active Pharmaceutical Ingredient (API)	0.3 g
Purified Water (Solvent)	10 mL
Flavor of Choice	3 mL
Simple Syrup	q.s. to 60 mL

Suggested Compounding Procedures

1. Dissolve API in solvent.
2. Add flavoring and shake well.
3. Q.S. to 60 mL with simple syrup and shake well.

Student Name: _____

Lab Partner: _____

Grade/Comments: _____

_____

_____

Student Comments: _____

_____

_____

---

*This formula is for TRAINING PURPOSES ONLY. Do NOT inject, ingest, or otherwise dispense this product.

FC0710

LAB 14-5: Compounding Exercise—Suspension

for training purposes only

0.5% API Suspension *

Suggested Formula for 2 oz

Active Pharmaceutical Ingredient (API)	0.3 g
Polysorbate 80	to wet
Flavor of Choice	3 mL
Simple Syrup	q.s. to 60 mL

Suggested Compounding Procedures

1. Using a mortar, wet the API with Polysorbate 80 until a smacking sound is created.
2. Slowly add simple syrup to the wetted API, up to 75% of the final volume.
3. Transfer volume to beaker or dispensing container.
4. Add flavoring and shake well.
5. Q.S. to 60 mL with simple syrup and shake well.

Student Name: _____

Lab Partner: _____

Grade/Comments: _____

_____

_____

Student Comments: _____

_____

_____

_____

*This formula is for TRAINING PURPOSES ONLY. Do NOT inject, ingest, or otherwise dispense this product.

FC0711

LAB 14-6: Compounding Exercise—Cream

for training purposes only

7.5% API Cream *

Suggested Formula for 60 Gm

Active Pharmaceutical Ingredient (API)	4.5 g
Polysorbate 80	3 mL
Lite Cream Base	55.5 g

Suggested Compounding Procedures

1. On an ointment slab, wet the API with Polysorbate 80.
2. Slowly levigate the API with the base.
3. Dispense the cream in an ointment jar.

Student Name: _____

Lab Partner: _____

Grade/Comments: _____

_____

_____

Student Comments: _____

_____

_____

---

*This formula is for TRAINING PURPOSES ONLY. Do NOT inject, ingest, or otherwise dispense this product.

FC0811

LAB 14-7: Compounding Exercise—Suppositories

for training purposes only

20 mg API Suppositories*

Suggested Formula for 12 suppositories

Active Pharmaceutical Ingredient (API)	0.24 g
Silica Gel	0.18 g
Fatty Acid	15 g

Suggested Compounding Procedures

1. Melt the fatty acid at 50 °C.
2. Triturate the API and silica gel in a mortar, using geometric dilution.
3. Sift the powders into the melted base and stir.
4. Turn off heat and stir until fully suspended.
5. Pour into molds (blue suppository mold) and allow to cool at room temperature.

Student Name: _____

Lab Partner: _____

Grade/Comments: _____

_____

_____

Student Comments: _____

_____

_____

*This formula is for TRAINING PURPOSES ONLY. Do NOT inject, ingest, or otherwise dispense this product.

FC0610

LAB 14-8: Compounding Exercise—PLO Gel

for training purposes only
25 mg/mL API PLO Gel*

Suggested Formula for 10 mL

Active Pharmaceutical Ingredient (API)	0.25 g
Lecithin Isopropyl Palmitate Solution	2.5 mL
Poloxamer 407 NF Gel 20% (refrigerated)	7.5 mL

Suggested Compounding Procedures

1. Remove the barrel of a 10 cc Leur-Lock syringe, attach a syringe cap, pour the API into the syringe, and replace the barrel.
2. Using a Leur-to-Oral connector, add the lecithing isopropyl palmitate solution to the API powder.
3. In a second Leur-Lock syringe, use a Leur-to-Oral connector and withdraw the Poloxamer 407 NF Gel 20% (refrigerated).
4. Connect both syringes using a Leur-to-Leur connector.
5. Push the API and lecithin mixture into the syringe containing the poloxamer gel.
6. Mix the ingredients by pushing the contents syringe to syringe. Approximately 15 times.
7. Push all contents into one of the two syringes, remove the Leur-to-Leur connector, and attach a syringe cap.

Student Name: _____

Lab Partner: _____

Grade/Comments: _____

_____

_____

Student Comments: _____

_____

_____

_____

---

*This formula is for TRAINING PURPOSES ONLY. Do NOT inject, ingest, or otherwise dispense this product.

FC0812

CHAPTER 14 *Introduction to Compounding*   **243**

CHAPTER 15
Introduction to Sterile Products

After completing Chapter 15 from the textbook, you should be able to:	Related Activity in the Workbook/Lab Manual
1. Outline and describe the key regulations and guidelines pertaining to sterile product preparations.	Review Questions, PTCB Exam Practice Questions
2. Identify and list the equipment and supplies used in preparing sterile products.	Review Questions, PTCB Exam Practice Questions, Activity 15-1, Activity 15-2, Activity 15-3, Activity 15-4, Lab 15-1, Lab 15-2, Lab 15-3, Lab 15-4, Lab 15-5, Lab 15-6, Lab 15-7, Lab 15-8, Lab 15-9, Lab 15-10
3. Demonstrate proper cleaning of laminar flow hoods.	Review Questions, PTCB Exam Practice Questions, Lab 15-2, Lab 15-3
4. List the routes of administration associated with sterile products.	Review Questions, PTCB Exam Practice Questions, Activity 15-1, Activity 15-2, Activity 15-3, Activity 15-4, Lab 15-4, Lab 15-5, Lab 15-6, Lab 15-7, Lab 15-8, Lab 15-9, Lab 15-10
5. List and describe key characteristics of sterile products.	Review Questions, PTCB Exam Practice Questions, Activity 15-3, Activity 15-4, Lab 15-7, Lab 15-8, Lab 15-9, Lab 15-10
6. Discuss special concerns regarding total parenteral nutrition (TPN).	Review Questions, PTCB Exam Practice Questions, Activity 15-2, Lab 15-10
7. Discuss special concerns regarding chemotherapy and cytotoxic drugs.	Review Questions, PTCB Exam Practice Questions, Activity 15-5
8. Demonstrate proper garbing procedures.	Review Questions, PTCB Exam Practice Questions, Activity 15-3, Lab 15-1
9. Demonstrate proper hand-washing techniques.	Review Questions, PTCB Exam Practice Questions, Lab 15-1
10. Demonstrate how to withdraw from a vial.	Review Questions, PTCB Exam Practice Questions, Lab 15-4
11. Demonstrate how to reconstitute a powder vial.	Review Questions, PTCB Exam Practice Questions, Lab 15-5
12. Demonstrate how to remove fluid from an ampule.	Review Questions, PTCB Exam Practice Questions, Lab 15-4

INTRODUCTION

Sterile compounding is the preparation of compounded medications using aseptic technique, or the process of performing a procedure under controlled conditions in a manner that minimizes the chance of contamination of the preparation. Following proper aseptic techniques ensures that all compounded products remain free of bacteria, fungi, pyrogens, infectives, and other microorganisms. To ensure sterility, these products are prepared in laminar flow hoods, including horizontal flow hoods and biological safety cabinets, which contain a high-efficiency particulate air (HEPA) filter.

Patients generally receive sterile products parenterally through various administration sites, such as veins (IV) and muscle tissue (IM). Other sterile products include total parenteral nutrition (TPN), as well as ophthalmic and otic preparations.

Sterile product preparation can be a complex, high-risk process in the health care setting. As a pharmacy technician with proper training, you can play an integral role in the procurement, storage, preparation, and distribution of sterile products.

REVIEW QUESTIONS

Match the following.

1. _____ antineoplastics
2. _____ intradermal
3. _____ infusion
4. _____ pH
5. _____ buffer capacity
6. _____ intramuscular
7. _____ isotonic
8. _____ precipitate
9. _____ intrathecal

a. a relatively large volume of solution given at a constant rate
b. parenteral injection into a muscle
c. containing the same tonicity as red blood cells
d. parenteral injection into the spine
e. medications to prevent the growth of malignant cells
f. parenteral injection into the skin
g. solid that forms within a solution
h. ability of a solution to resist a change in pH when either an acidic or an alkaline substance is added to the solution
i. the degree of acidity of a solution

Choose the best answer.

10. A bevel is:
    a. an angle cut to measure cc/mL.
    b. a rounded-edge needle.
    c. the sharp pointed end of a needle.
    d. the only part of a needle that can be touched.

11. Medication class which is used to treat cancer is called:
    a. antitoxin.
    b. chemotherapy.
    c. radiation.
    d. cytoblast.

12. Class 100 environment is:
    a. a classification of an airflow unit.
    b. a dimensional measurement of the floor plan.
    c. an airflow of 100 psi.
    d. the best level of sterility available.

13. HEPA refers to:
    a. patient privacy rights.
    b. a large insurance group.
    c. a type of air filter.
    d. the government group that inspects air filters.

Identify and indicate the parts of a needle.

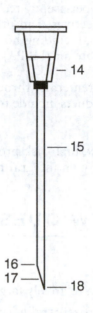

14. _____
15. _____
16. _____
17. _____
18. _____

Identify and indicate the parts of a syringe.

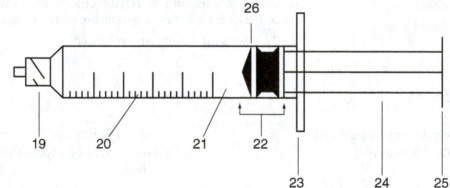

19. _____
20. _____
21. _____
22. _____
23. _____
24. _____
25. _____
26. _____

Identify and indicate the parts of an IV bag system.

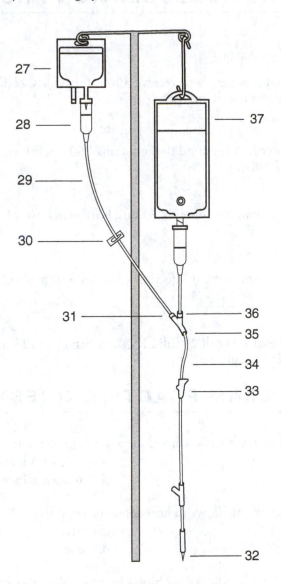

27. _____
28. _____
29. _____
30. _____
31. _____
32. _____
33. _____
34. _____
35. _____
36. _____
37. _____

CHAPTER 15 *Introduction to Sterile Products*

PHARMACY CALCULATION PROBLEMS

Calculate the following.

1. A medical order states that a patient is to receive 500 mL of 0.9% sodium chloride IV over two hours. How fast is the IV running in mL/hr?

2. A technician prepares a sterile compound that contains 100 mg/mL of active drug. How many mL are required for a dose of 800 mg?

3. If a bulk bottle of IV multivitamins contains 50 mL, how many 10 mL doses can be obtained from the bottle?

4. After reconstitution, ceftriaxone for IM injection contains 350 mg/mL. How many milligrams are in 2.5 milliliters?

5. A 1,000 mL bag of 5% dextrose with 20 mEq KCl is infusing at 125 mL/hr. How many hours will the bag last before it must be replaced?

PTCB EXAM PRACTICE QUESTIONS

1. When using a horizontal laminar airflow hood, how far should the technician work inside the hood?
   a. at least 2 inches
   b. at least 4 inches
   c. at least 6 inches
   d. at least 8 inches

2. In a laminar airflow hood, the air flows in how many direction(s)?
   a. four
   b. three
   c. two
   d. one

3. In horizontal laminar airflow hoods, the air blows in which direction?
   a. down toward the work area
   b. away from the operator
   c. toward the operator
   d. up toward the HEPA filter

4. Large-volume parenterals (LVPs) usually have what kind of infusion rates?
   a. intermittent
   b. rapid
   c. slow
   d. instantaneous

5. Vertical airflow hoods have what characteristic?
   a. vertical airflow down toward the product
   b. horizontal airflow away from the operator
   c. vertical airflow up toward the HEPA filter
   d. horizontal airflow toward the operator

ACTIVITY 15-1: Case Study—USP 797 and Training Personnel

Instructions: Read the following scenario and then answer the critical thinking questions.

All the sterile compounding areas in your facility have recently finalized plans to bring them up to USP 797 standards in the pending remodel. The rooms are constructed according to the guidelines and you have been placed in charge of providing the training to the certified pharmacy technicians who will be preparing sterile products in this area.

Your manager tells you that there are some training supplies left over in the pharmacy storage room and that you are welcome to look through it to find anything you could use for the training. The manager also states that a pharmacist will be available for any questions.

While searching through the storage room, you find a written manual that is 755 pages thick that appears to encompass numerous sterile preparation products. While continuing your search, you also find a sterile preparation workbook; however, it does not relate to the written manual you have already found. You also discover a video that you viewed when you were hired about nine years ago. You also discover a box of leftover products that contains various syringes, IV bags, packages, needles, dispensing pins, and gloves. You also find a poster, covered in dust, illustrating the steps for proper hand-washing techniques when preparing to compound a cream.

1. Which of the items found in the storage room do you think you could use for the current training?

   _____

   _____

   _____

   _____

2. Why did you choose to use or not to use each item?

   _____

   _____

   _____

   _____

3. What are the basic requirements for training personnel in sterile preparation, according to USP 797? Do you think these requirements are relevant for patient safety?

   _____

   _____

   _____

   _____

4. What are the barriers to USP 797 compliance in this scenario?

   _____

   _____

   _____

   _____

ACTIVITY 15-2: Case Study—IV Pump Machine and Shortcuts

Instructions: Read the following scenario and then answer the critical thinking questions.

Your 200-bed hospital incorporates automated sterile preparation pumps to help mix the large number of IV orders that arrive in your pharmacy each day. It is a very efficient system, which helps reduce errors, increases accuracy, and reduces time of preparation. Four pharmacy technicians are quite skilled at using these pumps, including for complicated orders such as the total parenteral nutrition (TPN) orders. Good aseptic technique is used in a USP 797-compliant sterile compounding area.

The process is simple: Pharmacy technicians prepare all the IVs according to the times they are due, then pharmacists check off the preparations when they are all finished. This is a round-the-clock operation broken up into eight-hour sections.

Time is of the essence for the new orders that arrive all day long. The same person must process these immediate requests along with the 24-hour IV orders. It can be quite hectic at times, and the staff is always looking for better ways to do things.

One such person is the pharmacy technician who is processing the TPNs for the day. The procedures clearly state that all the ingredients can be mixed through the machine with the exception of the potassium chloride. This must be added last, through a syringe, once the bag is detached from the automated sterile preparation pump.

To cut corners on a particularly busy day, the pharmacy technician decides to add the potassium chloride through the pump. The technician feels that this is acceptable because he is right there to watch and make sure the correct amount is added.

1. Why do you think the potassium chloride is not to be pumped along with the other ingredients?

   _____

   _____

   _____

   _____

2. Is it acceptable for the pharmacy technician to add the potassium chloride to the pump as long as he is standing right there?

   _____

   _____

   _____

3. Since the pharmacists check off the final product, are they at all liable for the shortcuts that the pharmacy technician took to make the TPN?

   _____

   _____

   _____

   _____

ACTIVITY 15-3: Case Study—IV Education and Skills

Instructions: Read the following scenario and then answer the critical thinking questions.

The IV pharmacy technicians at University Hospital where you work are at different levels of skill and experience in this area. All are learning, and the hospital provides ongoing training. Most of you take this position seriously, but unfortunately there are some who do not.

The majority of the IV staff follows the guidelines and utilizes resources provided by the pharmacy for the sterile preparations that come their way. Everything from small-volume reconstitution, piggybacks, and large-volume IVs are prepared by this staff. Different drugs require specific diluents based on compatibility, stability, and other factors.

As most of the IV pharmacy technicians have progressed in their skill, they also have helped other IV staff learn as well. They all realize that some people take a little longer than others to grasp ideas and sometimes need extra assistance—but how long is too long? For about six months now, most of the IV pharmacy technicians have used the resources mentioned. However, three continue to ask the same questions repeatedly without attempting to apply what they have learned.

1. What pharmacy resources might be available to the IV pharmacy technicians to assist them with preparation and drug knowledge?

   _____

   _____

   _____

   _____

2. What are the benefits of these resources?

   _____

   _____

   _____

   _____

3. How often do you think education and/or training should take place for IV pharmacy technicians? What medium or media would be good to utilize?

   _____

   _____

   _____

   _____

4. How would you address the problem with the IV pharmacy technicians who seem apathetic?

   _____

   _____

   _____

   _____

ACTIVITY 15-4: Case Study—Identifying Errors in Aseptic Technique

Read the following scenario and identify at least 10 aseptic errors that the pharmacy technician made. Describe ways to improve her technique.

As a student, you are assigned to observe the aseptic technique of the IV room technician. Mindy is scheduled to work in the IV room this morning, but she stayed up too late the night before and had to rush to get to work on time. Before leaving home, she quickly put on some makeup to cover up the circles under her eyes. After punching in late, she began by washing her hands for 10 seconds, missing the dirt she had under her fingernails. After drying her hands with a paper towel, she threw the towel away and then shut off the faucet with her right hand. Next, she put on her gloves, a face mask, and a gown.

Once gowned, Mindy began cleaning the laminar airflow hood with blue window cleaner, using paper towels. She randomly wiped down the hood in circular patterns, and then began preparations for compounding some IV orders. She piled several syringes and needles in the hood, as well as several vials of various medications for the prescriptions that had to be prepared.

At this point, Mindy told you she needed a cup of coffee to perk herself up, so she excused herself to grab some coffee in the break area. A few minutes later, she returned to the clean room with the coffee. She resumed preparing the IVs, selecting several small-volume bags that she would need for the medications. She put those in the hood next to the syringes and began removing the caps to the vials. She assembled a needle and syringe, pulled out the appropriate volume from one of the vials, and immediately injected it into a small-volume bag. It was at this point that you recognized she would need more aseptic training.

Critical Thinking Questions:

1. List at least 10 aseptic errors made in this scenario, then describe the correct solutions to the errors.

Mistake 1: _____

Correct Procedure: _____

_____

_____

_____

Mistake 2: _____

Correct Procedure: _____

_____

_____

_____

Mistake 3: _____

Correct Procedure: _____

_____

_____

_____

Mistake 4: _____

Correct Procedure: _____

_____

_____

_____

Mistake 5: _____

Correct Procedure: _____

_____

_____

_____

Mistake 6: _____

Correct Procedure: _____

_____

_____

_____

Mistake 7: _____

Correct Procedure: _____

_____

_____

_____

Mistake 8: _____

Correct Procedure: _____

_____

_____

_____

Mistake 9: _____

Correct Procedure: _____

_____

_____

_____

Mistake 10: _____

Correct Procedure: _____

_____

_____

_____

2. How could this pharmacy technician's negligent technique result in serious harm to a patient?

_____

_____

_____

_____

_____

ACTIVITY 15-5: Hazardous Drugs

As you learned in Chapter 15 of your textbook, health care personnel who work with chemotherapy and cytotoxic drugs face consequential damage to their own health unless they take the necessary precautions to protect themselves.

Part One

Find out more about hazardous drugs by discovering what some of the key terms mean. Use your text, a medical dictionary, or a reliable online resource to help you define the following terms.

antineoplastic

_____

_____

_____

_____

_____

_____

cytotoxic

_____

_____

_____

_____

_____

_____

genotoxicity

_____

_____

_____

_____

_____

_____

carcinogenicity

_____

_____

_____

_____

_____

_____

teratogenicity

_____
_____
_____
_____
_____
_____

Part Two

Visit the OSHA website (http://www.osha.gov/dts/osta/otm/otm_vi/otm_vi_2.html) and locate the OSHA Technical Manual, Section VI: Chapter 2. Then answer the following questions.

1. What are some examples of activities in the pharmacy that might cause splattering, spraying, or aerosolization of hazardous materials?

_____
_____
_____
_____
_____

2. What does the abbreviation HD mean?

_____
_____
_____
_____
_____

3. Why are horizontal airflow hoods inappropriate for use when preparing HDs?

_____
_____
_____
_____
_____

4. To prevent exposure of personnel who are working with HDs, what does OSHA require that every facility have on hand?

_____
_____
_____
_____
_____

LAB 15-1: Proper Hand Hygiene and Aseptic Gowning

Objectives:

Demonstrate the proper techniques for hand washing and aseptic gowning.

Explain why hand hygiene is a key component of aseptic technique.

Pre-Lab Information:

- Review Chapter 15 in your textbook.
- Go to www.usp.org and search for "General Chapter 797." You will find a document that explains all of the latest national guidelines for preparing sterile products. This bulletin is related to pharmaceutical compounding and sterile preparations and has specific information under "Personal Cleansing and Garbing."
- Gather the following materials:
- germicidal, microbial soap such as Hibiclens or chlorohexidene
- lint-free paper towels or gauze
- lint-free gowns, head/hair covers, shoe covers, gloves, and face masks

Explanation:

Proper hand hygiene and aseptic garbing are essential for maintaining cleanliness and sterility while preparing IV and other sterile medications in a clean room. All surfaces of our bodies have bacteria on them, called *normal bacterial flora*, which are harmless if we are healthy. However, patients who are ill or whose immune systems are not working properly (immunocompromised) can be harmed by these normal bacteria. Washing your hands with a germicidal, microbial soap before entering the clean room, after eating, performing personal hygiene, or doing anything that could cause contamination, is critical to maintaining asepsis.

When working in a sterile preparation area, you also need to wear the proper attire to maintain asepsis. At the minimum, this means clean hospital scrubs or surgical gowns, regardless of whether you are working under the hood or checking IVs. Proper garb also includes disposable hair and shoe covers, masks, and gloves. You will not necessarily need to wear all of these items every time. Your facility will have guidelines on what should be worn and when.

Activity:

Part 1

Review the information from the USP website, and then answer the following questions.

1. Chapter 797 suggests that hand washing should be done for how many seconds?
   _____
   _____

2. Describe the hand hygiene techniques discussed in the Chapter 797 bulletin.
   _____
   _____
   _____
   _____
   _____
   _____

3. Describe the order in which you should don your sterile garb and perform hand hygiene before working with sterile products.

_____

_____

_____

_____

4. What should you do if you accidentally touch your face after you have already cleansed yourself and dressed aseptically?

_____

_____

_____

_____

5. Describe the exiting or degarbing procedure when leaving the compounding area for the day.

_____

_____

_____

_____

6. Although Chapter 797 does not address this issue specifically, you should be able to apply its principles: After you wash your hands thoroughly, what do you feel would be the best method for turning off the faucet without risking recontamination?

_____

_____

_____

_____

Part 2

Now that you have reviewed the techniques for hand hygiene and gowning and degowning, it is time to practice each technique. Practice first with a lab partner. When you are ready, ask your instructor to observe.

Student Name: _____

Lab Partner: _____

Grade/Comments: _____

_____

_____

Student Comments: _____

_____

_____

LAB 15-2: The Horizontal Laminar Airflow Hood

Objective:

Review the technique involved in using a horizontal laminar airflow hood.

Pre-Lab Information:

- Read Chapter 15, "Introduction to Sterile Products," in your textbook.
- Visit the website http://www.globalrph.com/aseptic.htm

Explanation:

Nonhazardous sterile products are compounded inside a horizontal laminar airflow hood (LAH). The LAH contains a prefilter in the front of the hood that removes large contaminants from the air inside the room. After the air has been filtered by the prefilter, it travels to the back of the LAH, where it is filtered next by the HEPA filter. This removes particles that are two microns or larger (the size of most bacteria, fungi, and viruses). The filtered air is then blown back to the front of the hood. The LAH also maintains a constant airflow out of the hood which prevents the entry of contaminants. The hood must be turned on 30 minutes in advance of use in aseptic compounding.

If you perform aseptic compounding as a pharmacy technician, you must know how to clean and disinfect the LAH properly. At a minimum, the hood must be cleaned every eight hours, or sooner if it becomes dirty. To prevent cross-contamination of products, always wipe down the hood if you have finished compounding one product and need to switch to another.

Here are the steps for cleaning a LAH:

1. Turn on the LAH and allow the blower to run for 30 minutes.
2. Follow proper hand-washing procedure and technique and wear appropriate apparel. Keep your head on the outside of the hood to prevent contamination.
3. Wash the entire hood—all walls and surfaces—with sterile water to remove salt, starch, sugars, and/or proteins. Soak stubborn spots for 5 to 10 minutes, then wipe clean.
4. To disinfect, wipe all surfaces of the hood with 70% isopropyl alcohol, using a lint-free fabric such as special paper towels or gauze. Never use regular paper towels, as they produce lint and create particulates.
5. Clean the IV pole first, if applicable.
6. Second, clean the sides of the LAH, starting at the top and working side-to-side with overlapping strokes. Alternatively, the sides of the hood can be cleaned from top to bottom.
7. Last, clean the work surface, starting at the back and working side-to-side with overlapping strokes. Do not block airflow to or from the HEPA filter, and be careful not to contaminate any previously cleaned surface.
8. Dispose of the towels or gauze and document the hood cleaning.

Note that the prefilter is normally changed monthly, and the HEPA filter is tested every six months for efficiency.

Activity:

Part One

Review the technique for cleaning a LAH described in the preceding list and visit the website http://www.globalrph.com/aseptic.htm. Then, answer the following questions about the proper use of a horizontal laminar airflow hood.

1. What are the three functions of a horizontal laminar airflow hood?
   _____
   _____
   _____
   _____

2. What is the most important part of the horizontal laminar airflow hood?
   _____
   _____

3. What should be used to clean a horizontal laminar airflow hood?
   _____
   _____

4. Describe the technique used to disinfect the laminar airflow hood (e.g., where to start, what kind of motion to use, etc.).
   _____
   _____
   _____
   _____

Part Two

Now it is your turn to try cleaning a LAH. Review the procedure described earlier for cleaning a laminar airflow hood. Practice the technique with a partner, then perform the procedure for your instructor.

Student Name: _____

Lab Partner: _____

Grade/Comments: _____
_____
_____

Student Comments: _____
_____
_____

LAB 15-3: The Vertical Laminar Airflow Hood

Objective:

Review the technique involved in using a vertical laminar airflow hood.

Pre-Lab Information:

- Read Chapter 15, "Introduction to Sterile Products," in your textbook.
- Visit the website at http://orcbs.arizona.edu/biosafety

Explanation:

A vertical laminar airflow hood, also known as a chemo hood or biological safety cabinet (BSC), is used for compounding hazardous agents. A BSC has four sides with an 8- to 12-inch opening in the front, and a sliding glass door that can be brought down to the proper opening level. In a BSC, the room air enters the front opening and moves into the BSC grills, which are located in the front and back of the inside of the hood's work surface area. This air is then filtered and circulated to the HEPA filter, which filters the air to 0.3 micron. The filtered air is blown from the top of the hood vertically downward to the work surface area. The air is then filtered again and either eliminated back into the room air or to an outside vent.

Work with chemotherapy drugs or other sterile products using a vertical laminar airflow hood requires knowledge of proper techniques for cleaning and disinfecting the laminar airflow hood. The procedure for cleaning a BSC is essentially the same as the one used when cleaning a laminar airflow hood, although the class or level of the BSC may require some additional steps or precautions.

Activity:

Part One

Visit the website listed in the "Pre-Lab Information" section, then answer the following questions about the proper use and disinfection of a vertical laminar airflow hood.

1. In what ways does the BSC differ from the laminar airflow hood? Why do these differences make the BSC more appropriate for use with cytotoxic or hazardous agents?

   _____

   _____

   _____

   _____

2. What condition should never exist when operating a vertical laminar flow hood or biological safety cabinet?

   _____

   _____

   _____

   _____

3. When should you disinfect the BSC?

_____
_____
_____
_____

4. What are two appropriate disinfectants?

_____
_____
_____
_____

5. Biological safety cabinets are available in three different classes. Use the Internet to research the three different classes, then describe what you discover about each class and its different uses. Which one do you think you would be most likely to use in the pharmacy setting?

_____
_____
_____
_____

Part Two

Now it is your turn to try cleaning a BSC. Review the procedure described earlier for cleaning a laminar airflow hood. Practice the technique with a partner, then perform the procedure for your instructor.

Student Name: _____

Lab Partner: _____

Grade/Comments: _____
_____
_____

Student Comments: _____
_____
_____

LAB 15-4: Withdrawing Medication from a Vial or Glass Ampule

Objective:

Demonstrate the techniques involved in withdrawing medications from vials or glass ampules.

Pre-Lab Information:

- Review Chapter 15 in your textbook for review of aseptic compounding, needles, and syringes.
- Gather the following materials:
  - sterile vials and ampules of 0.9% sodium chloride
  - 10 mL syringes
  - 18 gauge, 1 1/2 inch needles
  - filter needles
  - gloves
  - alcohol swabs

Explanation:

You will learn the proper aseptic techniques for withdrawing medication from vials and glass ampules. If your instructor is unable to provide a lab component, your local hospital pharmacy may provide a demonstration for students upon request.

Activity:

Your instructor will take you through the proper procedures for withdrawing medication from vials and glass ampules. You will then have the opportunity to practice some of these techniques in class. If a laminar airflow hood is not available, you will need to use a little imagination regarding aseptic technique and the standards of USP 797.

Key points for working with vials:

1. Always observe the 6-inch rule and critical areas while you are working with sterile products in a laminar airflow hood.

2. Always disinfect the top of the vial with an alcohol swab. One single swipe in one direction should be adequate to disinfect the vial and its stopper. Wait a moment for the alcohol to evaporate before entering the vial with a needle.

3. Attach a needle to a syringe of appropriate size. Before entering the vial, always draw some air into the syringe, to a volume that is slightly less than what you want to withdraw from the vial. This extra air will be pushed into the vial before withdrawing the contents to help equalize the air pressure and make the withdrawal of the solution easier to accomplish.

4. Use care when entering the vial's stopper with the needle. Using too large a needle or the wrong entry technique could result in "coring" of the stopper. Coring could lead to small fragments of the rubber stopper in the medication vial. Adding too much air to the vial could also cause some of the medication to accidentally spray out or aspirate, reducing the required volume available for use as well as potentially contaminating the hood.

5. With the bevel of the needle facing upward, enter the vial's stopper by using a 60- to 90-degree angle entrance point. Press the needle into the middle of the stopper until it has completely broken the seal. Be careful not to interrupt any of the airflow between the hood and the entry point shared between the vial and the needle. This next process can be challenging for the beginner. Carefully reverse the vial and syringe while the needle is still inside the vial, to an upside-down position while maintaining aseptic technique. Gently push some of the air from the syringe into the vial. The syringe will usually start to withdraw some of the fluid on its own filling the syringe. Repeat the process until all the air is out of the syringe and you have withdrawn the correct amount of fluid.

6. The syringe is now ready either to be capped or to be added to an IV bag for an infusion.

Key points for working with glass ampules:

1. Always observe the 6-inch rule and critical areas while you are working with sterile products in a laminar airflow hood.

2. Always disinfect the narrow portion of the ampule with an alcohol swab.

3. Make sure that no liquid is trapped in the neck of the ampule. Gently tapping the top of the ampule with a finger usually will release any remaining liquid from the neck and allowing it to settle in the bottom of the ampule.

4. Break the ampule open at the weakest part around the neck, usually indicated by a dot or a stripe. Be sure to break it open toward the sides of the hood and not toward the back of the hood or toward yourself. Glass fragments can damage the HEPA filter.

5. When withdrawing a medication from a glass ampule, you must use a filter needle in order to filter out any glass particles and also any potential microbial contaminants that may have gotten into the medication. You do not need to withdraw air into the syringe before withdrawing medication from an ampule, because there is no longer a vacuum once you have broken open the ampule.

6. Using a filter needle attached to an appropriate syringe, tilt the ampule slightly in order to withdraw the amount of medication desired. You may need to adjust the volume in the syringe and repeat until you have the correct amount. Be careful not to push any air into the ampule container. Doing so may produce an aspirate and contaminate the airflow hood. If there is any excess liquid in the syringe carefully dispose of it onto a gauze pad or slowly push it back into the ampule.

7. If the contents of the syringe are to be added to an IV bag, you must first change to a new, nonfiltered standard needle. If you keep the same needle, all of the glass particles you may have trapped will be pushed into the IV bag along with the medication and potential microbial contaminants, negating the filtering process.

8. Alternatively, some technicians prefer to draw the medication from the ampule with a regular needle, and then change to a filter needle before injecting the medication into an IV bag. Either method will prevents glass particles from entering into the syringe or the IV bag.

Questions:

1. Why do you need to pull air into the syringe before withdrawing medication from a vial?

_____

_____

_____

2. Why do you need to swab off the top of a vial or a glass ampule with alcohol?

_____

_____

_____

3. Why is it important to use a filter needle when working with glass ampules?

_____

_____

_____

4. Why should you break open a glass ampule toward the sides of the hood instead of toward the back of the hood or toward yourself?

_____

_____

_____

5. Why do you not need to pull air into the syringe before withdrawing medication from a glass ampule?

_____

_____

_____

LAB 15-5: Reconstituting Sterile Dry Powder Medications

Objectives:
Determine the diluents and amount of diluents required to reconstitute sterile dry powder medications.

Determine the storage requirements for the reconstituted medication.

Pre-Lab Information:

- Reread Chapter 15 in your textbook for review of aseptic technique and sterile compounding.
- Gather the following materials:
  - miscellaneous package inserts from sterile powder medications that require reconstitution

Explanation:
Some drugs contained in vials are in powder form. Before they can be used in patient treatment, they have to be reconstituted, which simply means that one must add a diluent, like sterile water, to the vial to make a liquid. Every sterile drug that requires reconstitution contains directions for reconstitution either directly on the vial and/or on the package insert.

Activity:
Your instructor will provide you with miscellaneous package inserts that accompanied sterile dry powder medications. Read through the package inserts to see what kind of information is provided about the medication. Stability and reconstitution requirements are usually found toward the end of the insert.

Questions:
Find the following information from each of the inserts provided to you.

1. Drug name and strength (example: vancomycin, 1 g):
   _____
   _____

2. Preferred diluent(s) (examples: sterile water, 0.9% sodium chloride, etc.):
   _____
   _____

3. Amount of diluent needed (example: 20 mL):
   _____
   _____

4. Concentration of the medication after reconstitution (example: 50 mg/mL):
   _____
   _____

5. Stability of the reconstituted medication (example: 72 hours):
   _____
   _____

6. Storage requirements for the reconstituted medication (example: Keep refrigerated or at room temperature):

_____

_____

7. What do you think might happen if you were to reconstitute a medication with the wrong diluent?

_____

_____

_____

_____

8. When comparing the amount of diluent needed to the concentration obtained, did you notice any trends?

_____

_____

_____

_____

Student Name: _____

Lab Partner: _____

Grade/Comments: _____

_____

_____

Student Comments: _____

_____

_____

LAB 15-6: Transferring Liquid into an IV Bag

Objective:

Understand the technique involved in transferring liquid medication from a syringe into an IV bag so that you are able to apply the technique in a pharmacy setting.

Pre-Lab Information:

Review Chapter 15 in your textbook for information regarding aseptic technique and IV medications.

Explanation:

Many IV medications have to be further diluted before they are administered to patients. This process, also known as *sterile compounding*, is most often done with one or more syringes and an IV bag containing an isotonic fluid. In this activity, you will learn the proper aseptic technique for transferring solutions from a syringe into the IV bag, identify which port on the IV bag is used for the transfer, and learn how to add multiple products to the same bag.

Activity:

When compounding sterile products, follow these simple guidelines:

1. Read the prescription label to determine which products you need to use.

2. Select the correct IV bag and size (example: dextrose 5%, 100 mL) and the correct medication that will be transferred to this bag (example: diltiazem 125 mg/25 mL).

3. Remove the outer packaging and wipe down the entire bag with alcohol (in a clean room, parts of these processes may be done by a coworker).

4. Place the disinfected bag on a hanger in the laminar airflow hood.

5. Strip off the seal to the center port of the IV bag and disinfect the port with an alcohol swab. (The port is usually in the middle with a blue seal, but certain IV bags have more than one port for pharmacy use).

6. Prepare the medication for transfer to the IV bag. If it comes in a sterile powder, first follow the directions for reconstitution; then draw the appropriate amount of medication into a syringe, using aseptic technique.

7. Taking care to observe the critical areas of the hood and the 6-inch rule, insert the needle (which is still attached to the syringe of medication from step 6) straight into the center of the port. You will need to pass the needle through the outer core and through an inner membrane. Try to keep the needle straight so as not to puncture the side of the port or the bag. A puncture will void the sterility of all the products involved and you will have to start over with new supplies.

8. Once the needle has passed the inner membrane, gently push the fluid from the syringe into the bag; then carefully pull out the needle and the syringe.

9. If your pharmacist has not double-checked your work at this point, some pharmacies allow you to pull the empty syringe back with air to the volume that you placed in the bag, to indicate how much drug you used.

10. After your work has been checked by a pharmacist, place a cap or seal over the port you just used (this step may be omitted depending on the pharmacy). Remove the IV from the hook, gently shake the bag to distribute the drug, and then label the bag appropriately.

11. If multiple drugs are used in the same bag, gently shake the IV bag between medications to avoid possible precipitation. "Banana bags," which got their nickname from their yellow color, are a multivitamin/mineral infusion and are a good example of a prescription for which you would use more than one drug in a bag.

These step-by-step instructions can be used to prepare most sterile products that require further dilution in an IV bag. You or your instructor may be able to get permission from a local hospital to demonstrate these techniques or allow you to practice.

Questions:

1. What might happen if a punctured bag accidentally made it out of the pharmacy and were hung for a patient?

   _____

   _____

   _____

   _____

2. What might happen if you added several products to an IV bag without mixing in between additions?

   _____

   _____

   _____

   _____

3. Why is it so important to practice aseptic technique when preparing IV medications?

   _____

   _____

   _____

   _____

4. While you are performing a fluid transfer, you accidently lose your grip on the syringe and it falls onto the hood. You discover that the needle has touched the surface of the hood. What should you do?

   _____

   _____

   _____

   _____

LAB 15-7: Cefazolin

Order:
Patient: Judy Chambers Weight: 110 lb

Rx: cefazolin 1 g in 250 mL bag; dilute to 200 mg/mL

Supplies Needed
(1) Training Powder-Y Vial (cefazolin 1 g)

(1) Training Vial 50 mL (diluent)

(2) 5 cc Syringes

(1) IV Bag, 250 mL NaCl 0.9%

(3) Alcohol Swabs

Calculations

To dilute to 200 mg/mL – add 4.5 cc of diluent.

Stock	Needed
200 mg	1,000 mg
1 mL	X

5 mL of the reconstituted cefazolin is needed.

Procedure
1. Prepare yourself with proper garb and proper hand-washing technique.
2. Ensure the laminar flow hood has been running for 30 minutes and is cleaned.
3. Bring all necessary supplies into the flow hood. Open and clean appropriate items.
4. Open the syringe and draw up 5 cc of air.
5. Insert the syringe into the Training Diluent MDV and add the 5 cc of air.
6. Draw up 5 cc of diluent into the syringe and remove.
7. Insert the syringe into the Training Powder Y Vial and add the 5 cc of diluent using the milking technique.
8. Reconstitute the Training Powder Y by gently mixing the contents.
9. Withdraw 5 cc of the reconstituted cefazolin and add to the IV bag.
10. Inspect and label the IV bag.

Student Name: _____

Lab Partner: _____

Grade/Comments: _____

_____

_____

Student Comments: _____

_____

_____

LAB 15-8: Intropin

Order:

Patient: Susan Jones Weight: 147 lb
Rx: Intropin 400 mg in 1,000 mL bag

Supplies Needed

(1) Training Ampule (Intropin 160 mg/mL)

(1) 3 cc Syringe

(1) IV Bag, 1,000 mL NaCl 0.9%

(1) Filter Needle

(3) Alcohol Swabs

Calculations

Stock	Needed
160 mg	400 mg
1 mL	X

2.5 mL of the stock Intropin is needed.

Procedure

1. Prepare yourself with proper garb and proper hand-washing technique.
2. Ensure the laminar flow hood has been running for 30 minutes and is cleaned.
3. Bring all necessary supplies into the flow hood. Open and clean appropriate items.
4. Insert the syringe into the Training Ampule and draw up 2.5 cc of the Intropin.
5. Replace the needle with a filter needle.
6. Insert the syringe into the IV bag and add the Intropin.
7. Inspect and label the IV bag.

Student Name: _____

Lab Partner: _____

Grade/Comments: _____

_____

_____

Student Comments: _____

_____

_____

LAB 15-9: Methotrexate

Order:

Patient: Wesley Thompson Weight: 176 lb
Rx: methotrexate 0.05 mg/kg/day; dilute to 1 mg/mL

Supplies Needed

(1) Training Hazardous Powder Vial (methotrexate)

(1) Training Vial 20 mL (diluent)

(2) 10 cc Syringe

(1) IV Bag, 1,000 mL NaCl 0.9%

(3) Alcohol Swabs

(1) Chemo Pad

Calculations

To dilute to 1 mg/mL—add 10 cc of diluent—according to label instructions.

$176 \div 2.2 = 80$ kg.

80 kg $\times 0.05 = 4$ mg

Stock	Needed
1 mg	4 mg
1 mL	X

4 mL of the reconstituted methotrexate is needed.

Procedure

1. Prepare yourself with proper garb and proper hand-washing technique.
2. Ensure the laminar flow hood has been running for 30 minutes and is cleaned.
3. Bring all necessary supplies into the flow hood. Open and clean appropriate items.
4. Open the syringe and draw up 10 cc of air.
5. Insert the syringe into the Training Liquid Vial and add the 10 cc of air.
6. Draw up 10 cc of diluent into the syringe and remove.
7. Insert the syringe into the Training Hazardous Powder Vial and add the 10 mL of diluent using the milking technique.
8. Reconstitute the Hazardous Training Powder by gently mixing the contents.
9. When inserting a syringe back into the vial avoid going into the same hole.
10. Withdraw 4 cc of the reconstituted methotrexate (negative pressure) and add to the IV bag, then visually inspect the bag.

Student Name: _____

Lab Partner: _____

Grade/Comments: _____

_____

_____

Student Comments: _____

_____

_____

LAB 15-10: TPN

Order:

Patient: Eric Palms Weight: 4 lb

Rx:	Amino Acids 10%	100 mL	Use: Used IV bag
	Dextrose 50%	100 mL	Use: Used IV bag
	Na Acetate 4 mEq/mL	6 mEq	Use: Training Liquid Vial 2 mL
	Infivite Pediatric	5 mL	Use: Training Liquid Vial 5 mL

Calculations

Na Acetate

Stock	Needed
4 mEq	6 mEq
1 mL	X

1.5 mL of the stock Na Acetate is needed.

Procedure

1. Prepare yourself with proper garb and proper hand-washing technique.
2. Ensure the laminar flow hood has been running for 30 minutes and is cleaned.
3. Bring all necessary supplies into the flow hood. Open and clean appropriate items.
4. Use the lead(s) on the viaflex TPN bag to add the bases using the gravity method.
5. Add the Infuvite Pediatric to the TPN bag.
6. Add the Na Acetate to the TPN bag.
7. Disconnect all bags and close/lock all lead ports on the TPN bag.
8. Inspect and label the IV bag.

Student Name: _____

Lab Partner _____

Grade/Comments: _____

_____

_____

Student Comments: _____

_____

_____

Forms

The following forms are for use in logging aseptic technique practice and skill validations.

Aseptic Technique Training Log

Student Name	
Date	
Start Time	
End Time	
Contact Hour(s)	
Location	
Trainer's Name	
Trainer's Lic. #	
State of License	
Daytime Phone (trainer)	
Skill(s) Covered	

By signing below, I validate that the information listed above is complete and fully accurate.

_____   _____   _____   _____
Student Signature   Date   Trainer Signature   Date

Process Validation Record
Aseptic Hand-washing Technique

Student Name: _____ Date: _____

Procedure	Yes	No
Removed all jewelry, watches, and objects up to the elbow		
Did not have on acrylic nails or nail polish		
Starts water and adjusts to the appropriate temperature		
Avoided unnecessary splashing during process		
Used sufficient disinfecting agent/cleanser		
Cleaned all four surfaces of each finger		
Cleaned all surfaces of hands, wrists, and arms up to the elbows in a circular motion		
Did not touch the sink, faucet, or other objects that could contaminate hands		
Rinsed off all soap residue		
Rinsed hands holding them upright and allowing water to drip to the elbow		
Did not turn off water until hands were completely dry		
Turned water off with a clean, dry, lint-free paper towel		
Did not touch the faucet while turning off the water		

By signing below, I certify that the student has demonstrated 100% competency at the above task.

_____

Trainer Name (printed)

_____

Trainer Signature

_____   _____

Trainer Daytime Phone   Trainer's License #

_____   _____

Date   State Licensed

Process Validation Record

Horizontal Laminar Flow Hood

Student Name: _____   Date: _____

Procedure	Yes	No
Hood was turned on and running at least 30 minutes prior to preparation		
Followed proper hand-washing procedure and technique		
Wore appropriate apparel		
Used clean, sterile gauze/sponge and plenty of disinfectant to clean the hood		
Cleaned the IV pole first (if applicable)		
Cleaned the sides of the hood second, starting at the top and working side-to-side with overlapping strokes		
Cleaned the work surface last, starting at the back and working side-to-side with overlapping strokes		
Did not contaminate previously cleaned surfaces		
Did not block airflow from HEPA filter		
Did not utilize outer 6 inches of the hood opening		
Properly stood outside the hood without allowing the head to enter the inside		
Knows that hood certification is every six months, if moved, or if damaged		
Knows that prefilters should be changed monthly		

By signing below, I certify that the student has demonstrated 100% competency at the above task.

_____

Trainer Name (printed)

_____

Trainer Signature

_____   _____

Trainer Daytime Phone   Trainer's License #

_____   _____

Date   State Licensed

Process Validation Record
Vertical Laminar Flow Hood

Student Name: _____ Date: _____

Procedure	Yes	No
Hood was turned on and running at least 30 minutes prior to preparation		
Followed proper hand-washing procedure and technique		
Wore appropriate apparel		
Used clean, sterile gauze/sponge and plenty of disinfectant to clean the hood		
Cleaned the IV pole first (if applicable)		
Cleaned the sides of the hood second, starting at the top and working side-to-side with overlapping strokes		
Cleaned the back wall and inside the glass shield, starting at the top and working up and down with overlapping strokes		
Cleaned the work surface last, starting at the back and working side-to-side with overlapping strokes		
Did not contaminate previously cleaned surfaces		
Did not lower the glass shield more than 8 inches from the work surface prior to preparation		
Did not block airflow from HEPA filter or air intake grills at any time		
Did not utilize outer 6 inches of the hood opening		

By signing below, I certify that the student has demonstrated 100% competency at the above task.

_____

Trainer Name (printed)

_____

Trainer Signature

_____   _____

Trainer Daytime Phone   Trainer's License #

_____   _____

Date   State Licensed

Process Validation Record
Vial Preparation

Student Name: _____   Date: _____

Procedure	Yes	No
Followed proper hand-washing procedure and technique		
Wore appropriate apparel		
Followed proper procedure and technique in cleaning the hood		
Performed all necessary calculations correctly, prior to drug preparation		
Brought the correct drugs and concentrations into the hood for preparation		
Brought the correct supplies into the hood prior to preparation		
Inspected all products for particulate matter/contamination prior to use		
Removed dust covers and cleaned rubber diaphragms correctly		
Inserted needle correctly to prevent coring		
Used proper milking technique on venting device, and did not aspirate at any time		
Did not remove needle from vial until all air bubbles were removed and amount verified		
Removed air bubbles correctly and did not spill any liquid		
Withdrew needle correctly from vial to prevent spilling or aspiration		
Cleaned additive port on final container prior to injecting drug		
Did not core or puncture side of additive port when adding drug to the final container		
Properly mixed contents of container and inspected for incompatibilities or particulate matter		
Properly sealed additive port of container		
Did not contaminate the needle or syringe during preparation		
Did not contaminate the hood		
Did not block airflow from HEPA filter or air intake grills at any time		
Did not utilize outer 6 inches of the hood opening		
Properly discarded all waste, including sharps		

By signing below, I certify that the student has demonstrated 100% competency at the above task.

_____
Trainer Name (printed)

_____
Trainer Signature

_____   _____
Trainer Daytime Phone   Trainer's License #

_____   _____
Date   State Licensed

Process Validation Record
Ampule Preparation

Student Name: _____   Date: _____

Procedure	Yes	No
Followed proper hand-washing procedure and technique		
Wore appropriate apparel		
Followed proper procedure and technique in cleaning the hood		
Performed all necessary calculations correctly, prior to drug preparation		
Brought the correct drugs and concentrations into the hood for preparation		
Brought the correct supplies into the hood prior to preparation		
Inspected all products for particulate matter/contamination prior to use		
Ampule neck was cleared of fluid before breaking		
Ampule neck was cleaned correctly before breaking		
Ampule neck was wrapped correctly before breaking		
Ampule was broken correctly		
Attached filter device to syringe correctly		
Ampule was drawn up correctly, without spilling contents		
Filter needle was removed and replaced with new needle prior to injecting final container		
Drew up the correct amount of drug and checked measurement prior to injecting into container		
Cleaned additive port on final container prior to injecting drug		
Did not core or puncture side of additive port when adding drug to the final container		
Properly mixed contents of container and inspected for incompatibilities or particulate matter		
Properly sealed additive port of container		
Did not contaminate the needle or syringe during preparation		
Did not contaminate the hood		
Did not block airflow from HEPA filter or air intake grills at any time		
Did not utilize outer 6 inches of the hood opening		
Properly discarded all waste, including sharps		

By signing below, I certify that the student has demonstrated 100% competency at the above task.

_____

Trainer Name (printed)

_____

Trainer Signature

_____   _____

Trainer Daytime Phone   Trainer's License #

_____   _____

Date   State Licensed

Process Validation Record
Vial Preparation—Hazardous Drugs

Student Name: _____   Date: _____

Procedure	Yes	No
Followed proper hand-washing procedure and technique		
Wore appropriate apparel		
Followed proper procedure and technique in cleaning the hood		
Knew location of spill kit		
Knew location of eyewash station		
Performed all necessary calculations correctly, prior to drug preparation		
Placed prep-mat/paper drape correctly, prior to drug preparation		
Brought the correct drugs and concentrations into the hood for preparation		
Brought the correct supplies into the hood prior to preparation		
Inspected all products for particulate matter/contamination prior to use		
Removed dust covers and cleaned rubber diaphragms correctly		
Inserted needle correctly to prevent coring		
Used proper milking technique on venting device, and did not aspirate at any time		
Did not remove needle from vial until all air bubbles were removed and amount verified		
Removed air bubbles correctly and did not spill any liquid		
Withdrew needle correctly from vial to prevent spilling or aspiration		
Cleaned additive port on final container prior to injecting drug		
Did not core or puncture side of additive port when adding drug to the final container		
Properly mixed contents of container and inspected for incompatibilities or particulate matter		
Properly sealed additive port of container		
IV container was placed in a zip-lock bag before removal from the hood		
Used any and all appropriate hazardous labeling (for product and waste)		
Did not contaminate the needle or syringe during preparation		
Did not contaminate the hood		
Did not block airflow from HEPA filter or air intake grills at any time		
Did not utilize outer 6 inches of the hood opening		
Properly discarded all waste, including sharps		

By signing below, I certify that the student has demonstrated 100% competency at the above task.

_____

Trainer Name (printed)

_____

Trainer Signature

_____   _____

Trainer Daytime Phone   Trainer's License #

_____   _____

Date   State Licensed

CHAPTER 16
Basic Math Skills

After completing Chapter 16 from the textbook, you should be able to:	Related Activity in the Workbook/Lab Manual
1. Determine the value of a decimal.	Review Questions, Pharmacy Calculation Problems, PTCB Exam Practice Questions
2. Add, subtract, multiply, and divide decimals.	Review Questions, Pharmacy Calculation Problems, PTCB Exam Practice Questions, Activity 16-1
3. Recognize and interpret Roman numerals.	Review Questions, Pharmacy Calculation Problems, PTCB Exam Practice Questions
4. Change Roman numerals to Arabic numerals.	Review Questions, Pharmacy Calculation Problems, PTCB Exam Practice Questions
5. Change Arabic numerals to Roman numerals.	Review Questions, Pharmacy Calculation Problems, PTCB Exam Practice Questions
6. Describe the different types of common fractions.	Review Questions, Activity 16-4
7. Add, subtract, multiply, and divide fractions.	Review Questions, Pharmacy Calculation Problems, PTCB Exam Practice Questions, Activity 16-2
8. Define a ratio.	Review Questions, Activity 16-4
9. Define a proportion.	Review Questions, Activity 16-4
10. Solve math problems by using ratios and proportions.	Review Questions, Pharmacy Calculation Problems, PTCB Exam Practice Questions, Activity 16-3

INTRODUCTION

Knowledge of basic arithmetic is essential for today's pharmacy technician. You need basic math skills to understand and perform drug preparations. Nearly every aspect of drug dispensing requires a consideration of numbers. All advanced pharmacy calculations, which are explained throughout this text, rely on a solid understanding of basic math principles. Remember that Chapter 16 in your textbook is designed to serve as a review of these general principles and as an assessment of your basic math skills; the activities in this workbook/lab manual will provide you with additional review.

REVIEW QUESTIONS

Match the following.

1. _____ common fractions
2. _____ complex fractions
3. _____ cross-multiplication
4. _____ decimal fractions
5. _____ denominator
6. _____ fraction line
7. _____ improper fraction
8. _____ numerator
9. _____ proper fraction
10. _____ proportion
11. _____ ratio
12. _____ Roman numerals
13. _____ simple fractions

a. bottom value of a fraction; the number below the fraction line

b. setting up two ratios or fractions in relationship to each other as a proportion and solving for the unknown variable (X)

c. a symbol representing the division of two values; separates the numerator and denominator of a fraction

d. fractions written with a numerator separated by a fraction line from and positioned above a denominator

e. fraction in which both the numerator and the denominator are themselves fractions

f. fractions written as a whole number with a zero and a decimal point in front of the value

g. a fraction in which the value of the numerator is smaller than the value of the denominator

h. letters and symbols used to represent numbers

i. top value of a fraction; the number above the fraction line

j. expresses the relationship of two numbers, separated by a colon (:) between the numbers

k. proper fraction, with both the numerator and denominator reduced to lowest terms

l. fraction in which the value of the numerator is larger than the value of the denominator

m. two or more equivalent ratios or fractions that both represent the same value

Choose the best answer.

14. Which of these decimals has the highest value?
    a. 0.21
    b. 0.35
    c. 0.31
    d. 0.42

15. Which of these decimals has the highest value?
    a. 1.37
    b. 1.43
    c. 1.89
    d. 1.25

16. Add the following decimals: 14.25 + 36.75 =
    a. 55
    b. 51
    c. 21.5
    d. 60

17. Which of these decimals has the lowest value?
    a. 12.4
    b. 12.006
    c. 12.03
    d. 12.891

18. Which of these decimals has the lowest value?
    a. 0.15
    b. 0.16
    c. 0.016
    d. 0.22

19. Subtract the following decimals: 104.9 – 55.9 =
    a. 48
    b. 160.8
    c. 49
    d. 49.9

Multiply the following decimals.

20. 8.63 × 0.24 = _____

21. 6.583 × 2.26 = _____

22. 5.53 × 4.986 = _____

Divide the following decimals.

23. 0.98 / 40.3 = _____

24. 5.54 / 0.4 = _____

25. 6.04 / 0.66 = _____

Change these Roman numerals to Arabic.

26. XC _____

27. CL _____

28. XXI _____

29. LX _____

30. XXX _____

PHARMACY CALCULATION PROBLEMS

Calculate the following.

1. Add the following fractions: $\dfrac{2}{4} + \dfrac{1}{8} + \dfrac{3}{16} =$

2. Solve for X: $\dfrac{100}{2} = \dfrac{3}{X}$

3. Solve for X: $500 \text{ mg}/1 \text{ mL} = \dfrac{X}{5} \text{ mL}$

4. Solve for X: $1{,}000 \text{ mcg}/1 \text{ mL} = \dfrac{X}{2} \text{ mL}$

5. A physician writes an order for XL tablets. The patient's SIG states for the patient: 1 tab po × 10d. What will the day supply be for as it relates to the quantity being dispensed?

PTCB EXAM PRACTICE QUESTIONS

1. How many capsules will be taken in three days if a prescription order reads tetracycline 250 mg/capsule, one capsule qid?
   a. 16
   b. 12
   c. 3
   d. 6

2. Express 33.3% as a decimal:
   a. 33.3
   b. 0.333
   c. 3.33
   d. 333

3. What is 20% of 30?
   a. 6
   b. 60
   c. 3
   d. 300

4. Express 55 as a Roman numeral:
   a. LIXV
   b. XLV
   c. XXXXIX
   d. LV

5. Round 145.1155 to the nearest hundredth:
   a. 145.1
   b. 145.11
   c. 145.12
   d. 145.116

ACTIVITY 16-1: Case Study—How Much?

Instructions: Read the following scenario and then answer the critical thinking questions.

Ms. Kipsky is an elderly woman who is on a very tight budget. She has worked at the local fabric store on a part-time status since her children have all moved out of the home. In addition to this part-time job, she receives an overdue child support check that assists with her finances until the next payday. Luckily, she does not have any major health conditions or concerns that would require her to be on medication. She is very glad about her not having any major health conditions or concerns because she would not be able to afford medications along with her bills and the monthly bus fare that she spends on traveling to work every day.

It is deep into the winter season in the small town Ms. Kipsky works in. She comes into the independent pharmacy where you work and brings in a prescription that the health care team at the free clinic gave to her for an infection. They prescribed to her: amoxicillin 500 mg capsules and she is to take one capsule q8h until gone (for 10 days).

Unfortunately for Ms. Kipsky, her next payday is the following Friday and today is only Saturday. She brings the prescription to the pharmacy to be filled and asks you about the cost. You calculate the amount for her as $30.

1. Ms. Kipsky is uninsured and is paying cash. She asks you how much of the medication she will be able to purchase if she can only pay for 15 capsules right now.

   _____

   _____

   _____

2. Ms. Kipsky checks her purse and finds that she has only $5.00. She wants to know how many capsules that the $5.00 will buy. (Use the formula based on $30 for the entire prescription amount.)

   _____

   _____

   _____

   _____

3. She next asks you, how many capsules can she purchase for $10?

   _____

   _____

   _____

ACTIVITY 16-2: Case Study—A Tapering Dose

Instructions: Read the following scenario, and then answer the critical thinking questions.

Mr. Mindes is a regular customer at your retail pharmacy. His medication profile seems to be a who's who of allergy medicines. Your pharmacy typically begins to see Mr. Mindes in early spring when the rain slows down and the flowers start to bloom. He has tried a variety of medications to help relieve allergy symptoms, such as fexofenadine, chlorpheniramine, and loratadine. He also has a nasal spray that keeps his sinuses clear during allergy attacks.

In spite of Mr. Mindes's preparation for each spring's natural bounties, this year he finds that he has actually acquired an infection that makes it tough for him to breathe. He has an uncomfortable case of bronchitis. His provider is prescribing a course of prednisone to help reduce the inflammation in his lungs.

The prescription is as follows: five tablets daily for five days, then four tablets daily for five days, then three tablets daily for five days, then two tablets daily for five days, and then one tablet daily for six days.

1. What is the total number of tablets needed to fill the complete prescription?

   _____

   _____

2. At exactly halfway through his course of prednisone treatment, how many tablets will Mr. Mindes have left in the bottle?

   _____

   _____

3. With three days to the end of his treatment and last dose, how many tablets are left in his prescription bottle?

   _____

   _____

ACTIVITY 16-3: Case Study—Cream Compound

Instructions: Read the following scenario and then answer the critical thinking questions.

Sebastian, a very nice elderly man, has an irritating and unpleasant skin condition. For the past year, he has been uncomfortable with major constant itching and raised bumps that will not go away. Over the past year, he has tried a multitude of moisturizers, none of which seems to help keep his skin from getting the raised bumps that make him itch constantly.

Sebastian has put up with the skin condition for almost a year. His primary care physician (PCP) explained to Sebastian that it was not a condition such as psoriasis or eczema. Sebastian has tried a variety of home remedies and herbal concoctions to make the skin condition go away, but the skin condition is persistent. The active areas of his skin condition remains on his lower arms near the elbows.

Sebastian had an appointment with his PCP earlier in the day. He explained to his PCP that the rash has gotten a bit worse on his arms and that he is experiencing more uncomfortable itching. The PCP decides to try a compound of two ingredients that she thinks might help alleviate the itching and add more moisture to the skin. Sebastian brings the prescription to your pharmacy to have it filled. The prescription is for 60% of ingredient A and 40% of ingredient B. The total amount is 155 g.

1. How many grams of each ingredient will be used to make the compound?

   _____

   _____

   _____

   _____

2. If Sebastian wants to pick up only 80% of his prescription today, how many grams will he be receiving?

    _____

    _____

3. After you explain to Sebastian how much 80% of his prescription will cost him, he tells you that he only wants 50% of the prescription to be filled. How many grams will that be?

    _____

    _____

4. After you compound 50% of the prescription, Sebastian now has 3.5 refills on his prescription. After he is able to pay for the full amount of the prescription, he would like to know when he can pick up all of the remaining refills and how many grams of the cream will he be paying for.

    _____

    _____

ACTIVITY 16-4: Math Definitions

Match the math term in the left-hand column with its definition in the right-hand column.

Term	Definition
1. _____ proportion	a. can be expressed as one number that is set on a fraction line above another number
2. _____ common fraction	b. the value of the numerator is smaller than the value of the denominator
3. _____ improper fraction	c. expresses the relationship of two numbers
4. _____ simple fraction	d. two or more equivalent ratios or fractions that both represent the same value
5. _____ proper fraction	e. the value of the numerator is larger than the value of the denominator
6. _____ ratio	f. cannot be reduced to any lower terms

CHAPTER 17
Measurement Systems

After completing Chapter 17 from the textbook, you should be able to:	Related Activity in the Workbook/Lab Manual
1. List the three fundamental systems of measurement.	Review Questions, Pharmacy Calculation Problems, PTCB Exam Practice Questions
2. List the three primary units of the metric system.	Review Questions, Pharmacy Calculation Problems, PTCB Exam Practice Questions
3. Define the various prefixes used in the metric system.	Review Questions, Pharmacy Calculation Problems, PTCB Exam Practice Questions
4. Recognize abbreviations used in measurements.	Review Questions, Pharmacy Calculation Problems, PTCB Exam Practice Questions, Activity 17-1, Activity 17-2, Activity 17-3, Lab 17-1, Lab 17-2
5. Explain the use of International Units and milliequivalents.	Review Questions, Pharmacy Calculation Problems, PTCB Exam Practice Questions
6. Convert measurements between the household system and the metric system.	Review Questions, Pharmacy Calculation Problems, PTCB Exam Practice Questions, Lab 17-1
7. Convert measurements between the apothecary system and the metric system.	Review Questions, Pharmacy Calculation Problems, PTCB Exam Practice Questions
8. Perform temperature conversions.	Review Questions, Pharmacy Calculation Problems, PTCB Exam Practice Questions, Activity 17-3, Lab 17-2

INTRODUCTION

Three fundamental systems of measurement are used to calculate dosages: the metric, apothecary, and household systems. Most prescriptions are written using the metric system. Regardless of your practice setting as a pharmacy technician, you must understand each system and how to convert from one system to another. With practice, the conversions you need to calculate dosages will become second nature to you. Until that time, use the charts and formulas from Chapter 17 as a guide. Remember that although miscalculating a conversion may seem to be a minor issue, it could have irrevocable effects on a patient's health.

REVIEW QUESTIONS

Match the following.

1. _____ apothecary system
2. _____ avoirdupois system
3. _____ household system
4. _____ International Units
5. _____ metric system
6. _____ Celsius
7. _____ Fahrenheit
8. _____ grain
9. _____ milliequivalent
10. _____ gram
11. _____ liter
12. _____ meter

a. measures a drug in terms of its action not its physical weight
b. metric unit of length; (m), (cm), (mm)
c. the number of grams of a drug in 1 mL of a normal solution
d. metric unit of volume; (L), (mL)
e. international temperature unit
f. metric unit of weight; (kg), (g), (mg), (mcg)
g. more accurate than the household and apothecary systems
h. system based on 1 lb being equivalent to 16 oz.
i. old English system of measurement
j. American measurement of temperature
k. American measurement for weight
l. primary unit of weight in the apothecary system

Choose the best answer.

13. If you are denoting two-tenths of a milligram, you would write:
    a. 2/10 mg.
    b. 0.2 mg.
    c. 2 mg.
    d. .2 mg.

14. 4 g is equivalent to:
    a. 4,000 mg.
    b. 40,000 mg.
    c. 400 mg.
    d. 40 mg.

15. 8 oz. is equivalent to how many milliliters?
    a. 16 mL
    b. 24 mL
    c. 240 mL
    d. 160 mL

16. There are 16 oz. in a pint. How many milliliters is that?
    a. 480 mL
    b. 48 mL
    c. 4.8 mL
    d. 4,800 mL

17. If Mary is to take 3 teaspoonfuls twice a day for 10 days, how many milliliters will be dispensed?
    a. 30,000 mL
    b. 3,000 mL
    c. 300 mL
    d. 30 mL

Match the following.

18. _____ mg   **a.** microgram
19. _____ mL   **b.** milligram
20. _____ g   **c.** milliliter
21. _____ mcg   **d.** gram

PHARMACY CALCULATION PROBLEMS

Calculate the following.

1. An optometrist orders the medication latanoprost ophthalmic solution. The SIG is written as 1 gtt os qd. The bottle you have in stock is 2.5 mL. What is the total day supply for the order?

2. Metronidazole IV comes in a 500 mg/100 mL concentration. If the patient received 100 mL for eight doses, how many grams of metronidazole were given in total?

3. A prescription is written for 8 fl. oz. of guaifenesin a.c. syrup. If the patient is to take 10 mL po qid, what is the total day supply for the order?

4. A patient is to take 1 g valacyclovir po bid for five days. If the medication comes in 500 mg tablets, how many tablets will the patient need?

5. A 3 L TPN is ordered for a patient in ICU. The pump is to be programmed for 120 mL/hr. How many hours will the TPN last?

PTCB EXAM PRACTICE QUESTIONS

1. A prescription is written for a hydrocortisone 5% in zinc oxide compound. The total quantity to be dispensed is 50 g. On stock you have 50 mg of hydrocortisone tablets.

   How many hydrocortisone 50 mg tablets will you need to triturate for this compound?
   a. ½ tablet   c. 5 tablets
   b. 2.5 tablets   d. 50 tablets

2. KCl 30 mEq is to be given in 250 mL of IV fluid. Available vials contain 40 mEq/20 mL. What is the volume you require to fill the order?
   a. 1.5 mL   c. 60 mL
   b. 15 mL   d. 6 mL

3. You receive an order for 0.5 g of Tigan IM. You have a 5 mL vial labeled 100 mg/mL. What is the volume you will need to fill the order?
   a. 2 mL   c. 0.5 mL
   b. 5 mL   d. 0.02 mL

4. You check the pharmacy refrigerator and it is 40 °F. What is the temperature in degrees Celsius?
   a. 4 °C
   b. –4 °C
   c. 104 °C
   d. 72 °C

5. How many milligrams of phenobarbital are in one tablet of 2 grain phenobarbital?
   a. 65 mg
   b. 6.5 mg
   c. 13 mg
   d. 130 mg

ACTIVITY 17-1: Case Study—Kilograms

Instructions: Read the following scenario and then answer the critical thinking questions.

Mrs. Sarnoto is probably one of the world's best mothers. In addition to her three biological children, she has adopted four boys. Her days are full of chores, activities, driving, and homework, but many people say Mrs. Sarnoto would not have it any other way.

Mrs. Sarnoto also takes care of all the children's health care needs, from vaccinations to outbreaks of poison oak exposure. For this reason, she is a frequent visitor at the retail pharmacy where you work. Over the past five years alone, she has probably purchased at least half of the products in the pharmacy.

As luck would have it, five of the seven children have come down with a terrible bronchial infection. Everyone in the household is miserable, including Mrs. Sarnoto, who is also sick. She knows she has to be the strong one, though, and heads to the pharmacy to fill the amoxicillin prescriptions she has gotten for the family. Each person weighs a different amount, and the amoxicillin prescription doses are based on weight in the following formula: 40 mg/kg/day in divided doses every eight hours. The amoxicillin you have available in the pharmacy is 250 mg/5 mL.

1. One of the children weighs 28 lb. How much amoxicillin suspension (in milliliters) will this child receive for a seven-day course of treatment?

   _____
   _____
   _____
   _____

2. One of the children weighs 83 lb. How much amoxicillin suspension (in milliliters) will this child receive for each dose?

   _____
   _____
   _____
   _____

3. Mrs. Sarnoto has been prescribed amoxicillin capsules 500 mg three times daily, but she has a sore throat and wants the suspension. How much suspension (in milliliters) does she need to complete a 10-day course of treatment?

   _____
   _____
   _____
   _____

4. Mrs. Sarnoto had to travel 3 km to get to the pharmacy. How many miles is her round trip?

_____

_____

_____

_____

ACTIVITY 17-2: Case Study—Milliliters

Instructions: Read the following scenario and then answer the critical thinking questions.

Carlene is the most experienced IV pharmacy technician at the Children's Hospital on the hill. She has been making IVs of all types for more than 11 years. She is in charge of all the specialty formulations that require precise measuring of multiple ingredients. Carlene takes great pride in what she does and shares all the little tricks she knows with the other pharmacy technicians who mix IVs. She has found a way to manipulate fluids when measuring so that they come out with exactly the same volume the doctor has ordered, regardless of the IV contents. Some of the tricks she has learned include ways to use milliliters and liter measurements interchangeably, taking into account displacement of added items.

1. From a 2.5 L volume, Carlene removes 325 mL. What is the final volume in milliliters?

_____

_____

_____

_____

2. Carlene adds 6,700 mL to a volume of 2 L. How many total liters are there?

_____

_____

_____

_____

3. A formulation of 3.2 L requires Carlene to remove 1,600 mL of fluid. How many milliliters are left after this?

_____

_____

_____

_____

ACTIVITY 17-3: Case Study—Drug Storage

Instructions: Read the following scenario and then answer the critical thinking questions.

Note: False medication names are used in this case study.

Sam is an inventory pharmacy technician at one of the biggest compounding pharmacies in his home town. He is in charge of medication purchasing, rotation, budget, and destruction, to name just a few of his tasks. The medication inventory in the pharmacy is very large. The pharmacy has an inventory of more than 10,000 classifications of medications in their various dosage forms.

Many of the medications that are used for compounding in Sam's pharmacy are in raw and bulk forms. Proper storage of the bulk medications is very important in order to prevent the breakdown of the active components in each medication. With the volume of inventory Sam has to manage, it is challenging to recall the storage instructions for each medication or product. Sam periodically refers to the reference texts and tools in each section of the pharmacy.

In addition to counting all of the medications and products, Sam uses this time to ensure that all of the medications are stored within their optimum temperature ranges. For some of the medications, the manufacturers periodically issue updates on storage instructions and, where the medications should normally be stored when not in use.

1. The product ectium is a fine powder that must be kept in a temperature-controlled environment of 40–48 °F per the manufacturer's storage requirements. What is this temperature in degrees Celsius? Where is the ectium normally stored when not in use?

   _____

   _____

   _____

   _____

2. Another product, silicutitum, is composed of small 4 cm balls that will melt if it is stored at a temperature of above 55 °F, per the manufacturer's storage requirements. What is this temperature in degrees Celsius? Where is the silicutitum normally stored when not in use?

   _____

   _____

   _____

   _____

3. A liquid known as pasitoxel will release a vapor if it is stored in an area at a temperature above 3.333 °C per the manufacturer's storage requirements and warnings. What is this temperature in degrees Fahrenheit? Where is the pasitoxel normally stored when not in use?

   _____

   _____

   _____

   _____

4. The lab where the mixing takes place is kept at a steady 72 °F. When the staff needs to mix basculum, they have to drop the lab's temperature to 11.11 °C per the manufacturer's storage requirement. After the reduction in the lab's temperature occurs for mixing the basculum, what is the lab temperature in degrees Fahrenheit? Where is the basculum normally stored when not in use?

_____

_____

_____

_____

LAB 17-1: Measuring Liquids Using Different Measurement Systems and Units

Objectives:

Demonstrate the ability to measure liquids using common pharmacy measurement systems.

Describe the relationship between the metric and household systems.

Use ordinary kitchen tools to understand and visualize the relationship between the most common pharmacy measurement systems.

Pre-Lab Information:

- Review Chapter 17 in the textbook.
- Gather the following materials:
  - kitchen measuring spoons
  - kitchen measuring cup
  - 10 mL and 20 mL syringes
  - 100 mL graduated cylinder
  - container of water

Explanation:

It is important for you to understand the relationship between the different liquid measurements used in pharmacy. This exercise will help you visualize the differences and relate them to more familiar kitchen measurements. This knowledge will also help you assist your patients in understanding how to measure certain medications.

Activity:

Using the equipment you have collected, complete the following exercises.

1. Take the 10 mL syringe and draw up 5 mL of water.

2. Now use the 5 mL of water from the syringe to fill up the teaspoon.

3. How much of the water fits into the teaspoon? Describe the relationship between 5 mL and 1 teaspoon.

   _____

   _____

   _____

   _____

4. Take the 20 mL syringe and draw up 15 mL of water.

5. Now use the 15 mL of water to fill up the tablespoon.

6. How much of the water fits into the tablespoon? Describe the relationship between 15 mL and 1 tablespoon.

_____

_____

_____

_____

7. Add 2 tablespoons of liquid (water) to the 100 mL graduated cylinder.

8. Describe the relationship between 2 tablespoons and 1 fl. oz. (30 mL).

_____

_____

_____

_____

9. Using the 100 mL graduated cylinder from question 8, pour the liquid into the measuring cup.

10. Describe the relationship between 1 fl. oz. (30 mL) and 1 cup.

_____

_____

_____

_____

Student Name: _____

Lab Partner: _____

Grade/Comments: _____

_____

Student Comments: _____

_____

LAB 17-2: Measuring and Converting Temperatures

Objectives:

Demonstrate the ability to measure and convert temperatures between the two temperature scales.

Pre-Lab Information:

- Review Chapter 17 in the textbook about temperature conversions.
- Gather the following materials:
  - Three stock medications in the dosage forms of either a vial containing a liquid or a vial that requires a diluent. Please select two of the three medications which require refrigeration or freezing.
  - Calculator
  - Pencil
  - Temperature log from the instructor
  - Freezer/refrigerator thermometer(s)

Explanation:

Many medications have different storage requirements and temperatures in order to remain effective and safe for consumer use. A substantial number of medications are manufactured in other countries where the Celsius unit of temperature is common for the proper storage of those medications.

Activity:

Locate the storage requirements on each of the labels of the stock medications. With each of the stock medications, notate the required temperature or ranges of temperatures that have been established by the manufacturer for proper storage. Convert each of the medications temperatures from Celsius to Fahrenheit. After you have successfully converted the temperatures and checked your math with a teammate for accuracy, locate the freezer/refrigerator thermometer(s) and record on the temperature log the current temperatures. Next, compare the stock medications temperatures to the freezer/refrigerator thermometer(s) to check if the environment in the freezer/refrigerator is correct for proper storage of the medications.

Medication #1

Manufacturer's temperature: _____

Freezer/refrigerator thermometer(s): _____

Medication #2

Manufacturer's temperature: _____

Freezer/refrigerator thermometer(s): _____

Medication #3

Manufacturer's temperature: _____

Freezer/refrigerator thermometer(s): _____

Medication #4

Manufacturer's temperature: _____

Freezer/refrigerator thermometer(s): _____

Medication #5

Manufacturer's temperature: _____

Freezer/refrigerator thermometer(s): _____

Student Name: _____

Lab Partner: _____

Grade/Comments: _____

_____

_____

Student Comments: _____

_____

_____

CHAPTER 18
Dosage Calculations

After completing Chapter 18 from the textbook, you should be able to:	Related Activity in the Workbook/Lab Manual
1. Calculate the correct number of doses in a prescription.	Review Questions, Pharmacy Calculation Problems, PTCB Exam Practice Questions, Activity 18-1, Activity 18-2
2. Determine the quantity to dispense for a prescription.	Review Questions, Pharmacy Calculation Problems, PTCB Exam Practice Questions, Activity 18-1, Activity 18-2, Activity 18-3
3. Calculate the amount of active ingredient in a prescription.	Review Questions, Pharmacy Calculation Problems, PTCB Exam Practice Questions
4. Determine the correct days supply for a prescription.	Review Questions, Pharmacy Calculation Problems, PTCB Exam Practice Questions, Activity 18-1, Activity 18-2
5. Perform multiple dosage calculations for a single prescription.	Review Questions, Pharmacy Calculation Problems, PTCB Exam Practice Questions, Activity 18-2, Activity 18-3
6. Calculate accurate dosages for pediatric patients.	Review Questions, Pharmacy Calculation Problems, PTCB Exam Practice Questions, Activity 18-1, Lab 18-1, Lab 18-2
7. Convert a patient's weight from pounds to kilograms.	Review Questions, Pharmacy Calculation Problems, PTCB Exam Practice Questions, Activity 18-1, Lab 18-1, Lab 18-2
8. Perform dosage calculations based upon mg/kg/day.	Review Questions, Pharmacy Calculation Problems, PTCB Exam Practice Questions, Lab 18-1, Lab 18-2

INTRODUCTION

Proper dosing of medications is important to ensure patient safety. Dosage calculations include calculating the number of doses and dispensing quantities and ingredient quantities. These calculations are performed in the pharmacy on a daily basis. As a pharmacy technician, you must have a full working knowledge of how to perform these calculations. To perform dosage calculations, you will draw upon the knowledge you have mastered in previous chapters in the textbook, such as setting up ratios and proportions, keeping like units consistent, and cross-multiplying to solve for an unknown.

REVIEW QUESTIONS

Match the following.

1. _____ Clark's Rule
2. _____ dispensing quantity
3. _____ dose
4. _____ Fried's Rule
5. _____ days supply

a. pediatric dose based on age in months

b. how long the amount of medication dispensed will last if taken as directed

c. pediatric dose based on weight expressed in pounds

d. total amount of medication to be dispensed

e. amount of medication prescribed to be taken at one time

Write the correct sig codes.

6. every six hours _____
7. every day _____
8. four times daily _____
9. every other day _____
10. twice daily _____
11. every eight hours _____
12. as needed _____
13. every four hours _____
14. every 12 hours _____
15. every four to six hours _____
16. six times daily _____
17. three times daily _____
18. four to six times each day _____

Choose the best answer.

19. When calculating the quantity to be dispensed you should always:
    a. round up, so the patient gets enough medication.
    b. round down, so the patient will not overdose.
    c. dispense the exact quantity, including a tablet if necessary.
    d. not worry too much about quantity if the patient has refills.

20. A 5 mL bottle of eye drops will last for how long if the patient is using 1 gtt ou bid?
    a. 30   c. 20
    b. 25   d. 15

Fill in the blanks.

For questions 21–24:

21. Mr. Mestophel has a prescription for cephalexin 500 mg, #60, with the sig code "1 po bid ud."

22. The dose is _____ capsules.

23. The days supply is _____ days.

20. The daily dose is _____ mg.

20. The dispensing quantity is _____.

20. If Tyra's emergency inhaler contains 200 puffs and she uses 1 puff up to four times daily, how long should her inhaler normally last? _____

PHARMACY CALCULATION PROBLEMS

Calculate the following.

1. How many grams are in an 8 oz. bottle of levetiracetam 100 mg/mL oral solution?

2. A patient is prescribed 2 teaspoonfuls of citalopram hydrobromide 2 mg/mL. How many micrograms are in each dose?

3. A patient is prescribed, 4 mg/kg/day of a medication. The patient weighs 165 lbs. What is the final strength that the patient will receive?

4. A child needs a medication that does not have a pediatric formula available. The usual adult dosage for this medication is 800 mg. If the child weighs 60 lbs., how many milligrams would constitute a safe pediatric dose?

5. A patient weighing in at 220 lbs. is prescribed a medication that will be dosed at 10 mcg/kg/day in three divided doses. How many micrograms are in each of the doses?

PTCB EXAM PRACTICE QUESTIONS

1. A prescription reads: Amoxicillin 250 mg/10 mL, 1 tsp bid 10d. How many milliliters will you need to dispense?
   a. 50 mL   c. 150 mL
   b. 100 mL   d. 200 mL

2. The doctor orders vancomycin 10 mg/kg q12h IV for a toddler. The toddler weighs approximately 55 lbs. What is the strength that the toddler will receive per dose?
   a. 1,210 mg   c. 550 mg
   b. 250 mg   d. 500 mg

3. Calculate a single dose, in milliliters, for a 22-lb. child receiving gentamicin 2 mg/kg of body weight IVPB q8h. Gentamicin is available in 20 mg/2 mL concentration.
   a. 2 mL
   b. 10 mL
   c. 15 mL
   d. 20 mL

4. You have received a prescription for diphenhydramine 12.5 mg/5 mL, dispense 240 mL. The patient is to take 50 mg tid. What is the day's supply for this prescription?
   a. 60 days
   b. 12 days
   c. 20 days
   d. 15 days

5. A parent of a five-year-old child weighing 47 lbs. needs to give an oral dose of Tylenol elixir. The literature states that the dose for a child of this age and weight should not exceed 70 mg/kg/day. This daily maximum is to be divided into six doses. Tylenol elixir contains 125 mg/mL. How many teaspoonfuls would the parent give to the child for a single dose?
   a. 1 tsp.
   b. 1.25 tsp.
   c. 1.5 tsp.
   d. 2 tsp.

ACTIVITY 18-1: Case Study—Pediatric Dosing

Instructions: Read the following scenario and then answer the critical thinking questions.

Jimmy is an eight-year-old boy who weighs 55 lbs. and presents the typical symptoms of a cold. The primary symptoms he exhibits are a fever of 101 degrees and he is constantly tugging at his ears. The doctor has diagnosed Jimmy with acute otitis media and prescribes a seven-day course of amoxicillin capsules and acetaminophen tablets for fever. When Jimmy's mother hands the prescription to you, you notice that the doctor has forgotten to write in the dose for the amoxicillin.

1. What do the pharmacist and the technician need to know and do in order to dispense the correct doses and quantities of the amoxicillin and acetaminophen for Jimmy?

   _____
   _____
   _____
   _____

2. While turning the prescription in, the mother mentions that Jimmy's throat is very sore and he has had a hard time swallowing food and liquids. You realize that capsules and tablets will be too difficult for Jimmy to swallow. How is Jimmy going to take his medicine?

   _____
   _____
   _____

3. The ordered dose for the amoxicillin capsules turns out to be 500 mg three times daily (one capsule). If you were to dispense a suspension of 250 mg/5 mL, how much would Jimmy then receive per dose? How much would you need to dispense for the full seven days?

   _____
   _____
   _____

4. The ordered dose for the acetaminophen tablets is 250 mg for three days. However, the maximum total daily dose for a child less than 12 years old is 75 mg/kg/day, not to exceed 3,750 mg/day. What is the volume you would need to dispense if the order is now 10 mg/kg/dose every four to six hours as needed; do not exceed five doses in 24 hours?

_____

_____

_____

ACTIVITY 18-2: Case Study—Tablets

Instructions: Read the following scenario and then answer the critical thinking questions.

Ms. Kelsey, two-time award-winning journalist, has worked for the newspaper for more than 22 years. She absolutely loves her job because of the places it has taken her and the people she has met. Ms. Kelsey has interviewed so many different people that it truly has made her feel like she has lived a rewarding life.

Ms. Kelsey has taken one particular medication all through her life in tablet form. She has a form of asthma and this medication helps her breathe. In addition to this one tablet, she has a rescue inhaler. A few times in the past she has been treated with maintenance inhalers, but luckily does not have to be on them most of the time. The tablets seem to work very well. Occasionally, depending on age and situation, her doctor has increased or decreased the amount of medication in the tablets to prevent flare-ups.

1. In her 20s, Ms. Kelsey was instructed to take 3 tablets twice a day for 28 days at a time. How many tablets did she need to complete one course of treatment?

_____

_____

_____

2. When she turned 30 years of age, Ms. Kelsey was instructed to take 3.5 tablets three times a day for 28 days. How many tablets did she need for one course of treatment?

_____

_____

_____

3. Now that Ms. Kelsey is over 40 years of age, she is instructed to take 3.75 tablets twice a day for 34 days. How many tablets does she need to complete this course of treatment?

_____

_____

_____

4. When Ms. Kelsey turns 50 years old, she will need to take 272 tablets over 32 days with twice-daily dosing. How many tablets will she be taking per dose?

_____

_____

_____

ACTIVITY 18-3: Case Study—Cream

Instructions: Read the following scenario and then answer the critical thinking questions.

Note: False medication names are used in this case study.

Sharla is a very beautiful and active 16-year-old girl. She is captain of her high school cheerleading team, has played the lead role in three of the school's plays this year, and is taking classes for a future career in modeling. Sharla takes exceptionally good care of her body and skin from the inside out, so it was quite disturbing for her when one day she noticed that her slight acne had begun to worsen.

During her teenage years, Sharla has had periodic face and skin conditions resulting from sensitive skin. It turns out that she is very sensitive to detergents, soaps, lotions, and perfumes. It is very difficult for her to keep the rashes under control when she breaks the rules and wears perfume for special occasions such as school dances.

Sharla has received prescriptions from the compounding pharmacy for all types of perfume-free creams over the years. Almost all have helped, and she uses this pharmacy exclusively for all new formulations she is prescribed. She has received some prescriptions in heavy jars or small tubes depending on the area to be treated.

1. When Sharla had a round, mild rash on her bottom left cheek, she was prescribed listfal 34 g and palfite 16 g combined. How many milligrams is this?

   _____

   _____

   _____

   _____

2. When her legs were covered in a rash, Sharla was prescribed 12 lbs. of crexopen cream. How much is this in ounces?

   _____

   _____

   _____

   _____

3. For the mild hypersensitive reaction just under her ear, she was prescribed junisten 1.2 kg. How many ounces is this?

   _____

   _____

   _____

   _____

LAB 18-1: Converting Weights

Objective:

Demonstrate the ability to convert a patient's current weight from kilograms to pounds and pounds to kilograms

Pre-Lab Information:

- Review Chapter 18 in the textbook.
- Gather the following materials:
  - scale
  - calculator
  - pencil
  - paper

Explanation:

Converting a patient's weight from pounds to kilograms is sometimes required for the proper dosing of a prescribed medication therapy.

Activity:

Step on the scale to determine your current weight. Write down your current weight, and then convert the weight from pounds to kilograms. Next, talk with two family members or your lab partner and ask them to step on a scale to notate their current weight. One of the family members must be a child in order for you to weigh the child and record his or her current weight. Then convert his or her current weight from pounds to kilograms.

1) Your current weight in pounds: _____

   Your current weight converted to kilograms: _____

2) Your family member or lab partner's current weight in pounds: _____

   Your family member or lab partner's current weight converted into kilograms: _____

3) Your family member or lab partner's current weight in pounds: _____

   Your family member or lab partner's current weight converted into kilograms: _____

Student Name: _____

Lab Partner: _____

Grade/Comments: _____

_____

_____

Student Comments: _____

_____

_____

LAB 18-2: Pediatric Dosing

Objective:

Demonstrate the ability to convert a patient's current weight and factor the weight into a prescription order.

Pre-Lab Information:

- Review Chapter 18 in the textbook.
- Gather the following materials:
  - calculator
  - pencil
  - paper

Explanation:

Factoring a pediatric patient's current weight is often required from the technician in order to calculate the ordered strength of a medication.

Activity:

Using your child family member's weight from Lab 18-1 as a patient for this activity, please factor in his/ her weight to calculate the mg/kg/day. This will provide you a better perspective as to how accurate and careful you must be when calculating a pediatric dose for a patient. After you have calculated the accurate dose for the mg/kg/day of the child, validate your answer with your lab partner or the instructor.

1) The physician orders phenytoin 6 mg/kg/day for the pediatric patient as maintenance therapy. Calculate the new dose based on the child's weight. Verify the dose with another lab partner or the instructor and have them initial or sign below.

_____

New Dose: _____

Verified by: _____

Student Name: _____

Lab Partner: _____

Grade/Comments: _____

_____

Student Comments: _____

_____

_____

CHAPTER 19
Concentrations and Dilutions

After completing Chapter 19 from the textbook, you should be able to:	Related Activity in the Workbook/Lab Manual
1. Calculate weight/weight concentrations.	Review Questions, Pharmacy Calculation Problems, PTCB Exam Practice Questions
2. Calculate weight/volume concentrations.	Review Questions, Pharmacy Calculation Problems, PTCB Exam Practice Questions, Activity 19-1, Activity 19-2, Lab 19-1
3. Calculate volume/volume concentrations.	Review Questions, Pharmacy Calculation Problems, PTCB Exam Practice Questions, Activity 19-1, Lab 19-1
4. Calculate dilutions of stock solutions.	Review Questions, Pharmacy Calculation Problems, PTCB Exam Practice Questions, Lab 19-1, Lab 19-2

INTRODUCTION

Concentrations and dilutions, which can feel overwhelming and intimidating, are really no more than a series of simple ratios and proportions. Concentrations of many pharmaceutical preparations are expressed as a percent strength. Percent strength represents how many grams of active ingredient are in 100 mL. In the case of solids such as ointments, percent strength represents the number of grams of active ingredient contained in 100 g. Percent strength can be reduced to a fraction or to a decimal, which may be useful in solving these calculations. It is best to convert any ratio strengths to a percent. As a pharmacy technician, you will use concentrations and dilutions in a variety of pharmacy practice settings, so it is important that you master this skill.

REVIEW QUESTIONS

Match the following.

1. _____ concentration
2. _____ diluent
3. _____ percent strength
4. _____ % volume/volume
5. _____ % weight/volume
6. _____ % weight/weight

a. concentrations are those in which a liquid active ingredient is mixed with a liquid base

b. concentrations are those in which a solid active ingredient is mixed with a solid base

c. concentrations are those in which a solid active ingredient is mixed with a liquid base

d. the strength of active pharmaceutical ingredient in a medication

e. representation of the number of grams of active ingredient contained in 100 mL

f. a larger volume that you mix with the stock solution

True or False?

7. Grams and milliliters are used interchangeably in concentration problems, depending on whether you are working with solids in grams or liquids in milliliters, as they are considered equivalent measures.

   T   F

8. Concentration problems are classified into four categories.

   T   F

9. When mixing powders with liquids, the liquid (base) quantity is considered the total quantity, as the powder will either dissolve or suspend within the base liquid.

   T   F

Choose the best answer.

10. What is the first step when calculating a weight/weight concentration?
    a. add both the active and base quantities for the total quantity
    b. multiply the converted number by 100 to express the final
    c. set up a proportion with the amount of active ingredient listed over the total quantity, as grams over grams.
    d. convert the proportion to a decimal concentration as a percentage

11. How many 500 mg metronidazole tablets will be needed to compound the following prescription for a patient? "Metronidazole 3%, suspending agent 30%, simple syrup 40% qs ad H_2O to 150 mL."
    a. 9 tablets   c. 10 tablets
    b. 7 tablets   d. 18 tablets

12. You receive a prescription for "Amoxil 400 mg po tid × 10 days." Your pharmacy has in stock Amoxil oral suspension 250 mg/5 mL. What is the exact volume of medication you will need to correctly and completely fill the prescription for the patient?
    a. 150 mL   c. 240 mL
    b. 168 mL   d. 200 mL

13. How many grams of 2% silver nitrate ointment will deliver 1 g of the active ingredient?
    a. 25 g
    c. 50 g
    b. 4 g
    d. 20 g

14. What volume of 5% aluminum acetate solution will be needed if 120 mL of 0.05% solution are extemporaneously compounded?
    a. 12 mL
    c. 8.3 mL
    b. 1.2 mL
    d. 0.83 mL

15. Calculate the flow rate in drops per minute if a physician orders D5W/NS 2,000 mL to be run for 12 hours using an administration set that delivers 40 gtts/mL.
    a. 6,680 gtts/min
    c. 111 gtts/min
    b. 167 gtts/min
    d. 78 gtts/min

16. A bag of NaCl 0.45% in 500 mL has been ordered to be sent to the ER. What is the strength in gram weight of the bag?
    a. 45 g
    c. 0.0009 g
    b. 1,111 g
    d. 0.45 g

17. From the following formula, calculate in grams the quantity of miconazole needed to prepare 12 kg of powder.
    zinc oxide 1 part
    calamine 2 parts
    miconazole 1.5 parts
    bismuth subgallate 3 parts
    talcum 8 parts
    a. 15.5 g
    c. 1,161 g
    b. 0.09 g
    d. 1,548 g

18. Calculate the flow rate for an IV of 1,000 mL to run in over eight hours with a set calibrated at 20 gtt/mL.
    a. 42 gtt/min
    c. 125.1 gtt/min
    b. 17.36 gtt/min
    d. 50 gtt/min

PHARMACY CALCULATION PROBLEMS

Calculate the following.

1. How many grams of a drug are contained in 250 mL of a 20% solution?

2. A technician has an order to compound metoclopramide suspension 5 mg/5 mL, qs ad 100 mL. In stock, the technician has metoclopramide 10 mg tablets. How many tablets will the technician need to triturate for this compound?

3. What is the percent strength of a solution that is made by adding 150 mL of sterile water to 500 mL of a 50% solution?

4. If a technician is compounding a 5% hydrocortisone emulsion in 120 g of aquaphilic ointment, how many grams of hydrocortisone powder will the technician need to add to the compound?

5. How many grams of active ingredient are in 500 mL of a 1:20 solution?

PTCB EXAM PRACTICE QUESTIONS

1. You have 200 mL of a 30% solution. You dilute the solution to 600 mL. What is the percent strength of the final solution?
   a. 60%
   b. 30%
   c. 12%
   d. 10%

2. A solution of ampicillin contains 250 mg/mL. What is the percent strength of the solution?
   a. 2.5%
   b. 25%
   c. 12.5%
   d. 15.2%

3. What is the final volume when you dilute 50 mL of sorbitol 50% solution to a 20% solution?
   a. 150 mL
   b. 125 mL
   c. 250 mL
   d. 500 mL

4. Neostigmine is available in a 1:1000 concentration in a 20 mL vial. You have a prescription for 16 mg. How many milliliters are required?
   a. 1.6 mL
   b. 16 mL
   c. 12.5 mL
   d. 1.2 mL

5. Epinephrine is available as a 1:1000 w/v solution. If the patient dose is 0.2 mg IM, how many milliliters are needed?
   a. 2 mL
   b. 1 mL
   c. 0.2 mL
   d. 0.1 mL

ACTIVITY 19-1: Case Study—Dosing

Instructions: Read the following scenario, and then answer the critical thinking questions.

Wintertime brings a barrage of colds throughout the Hudson family. They are a very active family of Dad, Mom, two boys (11 and 14), and two girls (8 and 12). Each child participates in at least one winter sport, keeping them on the go. The children spend a lot of time riding to games with other families, and their parents think this makes it easier to pick up infections. Although they manage to avoid most ailments year round, three weeks in January of each year seem to bring an assortment of infection bugs to this household. This past winter was no exception.

When January rolled around, the infections hit this family like dominoes. The pattern is almost the same every year. Once everyone was sick at the same time, and everyone received treatments for different bacterial infections.

1. Dad received cefotetan in either 1 g or 2 g for IM injection. The 1 g vial would be mixed with 2 mL of sterile water and the 2 g would be mixed with 3 mL of sterile water. What is the concentration of the 1 g and the 2 g cefotetan with these diluent amounts?

_____
_____
_____
_____

2. Mom is going to receive a Zithromax suspension 500 mg/day for one day, then 250 mg/day for four days. The concentration available to you is 200 mg/5 mL. How many teaspoonfuls does Mom receive per dose on day 1? How many on day 2?

_____
_____
_____
_____

3. The eight-year-old girl weighs 42 lbs. and will receive Unasyn at 300 mg/kg/day. How much is her dose per day?

_____
_____
_____
_____

4. The 14-year-old boy is going to receive ceftriaxone 2 g IV daily for three days, to be infused over 30 minutes. For a 2 g dose, 19.2 mL of sterile water were added to the vial and the medication was then injected into a 100 mL bag of NS. How many milliliters per minute are infused if the total volume of the piggyback has to empty out over 30 minutes?

_____
_____
_____
_____

ACTIVITY 19-2: Case Study—Reconstitution

Instructions: Read the following scenario and then answer the critical thinking questions.

Jeremy is a recent graduate of the Pharmacy Technician Training program from the local community college. This is his first job as he is working in an independent closed-door pharmacy. Within six months of his hire date, he is already being trained to compound orders for small-volume parenteral admixtures in the sterile preparation area of the pharmacy. Training in this area begins with practicing reconstitution techniques for a month and then after specific competencies have been met per USP <797>, Jeremy will be compounding large-volume parenteral admixtures.

During each workday, Jeremy compounds about 30–50 small-volume parenteral admixtures that are less than 50 mL of total volume. The medications Jeremy works within this pharmacy use sterile water as the main diluent. Jeremy works with any number of powdered medications within vials, in which he is required to reconstitute to compound sterile admixtures.

1. Jeremy has a 1 g vial of vancomycin and adds 10 mL of sterile water. What is the final concentration of the vancomycin?

_____

_____

_____

_____

2. If Jeremy were to add 20 mL of sterile water to this vancomycin, what would be the final concentration?

_____

_____

_____

_____

3. What is the final concentration if Jeremy has 2 g of vancomycin and he added 20 mL of sterile water to this vial?

_____

_____

_____

_____

4. Jeremy has progressed with his skill sets so well that his supervisor would like for him to prepare a 500 mL bag of vancomycin. The order is prescribed for 500 mg vancomycin in 500 mL NaCl. As there is only the 1 g vial in stock, how much diluent will be needed to compound this medication?

_____

_____

_____

ACTIVITY 19-3 Case Study—Concentration

Instructions: Read the following scenario and then answer the critical thinking questions.

Note: False medication names are used in this case study.

Renee is a clinical pharmacy technician at a mid-sized hospital with about 120 patient beds. This bed count includes a small 20-bed unit that is for patients who require a little longer stay for rehabilitation purposes. Typically these patients are a little older and less mobile than patients who are in the hospital for routine surgical needs. Many of these patients move on to some sort of assisted living situation, such as community apartment homes where part-time nursing care is available.

Part of the care the nurses provide to these patients is the administration of medications such as IV infusions, insulin shots (for the squeamish), and other types of injections (such as cyanocobalamin). Other nurses occasionally have to do careful calculation and administration of pain medications in suspension or injectable forms.

Part of Renee's job is to help provide the medications to the nursing unit for patient administration; this includes mixing of unit-dose preparations such as injectables or oral liquids. In addition, Renee helps double-check all the calculations as part of a safety check. Because she works in pharmacy, she also knows what drug forms and strengths are immediately available.

1. Bascoletine is available as 30 mg/mL in a 15 mL vial. How many total milligrams are available in this vial?

   _____

   _____

   _____

   _____

2. If the nurse withdrew one-quarter of the vial contents for a dose, how many milligrams would be in that dose?

   _____

   _____

   _____

   _____

3. The doctor prescribes the entire vial of medication from question 1, divided into five equal doses. How many milligrams and milliliters would each dose have?

   _____

   _____

   _____

   _____

4. Using the medication information from question 1, how many milligrams are in 5 mL?

   _____

   _____

   _____

   _____

LAB 19-1: Working with Concentrations

Objective:

Demonstrate the ability to measure liquids and work with solutions of differing concentrations.

Pre-Lab Information:

- Review Chapter 19 in the textbook.
- Gather the following materials:
  - 20 mL, 50 mL, and 100 mL graduated cylinders
  - bottle of blue-colored water
  - bottle of red-colored water
  - bottle of distilled water
  - syrup/suspension medication bottles in 3 oz, 4 oz, and 6 oz sizes

Explanation:

It is important for pharmacy technicians to understand how to calculate the percent strength of solutions of varying concentrations. This exercise will give you the opportunity to experience working with solutions of different concentrations and the calculations involved.

Activity:

Use the materials in the preceding list to prepare the solutions as instructed; then answer the following questions about the resulting concentrations.

Assumptions:

- The blue-colored water solution should be considered a 100% solution (100 g/100 mL).
- The red-colored water solution should be considered a 100% solution (100 g/100 mL).
- The distilled water should be considered a 0% solution.

1. Measure 20 mL of the 100% red-colored water solution. Dilute the solution to 80 mL with the distilled water. What is the percent strength of the final solution?

   _____

   _____

2. Measure 55 mL of the 100% blue-colored water solution and mix it with 35 mL of the 100% red-colored water solution. What is the final percent strength of the blue-colored solution in the new red-colored water solution?

   _____

   _____

3. Using the solution from question 2, what is the final percent strength of the red-colored water solution in the new green-colored water solution?

   _____

   _____

4. Measure 60 mL of the 100% red-colored water solution and dilute it to 100 mL with distilled water. What is the percent strength of the resulting solution?

_____

_____

5. Make a 50% solution of red-colored water solution by mixing 25 mL of the red-colored water solution with 25 mL of distilled water. Take 30 mL of the diluted red-colored water solution (50%) and mix it with 20 mL blue-colored solution. How many grams of red-colored water solution are in the new mixture?

_____

_____

6. What is the percent strength of the diluted red-colored water solution juice in the solution from question 5?

_____

_____

Student Name: _____

Lab Partner: _____

Grade/Comments: _____

_____

_____

Student Comments: _____

_____

_____

LAB 19-2: Working with Dilutions

Objective:

Demonstrate the ability to measure diluents and work with solutions of differing concentrations.

Pre-Lab Information:

- Review Chapter 19 in the textbook.
- Gather the following materials:
  - 20 mL, 50 mL, and 100 mL graduated cylinders
  - bottle of blue-colored water
  - bottle of red-colored water
  - bottle of distilled water
  - syrup/suspension medication bottles in 3 oz, 4 oz, and 6 oz sizes

Explanation:

Just as it is important for pharmacy technicians to understand how to calculate the percent strength of solutions of varying concentrations, it is as equally important to understand how to calculate the amount of diluent for a stock solution. This exercise will give you the opportunity to experience working with diluents of different volumes and the calculations involved.

Activity:

Use the materials in the preceding list to prepare the solutions as instructed; then answer the following questions about the resulting concentrations.

Assumptions:

- The blue-colored water solution should be considered a 100% solution (100 g/100 mL).
- The red-colored water solution should be considered a 100% solution (100 g/100 mL).
- The distilled water should be considered a 0% solution.

1. If you diluted 90 mL of 10% of the blue-colored water solution to 8%, how much volume would there be?

   _____

   _____

2. How much of the 10% red-colored water solution will you need to produce 120 mL of a 5% solution?

   _____

   _____

3. How much 50% of the blue-colored water solution would you need to produce 30 mL of a 10% blue-colored water solution?

   _____

   _____

4. How much 5% red water solution can you make by diluting 500 mL of the 20% red water solution?

_____

_____

Student Name: _____

Lab Partner: _____

Grade/Comments: _____

_____

_____

Student Comments: _____

_____

_____

CHAPTER 20
Alligations

After completing Chapter 20 from the textbook, you should be able to:	Related Activity in the Workbook/Lab Manual
1. Understand when to use the alligation principle for calculations.	Review Questions, Pharmacy Calculation Problems, PTCB Exam Practice Questions, Activity 20-1, Activity 20-2, Activity 20-3, Lab 20-1
2. Calculate and solve a variety of alligation-related problems.	Review Questions, Pharmacy Calculation Problems, PTCB Exam Practice Questions, Activity 20-1, Activity 20-2, Activity 20-3, Lab 20-1

INTRODUCTION

The alligation method is used in the pharmacy when it is necessary to mix two products that have different percent strengths of the same active ingredient. The strength of the final product will fall between the strengths of each original product. Although these calculations can be confusing at first, once you master the alligation grid, you should be able to perform these calculations easily.

REVIEW QUESTIONS

Fill in the blanks.

1. Solvents and diluents such as water, vanishing cream base, and white petrolatum are considered a percent strength of _____.

2. Liquids, including solutions, syrups, elixirs, and even lotions, are expressed in _____.

3. Solids are expressed in _____. Examples of solids are powders, creams, and ointments.

4. The alligation formula requires that you express the strength as a _____ when setting up the problem.

5. When writing percentages or using decimals, always use a leading _____.

6. 1 fl. oz. is equal to _____ mL but it is commonly rounded to _____ mL.

7. 1 avoirdupois oz. is equal to _____ g but it is commonly rounded to _____ g.

8. The _____ strength goes in the top left box of an alligation grid.

9. The _____ strength goes in the bottom left box of an alligation grid.

10. The _____ goes in the center box of an alligation grid.

11. The allegation grid is also referred to as the _____ - _____ - _____
   _____.

Use the alligation method to answer the following questions.

You have in stock 1 gallon of silver nitrate 1% solution that you can dilute with distilled water. How many milliliters of each solution will you need in order to make 2 L of silver nitrate 0.5% solution?

12. _____ mL of the 1% stock solution

13. _____ mL of distilled water

You have in stock, hydrocortisone 10% ointment and hydrocortisone 2% ointment. How many grams of each ointment will you need in order to prepare hydrocortisone 5% ointment 120 g?

14. _____ g of the 10% ointment

15. _____ g of the 2% ointment

Prepare 480 mL of a 1:30 solution using a 1:10 solution and a 1:50 solution.

16. _____ mL of the 1:50 solution

17. _____ mL of the 1:10 solution

18. How many grams of 10% ointment should you add to 20 g of 2% ointment to make 5% ointment?
   _____ g

19. How many milliliters of water should you add to 50 mL of betadine 0.25% solution to prepare a betadine 1:1000 solution? _____ mL

20. How many grams of lidocaine 2% ointment should you mix with 22.5 g of lidocaine 10% ointment to prepare 2 oz of lidocaine 5% ointment? _____ g

21. Convert 25% to a ratio strength. _____

22. 1:2 is what percentage strength? _____

Fill in the blanks.

23. 1:2   50%   0.50   _____

24. _____   33%   0.33 $\frac{1}{3}$

25. 3:4   _____   0.75 $\frac{3}{4}$

26. 1:1   100%   _____   1

27. 1:4   _____   0.25   _____

PHARMACY CALCULATION PROBLEMS

Calculate the following.

1. A technician is going to compound 8 oz of zinc oxide 7.5% ointment. In stock, there is zinc oxide 20% ointment and petroleum jelly. How many grams of each medication will the technician need in order to make the compound?

2. A physician prescribes 3 L of a 4% solution. The pharmacy has a 12% solution and a 2% solution in stock. How many milliliters of each solution will be needed to make the final product?

3. You will need to prepare a 5% solution from the 15% solution and sterile water. The final volume of the solution will be 4 fl. oz. What are the volumes of each solution?

4. You will need 0.5 L of a 2.5% solution for a prescription. In stock there is a 1:5 solution and a 1:100 solution. How many milliliters of each solution will be required for this compound?

5. A doctor prescribes 30 g of a 20% ointment. In stock, there are a 15% ointment and a 30% ointment. How many grams of each available ointment will be required to prepare the ointment prescribed?

PTCB EXAM PRACTICE QUESTIONS

1. What volumes of a 50% dextrose solution and of water are needed to prepare 3 L of a 30% solution?
    a. 1,800 mL dextrose and 1,200 mL water
    b. 30 mL dextrose and 20 mL water
    c. 1,200 mL dextrose and 1,800 mL water
    d. 20 mL dextrose and 30 mL water

2. What volumes of a 15% solution of sodium chloride and of water should be used to prepare 1 L of a 0.9% solution of sodium chloride?
    a. 60 mL 15% and 940 mL water
    b. 940 mL 15% and 60 mL water
    c. 500 mL 15% and 500 mL water
    d. 200 mL 15% and 800 mL water

3. How many grams of 10% boric acid ointment should be mixed with petrolatum (0%) to prepare 700 g of a 5% boric acid ointment?
    a. 300 g petrolatum and 400 g 10%
    b. 200 g petrolatum and 500 g 10%
    c. 300 g 10% and 400 g petrolatum
    d. 350 g 10% and 400 g petrolatum

4. You are asked to prepare 2.5 L of a 1:20 solution from a 30% solution and water. What volumes of the 30% solution and of water are needed?
    a. 500 mL water and 2,000 mL 30% solution
    b. 417 mL 30% solution and 2,083 mL water
    c. 417 mL water and 2,083 mL 30% solution
    d. 2,000 mL water and 500 mL 30% solution

5. What volumes of a 50% dextrose solution and of a 10% dextrose solution are needed to prepare 4 L of a 20% solution?
   a. 3,000 mL 50% solution and 1,000 mL 10% solution
   b. 3,000 mL 10% solution and 1,000 mL 50% solution
   c. 3.0 mL 50% solution and 0.1 mL 10% solution
   d. 3.0 mL 10% solution and 0.1 mL 50% solution

ACTIVITY 20-1: Case Study—Cream

Instructions: Read the following scenario and then answer the critical thinking questions.

Jerry Rands is hypersensitive to numerous substances and frequently develops a small rash somewhere on his body. He is not even sure of all the things he is sensitive to! All he knows is that over the course of his lifetime, he has had a skin rash at least once a month somewhere on his body. He has been to the pharmacy to purchase anti-itch cream in many different brands and strengths. Jerry's doctor usually advises him to purchase the OTC or prescription-strength product known as hydrocortisone cream.

The time has come again when Jerry develops a small rash and asks the doctor which strength he will need to treat this one. Just like anybody else, Jerry has a small collection of these creams in his medicine cabinet that are still in date and available for use. The problem, however, lies in getting the correct strength when he has only certain amounts of certain strengths. It seems that he does not have enough of the strength the doctor ordered this time, so he wonders if he can mix them.

1. Jerry is to use hydrocortisone 1% cream. All he has available is 2.5% and 0.25%. How many grams of 2.5% hydrocortisone cream should be mixed with 240 g of 0.25% hydrocortisone cream to make 1% hydrocortisone cream?

   _____

   _____

   _____

   _____

2. The doctor tells Jerry to divide the total amount of cream calculated in question 1 into six even doses for application. How many grams are in each dose?

   _____

   _____

   _____

3. What is the total amount of 1% hydrocortisone cream Jerry mixed?

   _____

   _____

   _____

   _____

4. Jerry decides to divide the total amount of 1% hydrocortisone cream he has mixed into 2 oz jars. How many jars does he need?

_____

_____

_____

ACTIVITY 20-2: Case Study—Gelcaps

Instructions: Read the following scenario and then answer the critical thinking questions.

Maryann works in a mid-sized veterinarian compounding pharmacy. Each day brings something new and creative. She may receive an order for suppositories for medium-size rodents or syringes filled with antibiotics for baby birds. Maryann's job requires her to have solid math skills and excellent aseptic technique.

Compounding is used to formulate prescriptions when no commercial strength is available—and animal pharmaceuticals are a very narrow field. Compounding medications for animals fill a void in a world where little is known about what works on a grand scale for a general species. More and more information appears every week for new formulations and animal behavior. With these updates occurring constantly, Maryann must stay on top of her education and training to remain an asset to her chosen field.

A major part of Maryann's compounding is the creation of various gelcaps for various medications. It is a very convenient form for most animals, and flavoring is easily added to this drug form under most conditions.

1. The following formula is to make a total of 50 gelcaps. How much of each ingredient is needed to make only 10 gelcaps?

FORMULA

caffeine	0.6 g
aspirin	2 g
inert ingredient	0.25 g

_____

_____

_____

_____

2. How much is needed to make 15 capsules?

_____

_____

_____

3. What is the total number of grams of all 3 ingredients for 20 capsules?

_____

_____

_____

_____

ACTIVITY 20-3: Case Study—Bulk

Instructions: Read the following scenario and then answer the critical thinking questions.

Note: False names are used for the homeopathic substances in this case study.

A good part of the day at the homeopathic compounding pharmacy, where Lynette the lead pharmacy technician works, is spent mixing large batches of specialty gels for patients who require these compounds to effectively treat each of their specific conditions. A variety of herbs for compounding the gels is available to Lynette. Lynette has to wear all of the appropriate personal protective equipment, such as gloves, gowns, and masks due to the fact that the strength of some of these compounds can cause allergic/hypersensitive skin reactions.

Part of Lynette's duties includes the purchasing of the larger size containers, lids, and packaging tools. It is very common for Lynette to make a 2,000 g jar full of homeopathic gel for a patient's muscle aches and pains. All of the final compounds in this facility are composed of four different strengths.

1. Lynette is making histkatel crucious gel for a patient's muscle fatigue. The order is for a 10% final concentration. How many grams of 15% histkatel crucious gel should be mixed with 1,800 g of 6% histkatel crucious gel to make the 10% gel?

   _____
   _____
   _____
   _____

2. Convert the final volume of this compound to pounds.

   _____
   _____
   _____
   _____

3. Lynette is to repackage the bulk gel into 6 oz sealed jars. How many jars will she need?

   _____
   _____
   _____
   _____

LAB 20-1: Working with Alligations

Objective:

Use the alligation method to understand the relationship of measuring liquids while visualizing the different concentrations and volumes for each compound.

Pre-Lab Information:

- Review Chapter 20, "Alligations," in the textbook.
- Gather the following materials:
  - 20 mL, 50 mL, and 100 mL graduated cylinders
  - bottle of blue-colored water
  - bottle of cherry syrup
  - syrup/suspension medication bottles in 4 oz, 6 oz, and 8 oz sizes

Explanation:

While working in the community pharmacy setting, the technician may have to use the alligation method. When a prescription order is required to be compounded, the two products will have different percent strengths of the same active ingredient. This exercise will provide you the opportunity to experience working with liquids of differing concentrations while using the tic-tac-toe method.

Activity:

Use the materials in the preceding list to prepare the following prescription orders. The alligation table below is a guide to use in your processes.

Note: The percentage for each solution is fictitious; obviously, you will be using 100% blue-colored water and 100% cherry syrup. If cherry syrup is not available, then red-colored water may be substituted for the cherry syrup.

Sample Alligation Table

% High:		Parts High:
	% Desired:	
% Low:		Parts Low: Total Parts:

You may round your answers to the nearest whole number.

1. You are asked to prepare 150 mL of a 50% syrup solution. You have in stock, 90% cherry syrup and blue-colored water (0%). Using the alligation method, calculate the volume of each solution and then prepare the solution.

   a. 90% cherry syrup = _____ mL
   b. blue-colored water = _____ mL

2. You are asked to prepare 240 mL of a 30% syrup solution. You have in stock, 60% cherry syrup and 50% blue-colored water solution. Using the alligation method, calculate the volume of each solution and then prepare the solution.

   a. 50% blue-colored water = _____ mL
   b. 70% cherry syrup = _____ mL

3. You are asked to prepare 120 mL of a 1:8 solution. You have in stock a 40% blue-colored water solution and a 1:100 cherry syrup solution.

Note: You must convert the ratio to percentage to use the alligation table. Calculate the volume of each solution and then prepare the solution.

   a. 40% blue-colored water = _____ mL
   b. 1:100 cherry syrup = _____ mL

Student Name: _____

Lab Partner: _____

Grade/Comments: _____

_____

_____

Student Comments: _____

_____

_____

CHAPTER 21
Parenteral Calculations

After completing Chapter 21 from the textbook, you should be able to:	Related Activity in the Workbook/Lab Manual
1. Illustrate the principle of basic dimensional analysis.	Review Questions, Pharmacy Calculation Problems, PTCB Exam Practice Questions, Activity 21-1, Activity 21-3, Activity 21-4, Lab 21-1
2. Calculate flow duration for parenteral products.	Review Questions, Pharmacy Calculation Problems, PTCB Exam Practice Questions, Activity 21-1, Lab 21-1, Lab 21-2
3. Calculate the volume per hour for parenteral orders.	Review Questions, Pharmacy Calculation Problems, PTCB Exam Practice Questions, Activity 21-2, Activity 21-3, Activity 21-4, Lab 21-1, Lab 21-2
4. Calculate the drug per hour for parenteral products.	Review Questions, Pharmacy Calculation Problems, PTCB Exam Practice Questions, Activity 21-2, Activity 21-3, Activity 21-4, Lab 21-1, Lab 21-2
5. Calculate drip rates in both drops per minute and milliliters per hour.	Review Questions, Pharmacy Calculation Problems, PTCB Exam Practice Questions, Activity 21-2, Activity 21-3, Activity 21-4, Lab 21-1, Lab 21-2
6. Calculate TPN milliequivalents.	Review Questions, Pharmacy Calculation Problems, PTCB Exam Practice Questions, Lab 21-1, Lab 21-2

INTRODUCTION

The preparation and administration of parenteral products, such as IVs, infusions, TPN, and chemotherapy, require the performance of specific calculations. It is common for individuals to become overwhelmed and confused when approaching complex pharmacy calculations. The truth is, however, that although many pharmacy calculations appear to be complex, they are in actuality very simple. Often described as the most difficult and challenging calculations used in pharmacy, parenteral calculations, drip rates, and TPN milliequivalents are all solved with basic fundamental math and arithmetic skills. The use of proportions, cross-multiplication, and dimensional analysis will aid you in performing virtually all parenteral calculations that you will need to solve as a pharmacy technician.

REVIEW QUESTIONS

Match the following.

1. drop factor
2. drops per minute
3. milligrams per hour
4. flow rates
5. flow rate duration
6. hypertonic solutions
7. isotonic solutions
8. hypotonic solutions
9. IV infusion
10. micro drip
11. total parenteral nutrition
12. milliliters per hour

a. solutions that have osmotic pressure equal to that of cell contents

b. length of time for which an IV will be administered, or how long an IV bag will last before it must be changed

c. amount of fluid, or solution, that will be administered to the patient intravenously per hour

d. term used to describe a number of common pharmacy calculations used in the preparation of IV infusions

e. dosage, or amount of medication in milligrams, that will be administered per hour of infusion

f. solution made to supply many of the body's basic nutritional needs via parenteral administration

g. compounded solution that provides fluids, specific medications, nutrients, electrolytes, and minerals to a patient

h. the volume of medication to be administered each minute

i. solutions that have greater osmotic pressure than cell contents

j. solutions that have a lower osmotic pressure than cell contents

k. an abbreviated form referring to a specific drip rate

l. most commonly used drip rate, 60 gtts/mL

Solve the following problems.

13. A physician orders a 2 L IV bag to be administered at a rate of 250 mL/hr. How long will this IV bag last? _____

14. A physician orders a 3 L IV to be administered at a rate of 500 mL/hr. How long will the IV last? _____

15. A patient is set to start a 250 mL infusion of amoxicillin in lactated Ringers 5% at noon. The bag is to be administered at a rate of 100 mL/hr. At what time will the infusion be complete? _____

16. A physician orders three 500 mL IV bags that are to be infused at a rate of 150 mL/hr. How long will these three bags last? _____

17. A physician orders three 2 L IV bags containing ciprofloxacin and NS that are set to be administered at a rate of 250 mL/hr at 1:00 p.m. When will all three bags be completely administered? _____

18. A patient is to receive a 1,500 mL IV infused over five hours. What is the rate of infusion in milliliters per hour? _____

19. A physician orders 500 mL IV, containing 2 mg of Toradol, which is to be infused to the patient over 120 minutes. What is the rate of infusion in milliliters per hour? _____

20. A physician orders 500 mL of D5W containing 1 g of lidocaine hydrochloride that is to be infused to the patient over 250 minutes. What is the infusion rate in milliliters per hour? _____

PHARMACY CALCULATION QUESTIONS

Calculate the following.

1. How many hours will a 3 L bag of TPN last if it is scheduled to run for 100 mL/hr?

2. A bag of heparin IV with a concentration of 25,000 units/250 mL is ordered for a patient. How many units per hour will the patient receive if the solution is infusing at 50 mL/hr?

3. What will the flow rate be in milliliters per hour for vancomycin 1g/500 mL IV, if it is to be infused for 90 minutes?

4. What will the flow rate be in drops per minute for 150 mL of an antifungal medication that is to be administered over 60 minutes? The tubing is calibrated at 30 gtts/mL.

5. If a 1 L bag of D5NS with 20 mEq KCl is hung at 0700, when will the new bag be due if it is running at 125 mL/hr?

PTCB EXAM PRACTICE QUESTIONS

1. If an order for a 1 L bag of D5W is to be infused into a patient's arm for eight hours, what is the rate of infusion in milliliters per hour?
   a. 100 mL/hr
   b. 10 mL/hr
   c. 12.5 mL/hr
   d. 125 mL/hr

2. If an order for a 1,000 mL bag of normal saline is to run at 100 mL/hr, how long will the bag last?
   a. 8 hours
   b. 10 hours
   c. 12 hours
   d. 6 hours

3. If the infusion rate for an IV is 60 mL/hr and it is running for 4 ½ hours, how many milliliters will the patient receive?
   a. 13 mL
   b. 270 mL
   c. 240 mL
   d. 380 mL

4. How many drops per minute will a patient receive if the order for an IV infusion of 1,000 mL of 5% dextrose injection is run for six hours? The drip factor is 15 gtts/mL.
   a. 7 gtts/min
   b. 167 gtts/min
   c. 90 gtts/min
   d. 67 gtts/min

5. You receive an order for heparin IV to be infused at 1,000 units/hr. What will be the flow rate be in milliliters per hour for a 500 mL bag of D5W with 25,000 units of heparin?
   a. 5 mL/hr
   b. 10 mL/hr
   c. 8 mL/hr
   d. 1 mL/hr

ACTIVITY 21-1: Case Study—Iron Dextran

Instructions: Read the following scenario and then answer the critical thinking questions.

After arguing with his then-girlfriend of whom his family did not approve, Philip drove away from the house in an angry state. He is certain now that he was not in the right frame of mind to be driving that night. The car spun out of control on a fairly isolated road and hit a tree. Eventually, Philip made it out alive, but he spent 12 weeks in the hospital recuperating. He did not call his family as he probably should have, because the last time he spoke to them, things ended on bad terms. It has now been eight months since the accident, and Philip has not seen his family during that time. He is reuniting with them now to discuss the accident, because he had decided that it would help him heal emotionally.

Philip was lucky to have made it back to health. He suffered a concussion, a fractured arm, and multiple bruises. The doctors told him he lost a lot of blood, but he is not exactly sure from what part of his body or how much. Philip received excellent care at the major medical center where he recalls being on numerous medications. Now all his family members are sharing stories of various hospital stays, and the discussion turns to the medications they recall getting, especially the IVs that hung on the poles while they were inpatients. Philip recalls one, called iron dextran, being "really black."

1. The first dose of iron dextran that Philip received was a test dose of 25 mg in 100 mL NS infused over 20 minutes. What was the concentration of this piggyback?

   _____

   _____

   _____

   _____

2. What was the infusion rate per minute for this test dose of iron dextran?

   _____

   _____

   _____

   _____

3. Philip's total daily dose of iron dextran became 1 g, mixed in a 1 L bag of NS, and infused over eight hours. What was the rate per hour?

   _____

   _____

   _____

   _____

4. Using the same information as in question 3, how much iron dextran did Philip receive per hour?

_____

_____

_____

_____

ACTIVITY 21-2: The Delicate Art of TPN Compounding

TPN stands for total parenteral nutrition. It may also be referred to as parenteral nutrition or hyperalimentation. Regardless of what it is called in different parts of the country, a TPN is an intravenous infusion containing dextrose (carbohydrates), amino acids (protein), water, and sometimes lipids (fats). TPN provides nutrients to patients with medical conditions that prevent them from physically eating, absorbing nutrients via their gastrointestinal systems, or absorbing enough calories through normal eating. Special TPNs are also used for premature infants who have undeveloped digestive systems. Other additives can be mixed into a TPN, such as famotidine, insulin, multivitamins, and a variety of electrolytes.

TPNs can be very complex and require adherence to certain protocols and standards throughout the entire process, from when a physician writes an order to when a pharmacist or a technician compounds the product. Manually compounding a TPN the first few times can be frustrating however, as more practice and time that the technician takes part in with the process of manually compounding TPNs, the TPNs become less frustrating to compound.

Compounding a TPN

The proper procedures when preparing to compound a TPN must be in place and strongly adhered to. When the pharmacy receives a TPN order, the pharmacist needs to calculate the correct percentages of dextrose, amino acids, water, and on occasion lipids. The lipids are often given separately, mostly because of an increased risk of precipitation and other issues that may occur when the additives in a TPN are not compatible. The pharmacist will also calculate the amount of additional electrolytes to be added in the TPN in order to make sure that the patient is receiving the proper balance of an electrolyte. Examples of common electrolytes are potassium chloride, potassium phosphate, calcium gluconate, sodium acetate, and magnesium phosphate. Certain medications, such as insulin or ranitidine, can also be added to the TPN. Multiple vitamins and vitamins such as folic acid or thiamine as well as trace elements such as manganese or zinc may be added to the admixture as well.

Automated TPN Compounding

If a hospital or home infusion pharmacy compounds a high volume of TPNs every day, the pharmacy team may take advantage of automated compounding equipment to assist with their workflow. A pharmacist inputs the TPN's data into the compounder's computer, while a technician sets up the compounder with special tubing that connects all of the solutions to the compounder. The compounder is always operated in a horizontal laminar airflow hood while involving the principles of aseptic technique as it pertains to USP <797>. One type of compounding machine measures all of the main components (dextrose, water, and the amino acids), while another type measures out the electrolytes, vitamins, and other additives. The technician attaches a special tube from the bag to the compounder and then hangs the bag on a scale. Through the series of tubes and pumps, this sophisticated technology slowly fills the bag with the correct amount of each additive based on the specific gravity of each component. After it is finished, the TPN can be removed and labeled appropriately.

TPN compounders have many advantages. Only minimal handling of the fluids and additives is needed (except to change out empty bottles) for aseptic technique to be maintained. The compounders are very fast to where a customized TPN can be compounded in a few minutes. Most TPN compounder software has safety features in order to alert the pharmacist if there is too much of an additive and/or will alert the technician when a stock bottle needs to be changed.

However, there are a few disadvantages of TPN compounders. Automated compounding equipment is expensive. The compounder(s) also take up a lot of space, and a specific laminar airflow hood or hoods may be dedicated just to TPN compounding. The compounders are very sensitive as each fluid is measured by specific gravity; thus, you must be careful not to bump the bag that is being filled. If the scale accidentally gets bumped during the filling cycle, the compounder will usually stop in mid-fill. If this happens, the rest of the fill will have to be reprogrammed by a pharmacist, or you may have to start the entire process again from the beginning step.

Some pharmacies use a combination of automated and manual systems. The bulk fluids, such as dextrose and amino acids, may be run on a compounder, but all of the electrolytes may be drawn up separately by a pharmacist or a technician. The distinctions and tasks of automated and manual systems will depend upon the volume of TPNs that the pharmacy routinely compounds each day.

Manual Compounding of TPNs

In a smaller pharmacy where TPN compounding is too low to warrant expensive automated equipment, other options may be chosen. The pharmacy may incorporate "ready-to-use" TPN solutions that are premade by the manufacturer. These TPNs come with varying amounts of amino acids, dextrose, water, and sometimes electrolytes. With this type of system in place, it is sometimes challenging to compound customized TPNs. If the pharmacy does not use premixed TPNs, dextrose and amino acids can also be purchased separately in different concentrations and of different-sized bags. Depending on the order, various amounts of solutions can be manually transferred into one larger bag to compound the TPN. In either case, additives such as electrolytes and vitamins must be drawn up by either a pharmacist or a pharmacy technician manually via syringes to infuse into the TPN for a final admixture. This method can be time-consuming, especially when you are trying to do a custom TPN manually with up to 12 additives in different syringes.

A key point to remember when you are compounding TPNs manually is that the technician needs to take special care. The more manipulations that are done for a TPN, it may be more challenging to maintain aseptic technique principles as well as the standards set forth by USP <797>. As more products are added, the more likely it is that some of them will develop incompatibilities with other medications. A recommendation for you to prevent precipitation in the bag would be to gently shake the TPN bag in between additives to encourage a more uniform solution. However, if there are any protein additives, such as insulin in the TPN, the bag should not be shaken. Two types of additives should always be added as far apart from one another as possible will be; any electrolyte with a phosphate base can easily form precipitates when it comes in direct contact with a calcium additive. One good method is to add all of the phosphates first (such as potassium phosphate or sodium phosphate), then add the other noncalcium additives (such as multivitamins, insulin, or trace elements), and then add the calcium last (like calcium gluconate). Even when using this order of operations, it is a good idea to shake the bag gently in between additives.

Asepsis

Most patients who are prescribed a TPN are very sick and their immune systems may be functioning poorly; therefore, aseptic technique and the standards set forth by USP <797> must be in full practice. As there are many additives and fluid transfers with TPN compounding, it is vital that you do your best to keep the workflow area and the prescribed TPN compound free from all contaminates. If after compounding a TPN, you notice small white flakes in the TPN bag, which would resemble snow, a cloudy haze, or anything else unusual, notify a pharmacist and/or a pharmacy technician immediately. Precipitates may occasionally form even when the greatest of care has been taken. A TPN admixture should not be dispensed if any of these conditions are present. When lipids are added to the TPN, the likelihood of these problems will increase. As a technician, it is imperative to be attentive and also to learn what to look for. However, being proactive with your approach to TPN compounding is the best method for creating a stable TPN. If you are using proper aseptic technique and following USP <797> standards, shaking the TPN bag gently between additives, and separating a phosphate additive from a calcium additive, you will succeed in this delicate art of compounding a TPN.

Activity:

Now that you have learned more about TPN, answer the following questions.

1. List two advantages and two disadvantages of using automated compounding equipment to prepare TPNs?

_____

_____

_____

_____

2. List two advantages and two disadvantages of manually compounding TPNs?

_____

_____

_____

_____

3. Is it more or less challenging to compound a TPN manually? If so, why?

_____

_____

_____

_____

4. Which two electrolytes should be added apart from each other to avoid possible precipitation in a TPN?

_____

_____

_____

_____

5. Search the Internet to find news stories about automated compounding equipment for preparing TPNs and describe what information you find. Based on your research, discuss the importance of the role the pharmacy technician plays in preparing TPNs.

_____

_____

_____

_____

6. Research the electrolytes commonly used in a TPN. List each one and its average dose.

_____

_____

_____

_____

7. When should the TPN bag not be shaken?

_____

ACTIVITY 21-3: Case Study—IV Lipids

Instructions: Read the following scenario and then answer the critical thinking questions.

Melanie is an experienced pharmacy technician who has worked in a variety of hospital pharmacy settings. Her favorite setting and one in which she is quite proficient with is the IV sterile preparation setting. Over her 24-year career in pharmacy, she has worked in three different hospitals compounding sterile IV preparations. She notices that although each facility follows good aseptic technique guidelines, each facility may have different ways to go about their final outcomes.

For Melanie, this has been a real benefit to her, as she gets to see a variety of ways to perform her craft and can choose the best of each system. For example, the last hospital she worked at made its main TPNs with the lipids added—a mix that is commonly known as the "three-in-one" bag. This made the final product very heavy and milky white. Where she works now, the lipids are piggybacked during a TPN infusion. The average patient receives 250–500 mL of 10% or 20% lipids solution one to three times a week.

1. What are lipids?
   _____
   _____
   _____
   _____

2. To run a 20% 500 mL bottle of lipids over 12 hours would require what drip rate?
   _____
   _____
   _____
   _____

3. Refer to the lipid scenario in question 2. After three hours, another piggyback IV is run into the patient and the lipids are slowed down to a 14-hour rate. How much longer would the lipids run with what is left?
   _____
   _____
   _____
   _____

4. Is it necessary to "burp" a TPN bag with lipids? If so, why?
   _____
   _____
   _____
   _____

ACTIVITY 21-4: Case Study—IV Solution (TPN)

Instructions: Read the following scenario and then answer the critical thinking questions.

Madeleine is a TPN pharmacy technician at the 600-bed University Hospital. Working in such a large facility, she could easily prepare a total of up to 30 TPNs in any given day. The hospital deals with a lot of specialty cases; they see patients with all kinds of reasons for being on TPN. For example, some patients are in comas, others have swollen throats, and many others are in situations Madeleine might not get to see if she worked in a smaller pharmacy. Madeleine has learned a lot during her four years at this facility. The pharmacists and other pharmacy technicians are eager to share their knowledge whenever they discover a new technique or new medication.

TPNs are a specialty because they provide nutrition for patients who cannot receive it otherwise. This hospital is lucky enough to have a designated area in the pharmacy that is sufficiently sized for preparing TPNs. Ample storage in this area keeps all of the necessary ingredients close at hand, which helps cut down on the time it takes to prepare so many TPNs.

1. Once made and taken to the nursing area to await infusion, how is the TPN stored?
   _____
   _____
   _____
   _____

2. Is a filter needle required for infusion of a TPN, or just during preparation? What size needle would be used?
   _____
   _____
   _____
   _____

3. How long is a TPN good for at room temperature?
   _____
   _____
   _____
   _____

4. What are the key components of a TPN?
   _____
   _____
   _____
   _____

5. Madeleine carefully examines each TPN when she is finished. What is she looking for?
   _____
   _____
   _____
   _____

6. What are electrolytes and why are they important?
   _____
   _____
   _____
   _____

LAB 21-1: Calculating a TPN

Objective:

Calculate the milliliters of electrolytes and additives needed to prepare a TPN.

Pre-Lab Information:

- Review Chapter 21, "Parenteral Calculations," in your textbook.
- Review the information on TPNs contained in Activity 21-2, "The Delicate Art of TPN Compounding."
- Visit legitimate websites that will give you reliable information about TPN compounding, such as www .uspharmacist.com and www.ashp.org.

Explanation:

Depending on the career path you choose to take as a pharmacy technician, you may need to perform the calculations required to make a TPN. There is absolutely no room for error in TPN compounding, so all calculations are checked by at least one pharmacist; some hospitals require two different pharmacists to check calculations before a TPN is compounded.

Activity:

Part One

In the following exercise, you will be given several electrolytes and additives that must be added manually to a TPN. Calculate the milliliters needed to be drawn up in syringes for each additive and an appropriate order in which to insert the additives (to avoid precipitation) into the TPN bag. Round to the nearest tenth if necessary.

Additive	Concentration in Stock	Amount Needed for Order	Milliliters Needed
MVI (multiple vitamins, IV)	Not applicable	10 mL	
calcium gluconate	4.65 mEq/mL	45 mEq	
potassium phosphate	45 mmol/15 mL	30 mmol	
insulin R	100 units/mL	10 units	
magnesium sulfate	0.5 g/mL	5 g	
famotidine	10 mg/mL	20 mg	

Part Two

Visit an infusion pharmacy to witness firsthand how TPN compounding is done. This process is complex, but a demonstration may clear up some confusion.

Student Name: _____

Lab Partner: _____

Grade/Comments: _____

_____

Student Comments: _____

_____

_____

LAB 21-2: Working with IV Solutions

Objective:

To become familiar with reading labels on IM/IV vials of medications and logging the requirements for reconstitution as well as storage requirements

Pre-Lab Information:

- Review Chapter 21, "Parenteral Calculations," in your textbook.
- Gather four different vials of powdered and liquid IM/IV medications.

Explanation:

Manufacturers print the information for intramuscular/intravenous vials of medications in very small print. The technician is responsible for carefully reading and logging the concentration, the diluent amount required for reconstitution (if needed) and the storage requirements.

Activity:

Using the four different vials of IM/IV medications, log the concentration, the diluent amount required for reconstitution, if it is a powder, and the storage requirements.

1. _____
2. _____
3. _____
4. _____

When you are finished, prepare your sterile compounding area to draw up the medications in appropriate syringes. Using the powdered vials of IM/IV medications, reconstitute them per the manufacturer's recommendations. Using the liquid vials of IM/IV medications, draw up the amounts in which your instructor has decided upon as a mock emergency order from the "ER" department.

Have all of your syringes checked by your instructor.

1. _____
2. _____
3. _____
4. _____

Student Name: _____

Lab Partner: _____

Grade/Comments: _____

_____

_____

Student Comments: _____

_____

_____

CHAPTER 22
Business Math

After completing Chapter 22 from the textbook, you should be able to:	Related Activity in the Workbook/Lab Manual
1. Define and understand how to calculate cost, selling price, and markup.	Review Questions, Pharmacy Calculation Problems, PTCB Exam Practice Questions, Activity 22-1, Activity 22-2, Activity 22-3, Activity 22-4, Lab 22-1, Lab 22-2
2. Explain co-payments and average wholesale price (AWP).	Review Questions, Pharmacy Calculation Problems, PTCB Exam Practice Questions, Activity 22-1, Activity 22-2, Activity 22-3, Activity 22-4, Lab 22-1, Lab 22-2
3. Define and understand how to determine markup and markup percent.	Review Questions, Pharmacy Calculation Problems, PTCB Exam Practice Questions, Activity 22-1, Activity 22-2, Activity 22-3, Activity 22-4, Lab 22-1, Lab 22-2
4. Define and understand how to calculate gross profit and net profit.	Review Questions, Pharmacy Calculation Problems, PTCB Exam Practice Questions, Activity 22-1, Activity 22-2, Activity 22-3, Activity 22-4, Lab 22-1, Lab 22-2

INTRODUCTION

The goal of any business is to make a profit; pharmacy is no different. It is necessary to maintain enough profit in the business model to be able to take care of obligations such as rent and inventory expense and have a positive net income at the end of the fiscal year. Profits help pay salaries of employees, so it is important to keep a certain profit margin above supply costs so that the business can afford to keep and pay its employees.

REVIEW QUESTIONS

Fill in the blanks.

1. For every product sold in a pharmacy, it has three essential numbers—they're _____, _____, and _____.

2. Every product in a pharmacy, whether it is a bottle of prescription antibiotics or an over-the-counter (OTC) product, was purchased from a _____ or _____ for a _____ _____.

3. Whereas cost refers to the amount of money the pharmacy paid for a product, the selling price is the _____ the pharmacy receives for the sale of the product.

4. For prescription products, the _____ includes the amount to be paid by the third-party insurer and the patient's co-payment.

5. Calculating the amount an insurance company will contribute to the selling price of a product can be done so long as you are provided with the _____ and the _____.

PHARMACY CALCULATION PROBLEMS

Calculate the following.

1. What is the price that a bottle of vitamins be sold for if the acquisition cost is $7.99 and there is a $2.50 markup?

2. If a vial of insulin sells for $12.50 and a $2.10 markup is included, what is the invoice cost of the insulin?

3. If an erectile dysfunction device that costs $80.00 is marked up to $130.00, what is the markup percent?

4. If a prescription costs the pharmacy $17.95 and sells for $45.50, what is the amount of gross profit?

5. A bottle of OTC cough syrup sells for $10.95. The pharmacy paid $4.60 for the product and has $3.00 in associated overhead. What is the net profit?

PTCB EXAM PRACTICE QUESTIONS

1. All costs associated with a business is known as:
   a. overstock
   b. rent
   c. cost of goods sold
   d. overhead

2. What is the term that refers to the money left over after you pay invoice cost (cost of goods sold) and overhead?
   a. net income
   b. revenue
   c. net profit
   d. taxes

3. A 100 count bottle of atenolol 50 mg costs $29.99. The patient is prescribed 30 atenolol 1 tab qd and wants to pay cash for the medication. What is the amount the patient will pay?
   a. $9.01
   b. $8.99
   c. $2,999
   d. $899

4. Which of the following is an example of overhead?
   a. payroll
   b. inventory
   c. cost of goods
   d. markup

5. If an item that costs $80.00 is marked up to $120.00, what is the markup percent?
   a. 1.5%
   b. 5%
   c. 50%
   d. 12%

ACTIVITY 22-1: Case Study – Cost Concerns

Instructions: Read the following scenario and then answer the critical thinking questions.

A well-known patient comes into the pharmacy with a prescription for a medication. The medication is rather new on the market and has been advertised heavily in the media. The AWP from the manufacturer for this medication is approximately $500.00 for a 100 tablet count bottle. The dispensing fee for each prescription is $5.00. The patient has been prescribed a quantity of 60 tablets and the patient has an insurance plan with an open formulary. The prescribing physician has prescribed a few medications to the patient that is on the open formulary and the patient's co-pay is $25.00 for brand-name medications and $10.00 for generic medications. You process the prescription and adjudicate the claim as usual; however, the reject notice comes back as "NDC not covered."

While speaking to the pharmacist about this rejection notice, you both realize that there is no other medication on the market that is therapeutically equivalent to the one that this patient needs. As you speak with the patient about this situation, the patient tells you that "I guess I will have to pay cash." However, the patient is low on funds and would like to pay for a quarter of the quantity prescribed.

1. How much will the patient have to pay for the quarter of the prescribed quantity?

   _____

   _____

2. The patient has changed his mind and would like to pay for half of the prescribed quantity?

   _____

   _____

3. Is there an option or options that you could look into so that the patient does not have to pay cash for the medication? If so, what are they?

_____

_____

ACTIVITY 22-2: Case Study—Markups

Instructions: Read the following scenario and then answer the critical thinking questions.

The newest shipment of OTC products has arrived from your distribution center. The newest nonsedating antihistamine has just been approved by the FDA and is now available for consumers without a prescription in quantities of 7, 15, and 30 tablets. You have noticed that the pricing fees for each of the tablet counts are:

7 count—$10.99
15 count—$20.99
30 count—$41.98

The markup for these new products is $4.00

1. How much will each of the items be with the markup?

   _____

   _____

   _____

2. What is the percent markup for the products

   _____

   _____

   _____

3. What will be the gross profit for the products?

   _____

   _____

   _____

ACTIVITY 22-3: Case Study—The Bottom Line

Instructions: Review the income statement below and calculate the net profit to secure the bottom line.

Income	100%
Cost of goods sold	67%
Overhead and expenses	25%
Net profit	

ACTIVITY 22-4: Case Study—Reimbursement Rates

Instructions: Review the following examples and calculate the reimbursements for each example.

1. The AWP for a medication in a 100 tablet count bottle is $90.00—13% with a processing fee of $3.00.

   _____

   _____

2. The AWP for a medication in a 1,000 tablet count bottle is $110.99—15% with a processing fee of $2.50. The patient has been prescribed a quantity of 120 tablets.

   _____

   _____

3. The AWP for 480 mL of a cough syrup is $75.99 less 10% with a processing fee of $3.50. The patient has been prescribed a volume of 120 mL.

   _____

   _____

LAB 22-1: Product Pricing

Objective:
To understand that every inventory product must be priced accurately with operational calculations.

Pre-Lab Information:
Review Chapter 22, "Business Math," in the textbook.

Explanation:
The pharmacy technician is relied upon to accurately price all of the products in a pharmacy based upon a determined pricing from the manufacturer and the owners of the pharmacy.

Activity:
Calculate the cost of a blood glucose meter.

1. A blood glucose meter is sold for $99.99. The net profit on the strips is $25.00. The store's overhead per blood glucose meter is $6.00. What is the invoice cost for the meter?

   _____

Calculate the selling price of a bottle of vitamins.

2. The invoice cost for a bottle of vitamins is $6.74. The net profit on the vitamins is $1.35. The store's overhead per bottle is $0.18. What is the selling price for a bottle of vitamins?

   _____

Calculate the selling price of a pill container.

3. A pill container costs the pharmacy $0.86 to purchase. If the pharmacy marks up the pill container 25%, what is the selling price?

   _____

Student Name: _____

Lab Partner: _____

Grade/Comments: _____

_____

_____

Student Comments: _____

_____

_____

LAB 22-2: Profitability

Objective:

To understand that each item in a pharmacy is intended to make a profit and bring an income to keep the business running smoothly.

Pre-Lab Information:

Review Chapter 22, "Business Math," in the textbook.

Explanation:

The pharmacy technician is expected to understand that each item in the pharmacy is intended to bring in a profit for salaries to remain active and stable for the team as a part of the overhead.

Activity:

Calculate and determine the gross and net profits with each of the examples below.

1. Determine the cost for a product with a selling price of $45.55, overhead of $5.50, and net profit of $9.00. _____

2. Determine the gross profit for a product with a selling price of $98.99, cost of $47.00, and overhead of $8.50. _____

3. Determine the selling price for a product with a cost of $10.59, overhead of $3.69, and net profit of $3.50. _____

Student Name: _____

Lab Partner: _____

Grade/Comments: _____

_____

_____

Student Comments: _____

_____

_____

CHAPTER 23
The Body and Drugs

After completing Chapter 23 from the textbook, you should be able to:	Related Activity in the Workbook/Lab Manual
1. Explain the differences between pharmacodynamics and pharmacokinetics.	Review Questions, PTCB Exam Practice Questions, Activity 23-1, Activity 23-2
2. Understand the ways in which cell receptors react to drugs.	Review Questions, Lab 23-1, Lab 23-2
3. Describe mechanism of action and identify and understand its key factor.	Review Questions, Activity 23-3, Lab 23-2
4. Explain how drugs are absorbed, distributed, metabolized, and cleared by the body.	Review Questions, PTCB Exam Practice Questions, Activity 23-1, Activity 23-2, Activity 23-3, Lab 23-1, Lab 23-2
5. Explain the difference between fat-soluble and water-soluble drugs and give examples of each.	Review Questions, Lab 23-3
6. Identify and explain the effect of bioavailability and its relationship to drug effectiveness.	Review Questions, Activity 23-3, Activity 23-4, Activity 23-5
7. Understand addiction and addictive behavior.	Review Questions, PTCB Exam Practice Questions, Lab 23-1, Lab 23-3
8. Describe the role of the pharmacy technician in identifying drug-abusing patients.	Review Questions, Lab 23-1, Lab 23-3
9. List and identify some drugs that interact with alcohol.	Review Questions, Lab 23-1

INTRODUCTION

Pharmacology is the study of drugs, including their composition, uses, application, and effects. Although the pharmacist is responsible for using his or her specialized knowledge to provide pharmaceutical care to patients, pharmacy technicians too must understand the basics of pharmacology. *Pharmacodynamics* is the study of how drugs produce their effects on the desired cells, and how the drug is then processed by the body. *Pharmacokinetics* is the study of how the body handles drugs, how drugs are changed from their original form into something that the body can use, and how they are eliminated from the body.

REVIEW QUESTIONS

Match the following.

1. _____ absorption
2. _____ agonist
3. _____ bioavailability
4. _____ clearance
5. _____ dependency
6. _____ excretion
7. _____ metabolism
8. _____ addiction
9. _____ tolerance
10. _____ metabolites
11. _____ half-life
12. _____ distribution
13. _____ antagonist

a. the state of being dependent

b. a drug that does not produce any noticeable effect when it binds to a specific receptor on the cell

c. specific type of drug that produces a certain, predicted action when it binds to the correct receptor

d. the movement of an absorbed drug from the bloodstream into body tissues

e. the process by which drugs are eliminated from the body

f. pattern of compulsive substance abuse characterized by a continued psychological and physiological craving or need for the substance and its effects

g. any substance produced by the metabolic process

h. the time required for plasma serum concentration levels of an absorbed and distributed drug to decrease by one-half

i. process of transforming drugs in the body

j. when a person requires (psychologically or physiologically) larger doses of a drug to achieve the same effect

k. the degree to which a drug becomes available to body tissue(s) after administration

l. how a drug enters the body

m. the time it takes a drug to be eliminated from the body

Choose the best answer.

14. Pharmacodynamics can be described as the study of:
    a. how drugs produce their effects.
    b. what the body does to a drug.
    c. the process of drug interactions.
    d. how drugs are made on the desired cells.

15. How a drug works and produces its effect is called:
    a. effective distribution.
    b. chemical process.
    c. mechanism of action.
    d. potency.

16. Site of action refers to:
    a. the part of the body where a drug is injected.
    b. when the drug produces certain actions.
    c. the location where a drug will exert its effect.
    d. how the drug acts in the body.

17. ED50 refers to the:
    a. amount of a drug that produces half the normal response.
    b. binding medium used in compounding.
    c. effective drug at 50%.
    d. top 50 most effective drugs.

18. Once a drug is at a serum concentration of less than 3%, it is considered:
    a. nontoxic.
    b. out of range.
    c. eliminated.
    d. ineffective.

19. Which is not a form of excretion?
    a. breath
    b. sweat
    c. urine
    d. odor

20. Pinocytosis is a:
    a. form of transportation of drugs into cells.
    b. a medicinally powerful plant.
    c. a rare type of gum disease.
    d. none of the above.

14. The abbreviation for consumable alcohol is:
    a. ACh.
    b. EOH.
    c. ETOH.
    d. ISO.

22. The rate of administration of a drug is determined by the:
    a. prescriber.
    b. research and development process.
    c. chemical nature of the drug.
    d. health of the patient.

23. Addiction has how many criteria:
    a. 4
    b. 8
    c. 7
    d. 9

24. Which of these drugs may produce increased heart rate when mixed with alcohol?
    a. hydrocodone
    b. alprazolam
    c. metformin
    d. warfarin

25. Pharmacokinetics is a term for the study of:
    a. receptors producing a specific effect.
    b. the time course of a drug in the body.
    c. the process of drug interactions.
    d. how drugs are made.

True or False?

26. Salts do not matter if the active ingredient is the same.

    T   F

27. The absorption of a drug governs the bioavailability of that drug.

    T   F

28. Addiction is the same as chemical dependency.

    T   F

29. Pharmacokinetics involves absorption, distribution, metabolism, and elimination of a drug.

    T   F

30. Damaging consequences is not a characteristic of addiction.

    T   F

PHARMACY CALCULATION PROBLEMS

Calculate the following.

1. The physician ordered 500 mg tablets of a medication for a patient. The medication comes in a 250 mg tablet form. The patient was told to take the medication orally twice a day for 15 days. How many tablets are needed to fill this order?

2. A man has brought in a prescription for ranitidine 300 mg. The physician did not indicate Dispense As Written (DAW) on the prescription, but the customer insists on getting the brand-name drug. The insurance company will charge him the price of the co-pay, plus the difference in price between the generic and the brand. This is known as *difference pricing*. Calculate the cost to the customer if the generic price is $11.25 and the brand price is $27.95. His usual co-pay is $10.

   Hint: co-pay + (brand price − generic price) = cost

3. A customer wants to pay difference pricing for a prescription for nabumetone 500 mg. The price of the brand-name drug is $85.49, and the price of the generic drug is $17.99. His or her usual co-pay is $15. What will the insurance company charge the customer using difference pricing?

4. A pharmacy sets its retail prices as a 30% markup of cost. If a 100-count bottle of acetaminophen 325 mg costs the pharmacy $1.49, what will be the retail price for this item?

5. Conversion: 98 °F = _____ °C

PTCB EXAM PRACTICE QUESTIONS

1. Dopamine is a:
   a. hormone.
   b. catecholamine.
   c. neurotransmitter.
   d. all of the above.

2. Which organ is responsible for a drug's metabolism?
   a. kidney
   b. intestines
   c. lungs
   d. liver

3. All of the following drugs may be used to assist patients with smoking cessation *except*:
   a. nicotine patch.   c. Dilantin.
   b. Chantix.   d. Wellbutrin.

4. Which organ is responsible for the majority of a drug's excretion?
   a. kidney   c. lungs
   b. intestines   d. liver

5. Opiates fall under which schedule or category of controlled substances?
   a. C-I   c. C-III
   b. C-II   d. C-V

ACTIVITY 23-1: Common Drug Interactions

Look up http://www.mayoclinic.com/health/serotonin-syndrome/DS00860 on the Web. This problem—serotonin syndrome—occurs most frequently with combinations of drugs or herbal supplements that affect serotonin.

Perform a general Internet search on the phrase "herbal interactions." You should find many legitimate papers and documents regarding this specific type of interaction.

Although monitoring drug interactions is primarily the pharmacist's job, pharmacy technicians need to be aware of possible interactions and responsible when they encounter or learn of such possibilities. Many drug interactions tend to occur in older patients, as this population may have many different medical treatments for various maladies. As a person takes more and more medications for various illnesses (many take five or more different medications every day), the potential for drug–drug interaction increases. However, interactions do not occur only in the elderly.

With more medications being made available OTC, and the recent boom in herbal supplementation, many people treat themselves for various conditions without consulting a physician or a pharmacist. This factor increases the potential for serious drug–drug and drug–herb interactions. Most people are under the impression that herbal supplements are "natural" and that they have no side effects. This is not necessarily true, as you will learn. Certain herbal supplements can indeed cause interactions, and many also have side effects. St. John's wort, supposed to be a natural antidepressant, can interact badly if the patient is also taking prescription antidepressant medication. Those taking St. John's wort also experience photosensitivity and are easily sunburned. Dietary supplements, such as herbal remedies, are not regulated by the FDA as medications are. Therefore, different brands of the same supplement may not have the same potency or quality. For example, a customer who has not had a reaction to a drug changes to a higher potency supplement and thereby unknowingly triggers a drug–herb interaction.

Diet can also play a role in interactions. Patients taking warfarin as a blood thinner are advised to avoid green, leafy vegetables, and other foods that contain high amounts of vitamin K, because it is a natural coagulant. Because it has the opposite effect of warfarin, vitamin K will interfere with the blood-thinning properties of the warfarin. As you can see, it is important to be vigilant about possible interactions by educating yourself so that you can be responsive when you observe a potential for these interactions.

In pharmacy practice, computers are programmed with alerts that display when a potential drug interaction is found. This warning system is invaluable to pharmacy professionals and their customers. Nevertheless, pharmacy is a dynamic and changing environment. New drugs are introduced every year and updated information regarding current medications is not always available, so there may be times when the warning system does not have the information necessary to issue potential alerts. In addition, if a patient goes to multiple pharmacies, it is difficult to track likely drug interactions for all of the patient's medications.

Activity:

The following table lists some common drug–herb and drug–drug interactions, plus a simplified explanation of the effects of their interactions. Review the table, and then use it to answer the questions that follow.

Drug or Drug Class	Interacting Drug, Class, or Herb	Interaction
antidepressants (e.g., SSRIs, MAOIs)	St. John's wort	increased risk of serotonin syndrome
antiplatelets (e.g., aspirin, warfarin, clopidogrel)	gingko biloba	increased risk of bleeding
benzodiazepine hypnotics (e.g., alprazolam, diazepam)	antifungal agents ending in -azole (e.g., fluconazole)	increased benzodiazepine serum concentrations, resulting in excessive sedation
benzodiazepines, antipsychotics, alcohol	kava kava	increased sedation, lethargy, disorientation
digoxin	clarithromycin and erythromycin	increased digoxin levels, resulting in digoxin toxicity
fluoroquinolones (e.g., ciprofloxacin, levofloxacin)	antacids containing aluminum or magnesium compounds	decreased absorption of fluoroquinolones
MAO inhibitors (e.g., phenylzine, tranylcypromine)	anorexiants (e.g., phentermine, dextroamphetamine), decongestants (e.g., pseudoephedrine, phenylephrine), vasopressors (e.g., dopamine, ephedrine)	increased risk of serotonin syndrome or hypertensive event due to increased norepinephrine levels
nitrates (e.g., nitroglycerin, isosorbide)	sildenafil, tadalafil, vardenafil	increased risk of hypotension
oral contraceptives (estrogen–progestin combinations)	most antibiotics, rifampin	increased risk of contraceptive failure
SSRIs (e.g., escitalopram, fluoxetine, paroxetine)	MAO inhibitors	increased risk of serotonin syndrome
tetracyclines	penicillins, antacids, compounds containing iron	reduced absorption of tetracyclines
theophylline	fluoroquinolone antibiotics (e.g., ciprofloxacin, levofloxacin, fluvoxamine)	increased theophylline levels, resulting in theophylline toxicity
warfarin	aspirin, NSAIDs, antihyperlipidemics-fibric type (e.g., fenofibrate, gemfibrozil), thyroid hormones	increased risk of bleeding
warfarin	barbiturates (e.g., butalbital, phenobarbital), vitamin K (phytonadione), vegetables containing vitamin K	decreased anticoagulant effect

Questions:

1. What type of reaction might occur if a patient was taking paroxetine and St. John's wort?
   a. increased risk of bleeding
   b. increased risk of serotonin syndrome
   c. decreased absorption of paroxetine
   d. decreased absorption of St. John's wort

2. Which of the following can cause a drug–diet interaction?
   a. consuming antacids with ciprofloxacin
   b. taking antibiotics with oral birth control
   c. eating spinach while taking warfarin
   d. taking an iron supplement with tetracycline

3. What reaction might occur if a patient was taking nitroglycerin capsules and sildenafil?
   a. increased risk of hypotension
   b. increased risk of bleeding
   c. increased risk of contraceptive failure
   d. increased risk of serotonin syndrome

4. Many people feel that it is unnecessary to disclose to their physician all the dietary supplements they take. Could this common practice jeopardize their health? Explain your answer.

   _____

   _____

   _____

   _____

5. Go to the following website: http://www.mayoclinic.com/health/serotonin-syndrome/DS00860
   a. When does serotonin syndrome occur most frequently?

      _____

      _____

   b. What are the signs and symptoms of serotonin syndrome?

      _____

      _____

   c. Name five drugs that can lead to serotonin syndrome.

      _____

      _____

   d. What are ways to prevent serotonin syndrome?

      _____

      _____

6. What popular herbs or OTC products do you or your family use on a regular basis? Choose one and research common drug interactions with that herbal or OTC product.

   _____

   _____

   _____

   _____

ACTIVITY 23-2: Case Study—Identifying Drug Interactions

Instructions: Read the following scenario and then answer the critical thinking questions.

An 82-year-old woman brings four new prescriptions to the pharmacy, two from one physician and two from another physician. The first prescription is for ciprofloxacin 500 mg tablets and fluconazole 100 mg tablets. The second prescription is for theophylline 200 mg tablets and warfarin 2 mg tablets. While entering the new prescriptions, the technician notices that this patient has many medications in her patient profile and is confused about this patient's medication list. Upon further examination, the technician discovers that many of the medications are also from different physicians. For example the woman recently has had prescriptions filled for clonazepam, fenofibrate, magnesium oxide, levothyroxine, and sertraline. As the technician is processing the current orders for the patient, multiple drug–drug interaction alerts appear on the monitor. The technician asks her supervising pharmacist to review all of the alerts.

1. Using this customer's profile, list all the potential interactions between her existing medications and her new prescriptions.

   _____

   _____

   _____

   _____

2. As a technician, what is your responsibility and scope of practice ability to the patient and to the pharmacist after you have found out this information?

   _____

   _____

   _____

   _____

3. Do you think the customer's age could play a factor in potential drug–drug interactions? Explain.

   _____

   _____

   _____

   _____

ACTIVITY 23-3: Case Study—Calcium Bioavailability

Instructions: Read the following scenario and then answer the critical thinking questions.

Christina is a 48-year-old premenopausal woman with a busy lifestyle. She pops a vitamin every now and then, but she gleans most of her daily vitamins from eating a wide variety of foods. Although she is not a health nut, she has many female friends who are in tune with the nutritional needs of women as they age. One thing she knows for sure is that she needs to look at supplementing her diet with calcium for healthy bones as she ages.

Christina finds that many products claim to have better bioavailability than others. It is much too confusing because, as she discovers, each person you ask may give a different answer. Each of her friends seems to be taking a different type of calcium, and the products they use have a wide variety of pricing and claims.

Christina finally decides to research this on her own and make her own decision on which calcium supplement she will begin taking. The choices she encounters go by different names, and she does not know what this means. She finds calcium acetate, calcium citrate, calcium carbonate, calcium gluconate, calcium phosphate, calcium lactate, and eggshell calcium.

1. What is meant by the term *bioavailability*?
   _____
   _____

2. What are the differences between the calcium forms listed?
   _____
   _____
   _____

3. Which of these is a "better" calcium supplement? Which one has the best bioavailability?
   _____
   _____
   _____

4. Are there any special considerations when taking calcium supplements?
   _____
   _____
   _____

5. What information in this scenario makes you agree that now is a good time for Christina to begin taking a calcium supplement?
   _____
   _____
   _____

6. What substances interfere with calcium absorption?
   _____
   _____
   _____

360 **CHAPTER 23** *The Body and Drugs*

ACTIVITY 23-4: Case Study—Fastest Response

Instructions: Read the following scenario and then answer the critical thinking questions.

Charlie is a 72-year-old widower who leads a fairly sedentary lifestyle and smokes two packs of cigarettes a day. He takes occasional daily walks and trips to the grocery store. Almost every morning, Charlie takes his fox terrier mix for a five-block walk to meet some other friends at the local donut shop. In the early morning hours, the men talk and tell tales of what life was like when they were growing up. This all takes place over some delicious home-baked pastries and several cups of questionable-tasting coffee.

Charlie's medication profile resembles that of any man his age who has not lived a healthy life: some blood pressure problems, shortness of breath, and a heart condition or two. Charlie has seen some pretty scary times, medically speaking, in his life. For example, he has been the recipient of nitroglycerin many times. He has received it in a buccal extended-release tablet form, a sublingual tablet form, and an ointment form.

1. Describe an example of when Charlie would have received nitroglycerin buccal extended-release tablets. How long did the tablet take to work?

   _____

   _____

   _____

2. Describe an example of when Charlie would have used sublingual nitroglycerin tablets. How long did it take before Charlie felt the effects of the medication and then what was the duration of its effectiveness?

   _____

   _____

   _____

3. Describe an example of when Charlie would have used a nitroglycerin ointment.

   _____

   _____

   _____

4. How does nitroglycerin work?

   _____

   _____

   _____

ACTIVITY 23-5: Case Study—Time for Some Help

Instructions: Read the following scenario and then answer the critical thinking questions.

Marilyn is a 38-year-old, happily married housewife and mother. She has a wonderful husband and two beautiful children. She also has a small circle of friends whom she meets with on Saturday to shop or go on outings. She and her husband own a mid-sized auto repair shop that does moderately well. The shop specializes in American-made vehicles and has a staff of about 15 mechanics and office staff.

In addition to owning the shop, Marilyn's husband has volunteered through the national reserves since coming out of military service about 11 years ago. Unfortunately, the military has now called Marilyn's husband to active service, and he is to be deployed to a foreign country for a year or more. The family finds themselves in an emotional state about this recent news. Marilyn is very upset but knows she must support her husband, who feels it is his duty to serve.

As the date of her husband's deployment comes closer, Marilyn is consumed with the thought of being alone. She feels as if death is coming to the family and is also beginning to feel overwhelmed with the idea of managing the shop and taking care of her children without her husband. Marilyn's husband attempts to train her in all the things he does in the shop (outside of auto repair) in order to prepare her for his absence. To accommodate this extra time requirement, Marilyn no longer visits with her friends on the weekends.

One week away from her husband's deployment, Marilyn has reached a new low. She barely gets dressed, never visits anyone, and cries steadily. She is tense, irritable, as well as consistently complains of body aches. Her husband takes her to visit their family doctor, who examines her and prescribes the medication nortriptyline.

1. Is Marilyn encountering exogenous or endogenous depression?

   _____

   _____

2. What class of medication is nortriptyline?

   _____

   _____

   _____

3. What are some precautions with nortriptyline regarding dosage and use?

   _____

   _____

   _____

4. How long does it take for nortriptyline to take effect?

   _____

   _____

   _____

LAB 23-1: Web Research Activity—Understanding Addiction

Objective:

Learn about drug addiction by researching the topic at the Mayo Clinic website.

Pre-Lab Information:

- Review Chapter 23 in the textbook.
- Explore the following website: http://www.mayoclinic.com/health/drug-addiction/DS00183

Explanation:

This exercise will give you the opportunity to research and better understand drug addiction. As a pharmacy technician, you may encounter patients with drug addictions, and it is important to understand this disease.

Activity:

Using the Mayo Clinic website (http://www.mayoclinic.com/health/drug-addiction/DS00183), answer the following questions.

1. What are the six general characteristics that you might find with any drug addiction?

   _____

   _____

   _____

   _____

   _____

2. What are the five risk factors for developing an addiction?

   _____

   _____

   _____

   _____

3. What are the seven major complications associated with addiction?

   _____

   _____

   _____

   _____

   _____

   _____

4. After withdrawal treatment (detoxification), what are the three major categories of continued addiction treatment?

_____

_____

_____

5. What are the four steps listed in this article that parents can take to help children avoid addiction?

_____

_____

_____

_____

Student Name: _____

Lab Partner: _____

Grade/Comments: _____

_____

_____

Student Comments: _____

_____

_____

LAB 23-2: Web Research Activity: Agonists versus Antagonists

Objective:

Learn about drug agonists and antagonists by researching the topic using the Merck Manual website.

Pre-Lab Information:

- Review Chapter 23 in the textbook.
- Visit the website: http://www.merck.com/mmhe/sec02/ch012/ch012b.html

Explanation:

This exercise gives you the opportunity to explore the differences in how agonist and antagonist drugs affect the body. The following is a summary of the information you should study.

Drugs that target receptors are classified as either agonists or antagonists. *Agonist* drugs activate, or stimulate, their receptors, triggering a response that increases or decreases the cell's activity. *Antagonist* drugs block access by or attachment of the body's natural agonists, usually neurotransmitters, to receptors and thereby prevent or reduce cell responses to natural agonists.

Agonist and antagonist drugs can be used together in patients with asthma. For example, albuterol (Proventil or Ventolin) can be used with ipratropium (Atrovent). Albuterol, an agonist, attaches to specific (adrenergic) receptors on cells in the respiratory tract, causing relaxation of smooth muscle cells and thus widening of the airways (*bronchodilation*). Ipratropium, an antagonist, attaches to other (cholinergic) receptors, blocking the attachment of acetylcholine, a neurotransmitter, that causes contraction of smooth muscle cells and thus narrowing of the airways (*bronchoconstriction*). Both drugs work to widen the airways and thus make breathing easier, but they do so in different ways.

Beta blockers, such as propranolol (Inderal), are a widely used group of antagonists. These drugs are used to treat high blood pressure, angina (chest pain caused by an inadequate blood supply to the heart muscle), and certain abnormal heart rhythms, as well as to prevent migraines. They block or reduce stimulation of the heart by the agonist hormones epinephrine (adrenaline) and norepinephrine (noradrenaline), which are released during stress. Antagonists, such as beta blockers, are most effective when the concentration of the agonist is high in a specific part of the body. A roadblock stops more vehicles during the 5:00 p.m. rush hour than at 3:00 a.m.; similarly, beta blockers, given in doses that have little effect on normal heart function, may have a greater effect during sudden surges of hormones released during stress, and thereby protect the heart from excess stimulation.

Activity:

Using the Merck Manual website (http://www.merck.com/mmhe/sec02/ch012/ch012b.html) and the preceding summary, answer the following questions.

1. What effect does an agonist drug have on its respective receptor?

   _____

   _____

   _____

2. What effect does an antagonist drug have on its respective receptor?

   _____

   _____

   _____

3. Beta blockers are antagonist drugs. What effect do they have on the heart?

_____

_____

_____

4. Albuterol is an agonist drug. What effect does it have on the respiratory system?

_____

_____

_____

Student Name: _____

Lab Partner: _____

Grade/Comments: _____

_____

_____

Student Comments: _____

_____

_____

LAB 23-3: Fat-Soluble and Water-Soluble Drugs

Objective:

Explore the differences between fat-soluble and water-soluble drugs by researching the topic using the Merck Manual website.

Pre-Lab Information:

- Review Chapter 23 in the textbook.
- Explore the website at http://www.merck.com/mmhe/sec02/ch011/ch011d.html
- Review the following summary of the website material.

Drug distribution refers to the movement of drug to and from the blood and various tissues of the body (e.g., fat, muscle, and brain tissue) and the relative proportions of drug in the tissues.

After a drug is absorbed into the bloodstream, it rapidly circulates through the body. The average circulation time of blood is one minute. As the blood recirculates, the drug moves from the bloodstream into the body's tissues.

Once absorbed, most drugs do not spread evenly throughout the body. Drugs that dissolve in water (water-soluble drugs), such as the antihypertensive drug atenolol (Tenormin), tend to stay within the blood and the fluid that surrounds cells (interstitial space). Drugs that dissolve in fat (fat-soluble drugs), such as the anesthetic drug halothane, tend to concentrate in fatty tissues. Other drugs concentrate mainly in only one small part of the body (e.g., iodine concentrates mainly in the thyroid gland), because the tissues there have a special attraction for (affinity) and ability to retain the drug.

Drugs penetrate different tissues at different speeds, depending on the drug's ability to cross membranes. For example, the anesthetic thiopental (Pentothal), a highly fat-soluble drug, rapidly enters the brain, but the antibiotic penicillin, a water-soluble drug, does not. In general, fat-soluble drugs can cross cell membranes more quickly than water-soluble drugs can. For some drugs, transport mechanisms aid movement into or out of the tissues.

Some drugs leave the bloodstream very slowly, because they bind tightly to proteins circulating in the blood. Others quickly leave the bloodstream and enter other tissues, because they are less tightly bound to blood proteins. Some or virtually all molecules of a drug in the blood may be bound to blood proteins. The protein-bound part is generally inactive. As unbound drug is distributed to tissues and its level in the bloodstream decreases, blood proteins gradually release the drug bound to them. Thus, the bound drug in the bloodstream may act as a reservoir of the drug.

Some drugs accumulate in certain tissues, which can also act as reservoirs of extra drug. These tissues slowly release the drug into the bloodstream, keeping blood levels of the drug from decreasing rapidly and thereby prolonging the effect of the drug. Some drugs, such as those that accumulate in fatty tissues, leave the tissues so slowly that they circulate in the bloodstream for days after a person has stopped taking the drug.

Distribution of a given drug may also vary from person to person. For instance, obese people may store large amounts of fat-soluble drugs, whereas very thin people may store relatively little. Older people, even when thin, may store large amounts of fat-soluble drugs because the proportion of body fat increases with age.

Explanation:

This exercise gives you the opportunity to explore how the characteristics of drugs differ depending on whether the compound is water- or fat-soluble.

Activity:

Using the Merck Manual website (http://www.merck.com/mmhe/sec02/ch011/ch011d.html) and the preceding summary, answer the following questions.

1. What are the implications for a drug that is fat-soluble?

   _____

   _____

   _____

   _____

2. In what organs is a fat-soluble drug likely to accumulate?

   _____

   _____

   _____

   _____

3. What are the implications for a drug that is water-soluble?

   _____

   _____

   _____

   _____

Student Name: _____

Lab Partner: _____

Grade/Comments: _____

_____

_____

Student Comments: _____

_____

_____

LAB 23-4: Drug Dependency

Objective:

Learn about drug dependency by researching and visiting two of the most prominent worldwide nonprofit organizations called Alcoholics Anonymous (AA) and/or Narcotics Anonymous (NA).

Pre-Lab Information:

- Review Chapter 23 in the textbook.
- Explore the following websites: www.aa.org and/or www.na.org

Explanation:

This exercise will give you the opportunity to research and better understand drug dependency. As a pharmacy technician, you may encounter patients with dependency issues and it is important to understand these two diseases.

Activity:

Many medical students, as a part of their studies and residencies, are required to visit a meeting of AA and/or NA. The medical student does this so that he or she may further understand the elements of addiction and/or alcoholism as well as recovery options for a patient who may struggle with these two diseases.

Locate a meeting in your local area and plan on attending a meeting either in the daytime or evening hours. All meetings have a designation in their listings such as a men's meeting, a woman's meeting, LGBT meeting, book study, and so forth. However, both fellowships do welcome non-AA or non-NA guests in order for family members or members of the medical community and professions to be aware of and understand how the disease of addiction and/or alcoholism can affect everyone's life.

The positive transformations of an addict or alcoholic's life is what the fellowships of these meetings aspire to achieve through the daily application and practice of spiritual principles for the addicts and alcoholics in these meetings.

After the meeting is over, ask the meeting secretary to sign off on your attendance below with their initials.

Date: _____ AA/NA Secretary Initials: _____

Answer the following questions:

1. What is sponsorship?

   _____

   _____

   _____

   _____

2. What is clean time or sobriety?

   _____

   _____

   _____

   _____

3. What did you learn from attending this meeting?

_____

_____

_____

_____

Student Name: _____

Lab Partner: _____

Grade/Comments: _____

_____

_____

Student Comments: _____

_____

_____

CHAPTER 24
The Skin

After completing Chapter 24 from the textbook, you should be able to:	Related Activity in the Workbook/Lab Manual
1. List, identify, and diagram the basic anatomical structure of the skin.	Review Questions, PTCB Exam Practice Questions, Activity 24-1
2. Explain the function or physiology of the skin.	Review Questions, PTCB Exam Practice Questions, Activity 24-3, Activity 24-5
3. List and define common diseases affecting the skin and understand the causes, symptoms, and pharmaceutical treatments associated with each disease.	Review Questions, PTCB Exam Practice Questions, Activity 24-2, Activity 24-3, Activity 24-4, Activity 24-5

INTRODUCTION

The skin is the largest organ of the body. It consists of three main layers: the epidermis, the dermis, and the subcutaneous layer. Important functions of the skin include serving as a barrier to foreign organisms and debris, managing the regulation of body temperature, excreting salts and excess water, and acting as a "shock absorber" to protect the underlying organs. Unfortunately, the skin plays host to a wide variety of more than 1,000 medical conditions and diseases, ranging from minor irritations to severe infections. Although creams and ointments are widely used to treat skin conditions, treatment options also include oral and injectable medications. As a pharmacy technician, it is important for you to understand the basic anatomy and physiology of the skin and the conditions that affect it so that you have greater insight into how the drugs used to treat these conditions work.

REVIEW QUESTIONS

Match the following.

1. _____ acne
2. _____ sebum
3. _____ carcinoma
4. _____ pathogenic
5. _____ rosacea
6. _____ mitigate
7. _____ eczema
8. _____ bacteriostatic
9. _____ infection
10. _____ pigmentation
11. _____ bactericidal
12. _____ psoriasis
13. _____ rash
14. _____ parasite

a. oily substance produced by the sebaceous glands in the skin

b. an organism that lives on or inside another organism

c. a skin condition characterized by redness and inflammation

d. disease-causing microorganisms

e. kills microorganisms

f. inhibits the growth and/or reproduction of microorganisms

g. inflammatory skin condition characterized by itching, redness, blistering, and oozing

h. a bacterial infection accompanied by an overproduction of sebum

i. invasion of pathogens into the body; an infection occurs when a pathogenic microbe is able to multiply in the tissues (colonize)

j. malignant tumor

k. to lessen or decrease severity

l. a facial skin disorder accompanied by chronic redness and inflammation

m. color

n. a noncontagious, chronic immune disorder in which specific immune cells become overactive and release excessive amounts of proteins called cytokines

True or False?

15. The skin is the largest organ of the body.

    T   F

16. The outermost layer of the skin is the dermis.

    T   F

17. Cellulitis is caused by a fungus.

    T   F

18. Ringworm is an example of a bacterial infection.

    T   F

19. Greasy foods or chocolate may cause acne.

    T   F

Choose the best answer.

20. Normal body temperature regulated by the skin is:
    a. 98.6 °F.   c. 69.8 °C.
    b. 89.6 °F.   d. 98.6 °C.

21. Skin infections are not caused by which of the following?
   a. bacteria
   b. cancer
   c. fungi
   d. viruses

22. The most severe burn would be classified as:
   a. first degree.
   b. second degree.
   c. third degree.
   d. fourth degree.

23. The second most common skin cancer is:
   a. malignant melanoma.
   b. actinic keratosis.
   c. basal cell carcinoma.
   d. squamous cell cancer.

Fill in the blanks.

24. An acute, deep infection of the connective tissue is called _____.

25. Small red bumps and intense itching caused by mites is known as _____.

26. A chronic disorder of unknown cause, with symptoms including pimples, lesions, and redness, is known as _____.

27. The color of the skin is caused by the amount of _____.

28. If a person sustained burns to the leg, groin, and abdomen, he would be burned over _____% of his body.

Match the following ulcer descriptions with their classifications.

29. _____ Stage I   a. lesion extending through skin to the bone
30. _____ Stage II   b. crater-like lesion extending through tissue
31. _____ Stage III   c. reddening of unbroken skin
32. _____ Stage IV   d. abrasion or blister

PHARMACY CALCULATION PROBLEMS

Calculate the following.

1. A prescription reads: "Clindamycin 2% in aquaphilic ointment; 60 g. Apply to affected body part twice daily." The pharmacy stocks clindamycin 150 mg capsules. How many capsules will be needed to prepare this compound?

2. A physician has requested a compound for lidocaine 3% in 120 mL calamine lotion. How many milligrams of lidocaine powder must be added to the calamine lotion for the compound?

3. A compound is to contain equal parts nystatin cream, clotrimazole 1% cream, and triamcinolone 0.05% cream. How many grams of each product will be required to make 4 oz?

4. A physician wants to dilute 100 mL of a 10% topical solution to a 4% solution with sterile water. How many milliliters of sterile water will you need?

5. Conversion: 144 lbs = _____ kg

PTCB EXAM PRACTICE QUESTIONS

1. Which is the middle layer of the skin?
   a. subcutaneous
   b. epidermis
   c. dermis
   d. adipose

2. What is an acute, deep infection of the skin and connective tissue accompanied by inflammation?
   a. basal cell carcinoma
   b. eczema
   c. psoriasis
   d. cellulitis

3. Which drug is used to treat psoriasis?
   a. Enbrel
   b. clofibrate
   c. Restasis
   d. Silvadene

4. What disease is caused by bacteria and an overproduction of sebum?
   a. eczema
   b. acne
   c. psoriasis
   d. cellulitis

5. What kind of skin infection is described as a mycosis?
   a. fungal
   b. bacterial
   c. viral
   d. parasitic

ACTIVITY 24-1: Anatomy Worksheet—The Skin

Label the following illustration of the skin.

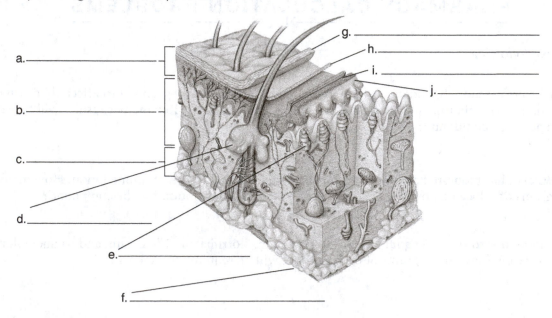

a. _____
b. _____
c. _____
d. _____
e. _____
f. _____
g. _____
h. _____
i. _____
j. _____

ACTIVITY 24-2: Case Study—Morgellons

Instructions: Read the following scenario and then answer the critical thinking questions.

Note: Based in part on a true situation.

Mark and his wife Carol built a home in the suburbs three years ago and have been very happy. One day, however, when Mark is working in the den, he begins screaming out his wife's name. Carol runs to him and Mark keeps saying that it feels as if little "bugs" are crawling all over him. He is itching uncontrollably and has a burning sensation. Carol takes Mark to the doctor, who finds nothing, but advises Mark to use an OTC anti-itching cream.

These symptoms continue for weeks with the addition of constant fatigue. Convinced that the doctor's diagnosis was correct, Mark tries every type of cream and anti-itch product available trying to get control of his symptoms.

Like something out of a science fiction movie, soon Mark develops painful sores all over his body, which ooze blue fibers, white threads, and black specks of sand-like material. Frightened by this, Mike and Carol head to the emergency room. Upon examination, Mike is diagnosed with delusional parasitosis. Mike is convinced that his body has been invaded by some type of parasitic bug, but cannot convince the doctor, who has found no such evidence of parasites. The doctor ignores the small bundles of fibers oozing from the sores and advises Mark to use an OTC antifungal cream.

A few days later, Mark is watching a popular morning news show that discusses a strange skin condition with symptoms exactly like Mark's. They name this condition *Morgellons*. The program states that there are a few cases in the United States, and that the Centers for Disease Control and Prevention is currently investigating. It is not yet known what it is or what might cure it. Health care providers have seen a higher incidence of Morgellons patients who also have fibromyalgia, attention deficit/hyperactivity disorder (ADHD), and chronic fatigue syndrome.

Mark makes an appointment with a dermatologist after viewing the TV program and has a sample of his fibers taken and sent to a forensic lab. Results show that the fibers are not related to anything in the national database; it is determined that the fibers are not manmade and do not come from a plant.

1. Patients who present to dermatologists with Morgellons are classified as having delusional parasitosis in more than 95% of cases, which unfortunately does nothing for the sores or fiber extrusion. What is delusional parasitosis? Search the Internet or use other references to find out.

_____

_____

_____

_____

2. Why do you think a high percentage of these patients are diagnosed with delusional parasitosis?

_____

_____

_____

_____

3. What could Mark pick up at the pharmacy that would help his skin condition?

_____

_____

_____

_____

4. What do you think is the likely psychological impact of this condition on Mark and his family?

_____

_____

_____

_____

ACTIVITY 24-3: Case Study—A Skin Infection

Instructions: Read the following scenario and then answer the critical thinking questions.

Mr. Tuttle has been coming to the retail pharmacy where you work for four years, ever since his daughter, Laura, was born. You have seen Laura grow from birth to a preschooler. Mr. Tuttle brings Laura, now four years old, with him to the pharmacy today and asks for any type of cream that would help heal her skin rash. The pharmacist talks to Mr. Tuttle, who repeats his request for a recommendation and lifts Laura's sleeve to reveal the rash. There are no lesions anywhere else on her body. Laura has several reddish, round lesions on her arm that are slightly raised and scaling. Pinpoint pustules around the edges of the lesions accompany these. Laura has no fever or any other symptoms. The pharmacist refers Mr. Tuttle to a doctor.

1. What was the rash on Laura's arm?

_____

_____

2. What is the treatment for Laura's rash?

_____

_____

3. Is Laura's condition considered contagious? If so, where might she have contracted it?

_____

_____

ACTIVITY 24-4: Case Study—A Skin Condition

Instructions: Read the following scenario and then answer the critical thinking questions.

Mrs. Cortez, a Hispanic woman, brings her 13-year-old daughter, Sarah, with her to the retail pharmacy where you work. She purchases a variety of skin care creams from the cosmetic section. Sarah has what appears to be uneven skin coloring on her face, particularly close to her nose. It is nothing significant, but Sarah is getting to an age at which she is more concerned about her appearance.

Mrs. Cortez returns after a week and asks to talk to the pharmacist about Sarah's skin spots. She explains to the pharmacist that Sarah has been using cold cream, but has noticed that the spots are changing in size. She is wondering if the cold cream is the cause of the change, or if Sarah might have cancer. Mrs. Cortez continues, saying that Sarah has a few of these symmetrical spots on her body, but the condition is now appearing on her face and she thinks it is spreading. Mrs. Cortez also adds that Sarah has become extremely sensitive to the sun.

No one else in the family has this condition. Sarah is referred to her doctor.

1. What is the name of the skin condition Sarah has?
   _____
   _____

2. Is there a cream in the pharmacy that could help with this condition?
   _____
   _____

3. What are some treatments for Sarah's condition?
   _____
   _____

4. How would the emotional impact of this condition be different for Sarah than for an adult?
   _____
   _____
   _____
   _____

ACTIVITY 24-5: What is Chemical Photosensitivity?

As you have learned, drugs sometimes interact with each other to cause unwanted consequences. Sometimes drugs or other chemical substances can interact with sunlight in a condition called *chemical photosensitivity*. Go online to learn more about chemical photosensitivity, and then answer the following questions.

1. What are photosensitizers? Give five examples of substances that might contain photosensitizers.
   _____
   _____
   _____
   _____
   _____

2. Name five short-term effects of exposure to photosensitizers.
   _____
   _____
   _____
   _____
   _____

3. Name five long-term effects of exposure to photosensitizers.

_____

_____

_____

_____

_____

4. Describe the difference between a photoallergic reaction and a phototoxic reaction. Which type of reaction is more common? Which type of reaction is harder to diagnose, and why?

_____

_____

_____

_____

5. Will using a sunscreen protect a person who is photosensitive?

_____

_____

_____

_____

6. Name five common OTC drugs and five prescription drugs that are known to cause chemical photosensitivity in some patients.

_____

_____

_____

_____

_____

7. Did anything you learned about chemical photosensitivity surprise you? If so, what?

_____

_____

_____

_____

CHAPTER 25
Eyes and Ears

After completing Chapter 25 from the textbook, you should be able to:	Related Activity in the Workbook/Lab Manual
1. List, identify, and diagram the basic anatomical structure and parts of the eye and ear.	Review Questions, PTCB Exam Practice Questions, Activity 25-1
2. Describe the function or physiology of the ears and eyes.	Review Questions, PTCB Exam Practice Questions
3. List and define common diseases affecting the eyes, and understand the causes, symptoms, and pharmaceutical treatments associated with each disease.	Review Questions, PTCB Exam Practice Questions, Activity 25-2, Activity 25-3, Activity 25-5
4. List and define common diseases affecting the ears, and understand the causes, symptoms, and pharmaceutical treatments associated with each disease.	Review Questions, PTCB Exam Practice Questions, Activity 25-1, Activity 25-4

INTRODUCTION

Seeing and hearing are two of our basic senses. Although both the eyes and the ears are susceptible to a variety of disorders, these maladies can normally be prevented, controlled, or reversed with treatment, except in rare cases. A wide variety of treatment modalities is available to treat eye disorders. However, it is important that ophthalmic products be used safely and properly, because they are sterile. One of your most important responsibilities as a pharmacy technician is to thoroughly understand the basics of safe using of ophthalmic remedies. As a pharmacy technician, it is important for you to understand the basic anatomy and physiology of the eyes and ears and the conditions that affect them so that you have greater insight into how the drugs used to treat these conditions work.

REVIEW QUESTIONS

Match the following.

1. _____ humor
2. _____ asymptomatic
3. _____ blepharitis
4. _____ hordeolum
5. _____ cataract
6. _____ cycloplegic
7. _____ conjunctivitis
8. _____ tinnitus
9. _____ glaucoma
10. _____ photoreceptors
11. _____ iridotomy
12. _____ retinopathy
13. _____ mucopurulent
14. _____ otitis media
15. _____ mydriatic
16. _____ ophthalmic
17. _____ eustachian tube

a. rods and cones
b. a group of eye diseases characterized by an increase in intra-ocular pressure
c. a noninflammatory disease in which the retina of the eye is damaged
d. pertaining to the eye
e. causing relaxation and paralysis of the intraocular muscles
f. containing or composed of mucus or pus
g. acute or chronic inflammation of the eye conjunctiva
h. showing no evidence of disease or abnormal condition
i. causing dilation of the pupil of the eye
j. an ocular opacity or obscurity in the lens of the eye
k. a body fluid
l. inflammation of the eyelid margins accompanied by redness
m. infection and inflammation of the middle ear
n. ringing or buzzing in the ear that is not caused by an external source; may be caused by infection or a reaction to a drug.
o. an incision made in the iris of the eye to enlarge the pupil
p. an infection of one (or more) of the sebaceous glands of the eye
q. connects the middle ear with the nasopharynx of the throat

Choose the best answer.

18. The _____ is often referred to as the "film" of the camera.
    a. pupil
    b. cornea
    c. iris
    d. retina

19. The visual pathway for electrical impulses to the brain is the:
    a. cornea.
    b. sclera.
    c. iris.
    d. optic nerve.

20. The likely culprit of a stye is:
    a. *Staphylococcus aureus.*
    b. *Lactobacillus Casei.*
    c. *Streptococcus meningitis.*
    d. *Staphylococcus epidermis.*

21. Which of the following would not be appropriate for treating a stye?
    a. Augmentin 500 mg po q8h
    b. dicloxacillin 250 mg po q6h
    c. erythromycin 250 mg po qid
    d. tetracycline 250 mg po qid

True or False?

22. Conjunctivitis is most commonly known as red eye.

    T   F

23. Most glaucoma is of the open-angle or wide-angle type.

    T   F

24. Oral medications that are used for hypertension can cause problems in patients with glaucoma.

    T   F

25. Cataracts are chronic and cannot be reversed.

    T   F

26. Looking directly into the sun may cause solar retinopathy.

    T   F

Fill in the blanks.

27. The snail-shaped part of the ear is called the _____.

28. _____ drops may be placed in the ear, but _____ may not be placed in the _____.

PHARMACY CALCULATION PROBLEMS

1. A 5 mL bottle of olopatadine, 0.1%, is dispensed for allergic conjunctivitis. If the patient uses 1 gtt ou q8h, how many days will the bottle last?

2. How many milligrams of pilocarpine are in a 10 mL bottle of pilocarpine 6% ophthalmic gel?

3. Azithromycin 100 mg/5 mL suspension is prescribed for a child's inner-ear infection. If the patient is to receive 100 mg on day 1 and 50 mg on days 2–5, how many milliliters will the patient need for the entire course?

4. If cephalexin 250 mg is prescribed to a child one capsule qid for seven days, what is the total strength for the course of therapy that the child will receive? How many capsules will be dispensed?

5. Conversion: 1 pt. = _____ mL

1. What disease of the eye is characterized by increased intraocular pressure?
   a. conjunctivitis
   b. cataract
   c. glaucoma
   d. macular degeneration

2. What is a condition of the eye in which the lens becomes opaque and interferes with clear vision?
   a. conjunctivitis
   b. cataract
   c. glaucoma
   d. macular degeneration

3. All of the following antibiotics must be monitored closely to avoid damage to the ear and possible hearing loss, *except*:
   a. gentamicin.
   b. amikacin.
   c. tobramycin.
   d. Protonix.

4. Which common infection of the eye is most commonly referred to as "pinkeye?"
   a. conjunctivitis
   b. cataract
   c. glaucoma
   d. macular degeneration

5. A patient may experience ototoxicity if he or she is prescribed:
   a. amoxicillin.
   b. hydrochlorothiazide.
   c. gentamicin.
   d. celecoxib.

ACTIVITY 25-1: Anatomy Worksheet

The Eye

Label the following illustration of the eye.

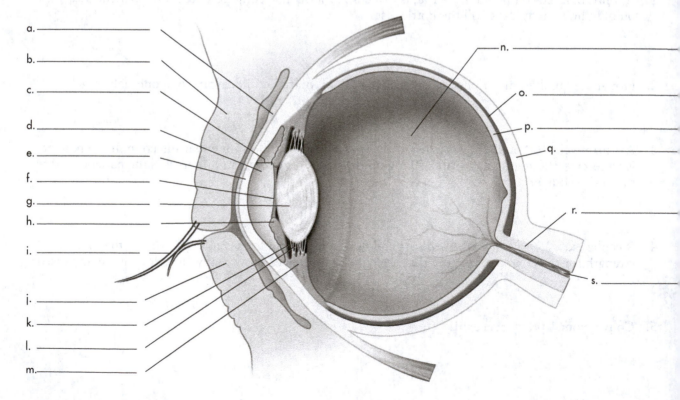

a.

b.

c.

d.

e.

f.

g.

h.

i.

j.

k.

l.

m.

n.

o.

p.

q.

r.

s.

The Ear

Label the following illustration of the ear.

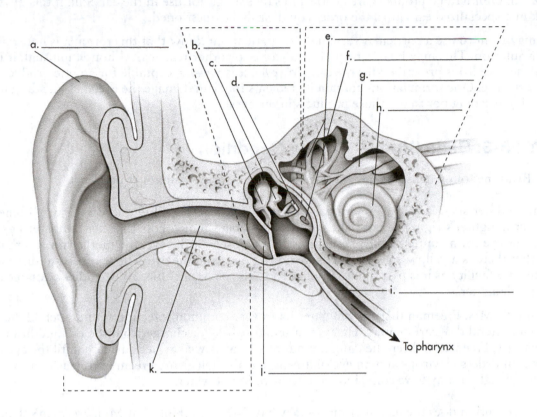

a. _____

b. _____

c. _____

d. _____

e. _____

f. _____

g. _____

h. _____

i. _____

To pharynx

k. _____

j. _____

ACTIVITY 25-2: Case Study—An Unusual Prescription

Simon, a CPhT, received a questionable prescription in the pharmacy today. Something didn't seem right to him at first. Take a look at the prescription.

1. What did you find unusual about the prescription?

_____

_____

_____

2. Do you think there is an error in this prescription?

_____

_____

_____

3. Why would a physician write a prescription such as this?

_____

_____

_____

A Closer Look

We hope that you observed from the data on the prescription that it is acceptable to order ophthalmic drops for the ear. Ophthalmic products are gentle and safe enough for use in the ear. Still, if this physician did not work in a specialized ear clinic, the order could easily be questioned.

A physician may want to use a particular formula for a patient but know that this formula is not available in an otic formulation. This may be due to patient allergies or other reasons. Although unusual, it is not uncommon to see eyedrops prescribed for the ear. However, it is *never* acceptable for an otic product to be prescribed for the eye. Otic formulations contain ingredients that can damage the eye, and otic drug inserts contain a specific warning not to use those products in the eyes.

ACTIVITY 25-3: Case Study—An Eye Condition

Instructions: Read the following scenario and then answer the critical thinking questions.

Mrs. Freeman and her six-year-old daughter are leaving the day care facility and on the way home. She notices that her daughter's right eye is bright red. Mrs. Freeman remembers that her daughter has been scratching at this eye for a couple of days. When she looks closely at the eye, the mother notices that it is swollen and that there is a yellow-colored discharge oozing out from the eye. They proceed to drive to the nearest urgent care facility as it is past 5 p.m. Upon arrival, the physician on staff is readily available to see Mrs. Freeman's daughter.

The physician tells Mrs. Freeman that her daughter has a very common infection found in children, especially those who attend day care centers. He takes a sample of the discharge from the eye and has it analyzed. He asks Mrs. Freeman to keep the daughter out of school as well as her day care until the eye clears up. The physician orders eyedrops and an eye ointment. He also tells Mrs. Freeman to wash all towels or clothes that her daughter may have come into contact with in hot water.

1. What eye condition does the daughter most likely have? Do you think that Mrs. Freeman's daughter has a contagious eye condition?

   _____

   _____

2. Why did the doctor ask Mrs. Freeman to keep the daughter out of school and day care?

   _____

   _____

   _____

   _____

3. What is the proper way to instill eyedrops for this six-year-old child?

   _____

   _____

   _____

   _____

4. What is the proper way to apply an eye ointment for a child?

   _____

   _____

   _____

   _____

ACTIVITY 25-4: Case Study—An Ear Condition

Instructions: Read the following scenario and then answer the critical thinking questions.

Jarred is a healthy 17-year-old high school senior and ranks very high of the swimming team at his high school. He has won many district competitions to where many college recruiters are monitoring his progress; Jarred believes that he may be able to obtain an athletic scholarship. He is in the water practicing seven days a week. In addition to his swimming, Jarred also competes in track and tennis.

With the exception of a badly sprained ankle last year and a few times where he had athlete's foot, overall Jarred has been in good health. Occasionally, Jarred has moderate ear pain during swimming practice and experiences intermittent pressure in his ears. Often the pressure relieves itself within a few minutes. However, there are times when the pressure does not go away. As of late, the pressure has become quite consistent and also very painful. He asks his mother to look inside his ear because it has become increasingly itchy and hurts when he chews on the same side of his mouth as the sore ear. When his mother takes a look, she sees that the outer ear canal is swollen and red.

Jarred's mother takes him to their family physician; the physician also notices an eczema-like skin condition surrounding the ear.

1. What condition do you think that the physician will diagnose Jarred with?

   _____

   _____

2. Given the facts of the scenario, what is the probable cause of Jarred's condition and diagnosis?

   _____

   _____

   _____

   _____

3. What is the first-line treatment for this type of condition?

   _____

   _____

   _____

   _____

4. Should Jarred continue his seven-day schedule of being in the water?

   _____

   _____

   _____

   _____

ACTIVITY 25-5: Case Study—Eye Trouble

Instructions: Read the following scenario and then answer the critical thinking questions.

Mr. Gaines is a 49-year-old African-American male who has been waking up every morning with a headache for more than a week. It has become so annoying that he is taking two aspirin before going to bed in the hopes that he will not wake up with a headache the next morning. Sometimes, he gets lucky.

Because he is nearly 50 years old, when Mr. Gaines begins having vision problems he shrugs it off, attributes them to middle age, and makes an appointment with his ophthalmologist. However, as the weeks and months go by, the problem gets much worse. His vision is blurry quite frequently and he sees "clouds" or "halos" most of the time. He also notices that his eyes become much more painful when doing ordinary things such as reading or watching television. He realizes that his problem is not just a need for glasses, so he makes an appointment with his primary care physician.

In the meantime, Mr. Gaines sees his ophthalmologist again, who conducts a routine test that diagnoses the condition that is giving him so much trouble.

1. What diagnosis did Mr. Gaines's ophthalmologist make?

   _____
   _____

2. Is the routine test given by the ophthalmologist done for all patients or only those who have symptoms similar to those experienced by Mr. Gaines?

   _____
   _____
   _____
   _____

3. What contributing factors put Mr. Gaines into a high-risk category for this condition?

   _____
   _____
   _____
   _____

4. What is the goal of treatment for this condition?

   _____
   _____
   _____
   _____

5. What pharmaceutical treatments are available for this condition?

   _____
   _____
   _____
   _____

6. Is this condition curable?

   _____
   _____
   _____
   _____

After completing Chapter 26 from the textbook, you should be able to:	Related Activity in the Workbook/Lab Manual
1. Identify the basic anatomical and structural parts of the digestive system.	Review Questions, PTCB Exam Practice Questions, Activity 26-1
2. Describe the physiology of the digestive system.	Review Questions, PTCB Exam Practice Questions, Activity 26-2, Activity 26-3, Activity 26-4
3. List and define common diseases affecting the gastrointestinal system and understand the causes, symptoms, and pharmaceutical treatments associated with each disease.	Review Questions, PTCB Exam Practice Questions, Activity 26-2, Activity 26-3, Activity 26-4, Lab 26-1, Lab 26-2
4. List and describe the three main categories of nutrients.	Review Questions, PTCB Exam Practice Questions, Activity 26-2, Activity 26-3, Activity 26-4
5. Identify the functions and AMDR of the macronutrients.	Review Questions, PTCB Exam Practice Questions, Activity 26-2, Activity 26-3, Activity 26-4
6. State the difference between essential and nonessential amino acids.	Review Questions, Activity 26-2, Activity 26-3, Activity 26-4
7. Identify the functions, symptoms of deficiencies, and RDIs of the micronutrients.	Review Questions
8. Understand the importance of water to the body.	Review Questions, Activity 26-2, Activity 26-3, Activity 26-4, Lab 26-2

INTRODUCTION

The gastrointestinal system manages digestion in the body. Food is broken down, absorbed, or chemically modified into substances that are required by the cells to survive and function properly. Waste products that the body cannot use are eliminated. The gastrointestinal system extends from the mouth to the anus. Its six main parts are the mouth, esophagus, pharynx, stomach, and small and large intestines. Various supportive structures, accessory glands, and accessory organs also help to make up the complete digestive system. The main purpose of the digestive system is to fuel the body by taking in and metabolizing nutrients.

An estimated 70 million Americans suffer from one or more digestive disorders; this accounts for 13% of all hospitalizations. As a pharmacy technician, you should be aware of the most common digestive disorders that require pharmacological treatment, including conditions treated with OTC drugs.

REVIEW QUESTIONS

Match the following.

1. _____ chyme
2. _____ mastication
3. _____ protease
4. _____ lipid
5. _____ monosaccharide
6. _____ μg
7. _____ pepsinogen

a. fat
b. microgram
c. enzyme that begins protein breakdown
d. simplest form of carbohydrate
e. chewing
f. precursor to pepsin
g. liquid that food turns into before entering the small intestines

Choose the best answer.

8. Which of the following refers to LDL?
   a. bad cholesterol
   b. low-density lipoprotein
   c. a and b
   d. good cholesterol

9. Kilocalories (kcal) refers to:
   a. bad calories.
   b. food energy.
   c. good calories.
   d. a 1,000-calorie meal.

10. Good cholesterol is referred to as:
    a. high-density lipoprotein.
    b. DRI.
    c. HDL.
    d. a and c.

11. DRI stands for:
    a. dietary restriction information.
    b. diet reference index.
    c. dietary reference intakes.
    d. dietary recommendation index.

Fill in the blanks.

12. An added nutrient for enrichment is known as _____.

13. The liver produces _____, which is stored in the gallbladder.

14. As chyme enters the duodenum, it must be neutralized by bicarbonate; otherwise, a _____ ulcer will result.

15. _____ are nutrients needed by the body in larger quantities.

16. The only vitamin the body produces itself is vitamin _____.

Match the following.

17. _____ cecum   **a.** an accessory organ

18. _____ tongue   **b.** a part of the small intestine

19. _____ pharynx   **c.** a part of the large intestine

20. _____ ileum   **d.** part of main digestive system

True or False?

21. GERD occurs because the lower esophageal sphincter relaxes when it should contract.

    T   F

22. Ginger root is an herb that is known to combat nausea and vomiting.

    T   F

23. NSAIDs block the effect of the enzyme cyclooxygenase.

    T   F

24. Carbohydrates are bad for our health.

    T   F

Match the following drugs with a corresponding disease, condition, or treatment.

25. _____ Reglan   **a.** double drug theory/therapy for *H. pylori* infection

26. _____ Transderm-scop   **b.** postoperative vomiting drug

27. _____ CTZ   **c.** nonsteroidal anti-inflammatory drug

28. _____ Zofran   **d.** antihistamine used as an antiemetic

29. _____ Compazine   **e.** PPI drug used for ulcer treatment

30. _____ ibuprofen   **f.** overproduction of acid

31. _____ lansoprazole + amoxicillin **g.** postemetogenic nausea

32. _____ Prilosec   **h.** a type of laxative

33. _____ emollient   **i.** promotes proper sphincter function

Match the following vitamins with their names.

34. _____ vitamin A   **a.** niacin
35. _____ vitamin D   **b.** pantothenic acid
36. _____ vitamin C   **c.** thiamine
37. _____ vitamin K   **d.** folic acid
38. _____ vitamin B1   **e.** phytonadione
39. _____ vitamin B2   **f.** cyanocobalamin
40. _____ vitamin B3   **g.** retinol
41. _____ vitamin B5   **h.** pyridoxine
42. _____ vitamin B6   **i.** ascorbic acid
43. _____ vitamin B9   **j.** riboflavin
44. _____ vitamin B12   **k.** ergocalciferol

PHARMACY CALCULATION PROBLEMS

1. You need to dispense omeprazole for a pediatric patient. The patient weighs 55 lbs. and the recommended dosage is 20 mg/kg. The dosing for this medication in the pediatric population is 20 mg if the patient is over 20 kg. Is this dosage safe for the patient to take?

2. Sucralfate comes in a concentration of 1 g/10 mL. If a patient is receiving 10 mL qid, how many milligrams of sucralfate is the patient receiving daily?

3. A 65-year-old woman weighing 156 lbs. is to receive a midazolam IVP dosed at 0.02 mg/kg prior to her colonoscopy. If midazolam contains 1 mg/mL, how many milliliters will the patient receive?

4. A standard pantoprazole drip at a hospital pharmacy contains 80 mg in 250 mL of 0.9% sodium chloride. If the patient is to receive 8 mg/hr, how many milliliters will be infused over each hour?

5. Conversion: 2.5 lb. = _____oz.

PTCB EXAM PRACTICE QUESTIONS

1. Where in the gastrointestinal system are oral drugs absorbed?
   a. stomach   c. large intestine
   b. small intestine   d. mouth

2. The colon is composed of how many areas?
   a. three   c. four
   b. seven   d. two

3. A major cause of peptic ulcers is infection by which of the following bacteria?
   a. *Staphylococcus aureus*
   b. MRSA
   c. *Escherichia coli*
   d. *Helicobacter pylori*

4. All of the following drugs are used to treat postemetogenic nausea *except:*
   a. Zofran.
   b. Colace.
   c. Kytril.
   d. Anzemet.

5. A commonly prescribed evacuant laxative for examinations is:
   a. Colace.
   b. CoLyte.
   c. Cephulac.
   d. Citrucel.

ACTIVITY 26-1: Anatomy Worksheet—The Digestive System

Label the following illustration of the digestive system.

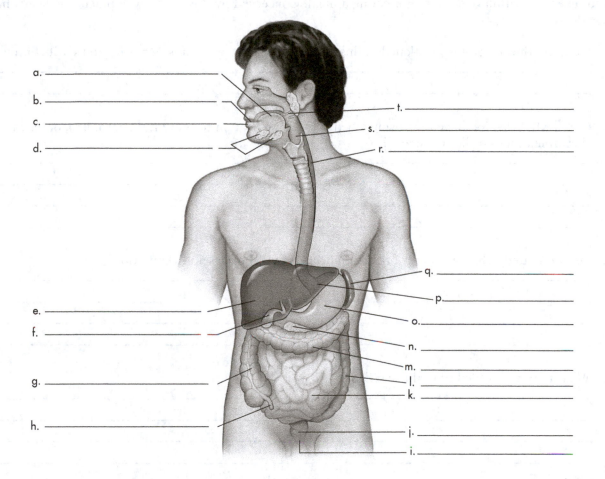

a. _____

b. _____

c. _____

d. _____

e. _____

f. _____

g. _____

h. _____

t. _____

s. _____

r. _____

q. _____

p. _____

o. _____

n. _____

m. _____

l. _____

k. _____

j. _____

i. _____

ACTIVITY 26-2: Case Study—Heartburn

Instructions: Read the following scenario and then answer the critical thinking questions.

Mr. Selescion is a 53-year-old executive who works out regularly. In addition to jogging, he swims, hikes, and lifts weights. Mr. Selescion does not always watch what he eats and has been known to indulge about once a week at a local Mexican restaurant. He loves their tamales, and sometimes buys enough to have leftovers for the next day. He drinks a lot of water and has wine on occasion with dinner.

The only problem he has ever encountered with his body has been stomach aches now and then, which he has had for years. Mr. Selescion began by taking OTC chewable tablets to help quell the "butterfly" feeling he had. He also remembers, a while back, buying a liquid antacid that tasted awful but seemed to work. Unfortunately, he did not think this was good, because he had to buy so much more than the chewable tablets to get the same relief. He often drank way too much of the liquid antacid with no relief.

Mr. Selescion visits his doctor, who prescribes omeprazole to control the heartburn this patient experiences at least two to three times a week. As the weeks pass, the omeprazole does not seem to work. Mr. Selescion begins experiencing chest pain and tasting a very sour/bitter acid in the back of his throat. He also finds he cannot exercise within one hour after eating a meal. Concerned by this new development, he heads back to the doctor.

1. Based on the symptoms mentioned in this scenario, what do you think Mr. Selescion's affliction is?
   _____
   _____

2. Could Mr. Selescion have been using a better OTC medication to prevent this problem, other than chewable tablets or liquid antacid?
   _____
   _____
   _____
   _____

3. Left untreated, what are some of the complications of Mr. Selescion's condition?
   _____
   _____
   _____
   _____

4. What tests are needed to evaluate GERD?
   _____
   _____
   _____
   _____

ACTIVITY 26-3: Case Study—Bowel Trouble

Instructions: Read the following scenario and then answer the critical thinking questions.

Jill is a 47-year-old, slightly overweight woman who has had periodic episodes of constipation during the past eight years. The episodes have not been that much of an inconvenience to Jill as they usually occur after Jill eats certain foods such as bananas or cheese. Jill also has a healthy intake of water, which helps to reduce the episodes of her constipation.

Jill also experiences intermittent diarrhea aside from her episodic constipation. Occasionally, she also experiences bloating and abdominal pain that accompanies the diarrhea. As time progresses, when Jill eats—whether it is a snack or an entire meal—she is frequently experiencing these uncomfortable symptoms. They seem to only go away when she is able to have a bowel movement.

Three months later, Jill's condition has progressed into a more complicated state. If she is not actually having a bowel movement, she is experiencing the urge to do so. Jill is also experiencing consistent abdominal pain that is much stronger during the morning after she wakes up. When Jill has the urge to have a bowel movement, there is little time for her to get successfully to the toilet. If there is work or any activity that lasts more than about 30–60 minutes, Jill feels that the risk of her not making it to a bathroom in time may be consequential for her.

Jill makes an appointment with her physician. During the encounter, they both discuss her medical history. Jill apprised her physician that she takes Excedrin for occasional headaches. She also apprises him that she was using laxatives for her constipation. Other than that, she is healthy. The physician orders both blood tests and a colonoscopy to where nothing significant is found with her intestinal tract.

1. What condition is Jill most likely experiencing?

   _____

   _____

2. Why was the physician not able to find anything significant with Jill's blood test or colonoscopy?

   _____

   _____

   _____

   _____

3. Will eating certain foods, such as bananas or cheese, further exacerbate Jill's condition?

   _____

   _____

   _____

   _____

4. Is there a treatment option for Jill's condition? Could her current condition lead to other, more serious conditions?

   _____

   _____

   _____

   _____

ACTIVITY 26-4: Case Study—A Liquid Diet

Instructions: Read the following scenario and then answer the critical thinking questions.

Ms. Ferrous is a mildly overweight, 33-year-old, Indian woman who had a baby two months ago. She is not happy with the fact that she is still a bit overweight, because she wants to fit into the clothes she wore before becoming pregnant. Ms. Ferrous feels that she needs to lose weight—fast. She decides to go on a liquid diet, one of those "meal in a can" types. There are lots of flavorful choices, and she does not find it difficult to stick to the plan, which includes three cans of fluid per day, lots of water, and an occasional low-calorie snack bar.

Ms. Ferrous starts having stomach pains, so she chews Tums as if they are going out of style. When her friends tell her that she takes too many of them, she replies that she needs the calcium.

Occasionally, Ms. Ferrous's stomach pain becomes so intense that she needs to lie down for a little while and she also becomes nauseated. She begins to experience heartburn that increasingly worsens. It seems like every passing day she encounters a new pain—abdominal pain, shoulder pain, chest pain, and now the constant heartburn. Occasionally, her stomach becomes so upset that she vomits. When she does vomit, she drinks another liquid meal because she is determined to lose the weight.

One morning, as she is bathing her baby, she has an excruciating, sharp pain in the chest area. It feels like intense heartburn, and she begins to beat on her chest. Convinced that she is experiencing a heart attack, she manages to call 911. When the ambulance arrives 45 minutes later, she is hunched over on the floor from the pain in her chest.

Once at the hospital, she vomits when they give her a liquid medicine to numb her throat. After the doctor asks about her symptoms, he or she orders an ultrasound and blood tests.

1. Why did the doctor order an ultrasound when he or she discovered that Ms. Ferrous was having chest pain?

   _____

   _____

   _____

   _____

2. Once the ultrasound results are read and the condition is confirmed, what is the treatment?

   _____

   _____

   _____

   _____

3. For severe cases of this condition, what can be done to help prevent future attacks?

   _____

   _____

   _____

   _____

LAB 26-1: Treating GERD

Objective:

To understand the differences and protocols of various treatment options associated with gastrointestinal reflux disorder.

Pre-Lab Information:

• Review Chapter 26 in the textbook.

Explanation:

This exercise will help you to understand the protocol of therapies and treatment options that are most commonly prescribed for GERD.

Activity:

Using the WebMD website (http://www.webmd.com/ahrq/gerd-acid-reflux-treatments#top), please answer the following questions.

1. What is the very first type of treatment that a patient can invest in to quickly relieve the symptoms of GERD? Does this treatment require a prescription?

   _____
   _____
   _____
   _____
   _____
   _____

2. If the first line or type of treatment is not successful for a patient with relieving his or her GERD, what is the second type of treatment option that he or she can invest in to relieve the symptoms of GERD? Does this treatment option require a prescription?

   _____
   _____
   _____
   _____

3. If the second line or type of treatment is not successful for a patient with relieving his or her GERD, what is the third treatment option that he or she can invest in to relieve the symptoms of GERD? Does this treatment option require a prescription?

   _____
   _____
   _____
   _____

4. After these three prescribed and unprescribed treatment options have been proven to be ineffective for a patient, what is the final treatment option for a patient to consider in order to successfully alleviate his or her symptoms of GERD?

_____
_____
_____
_____

Student Name: _____

Lab Partner: _____

Grade/Comments: _____

_____
_____

Student Comments: _____

_____
_____

LAB 26-2: Treating Diarrhea

Objective:

To understand the role that probiotics have as a treatment option for diarrhea.

Pre-Lab Information:

- Review Chapter 26 in the textbook.

Explanation:

This exercise will help you to understand how probiotics can effectively treat diarrhea when the condition is brought on by the contributing use of an antibiotic.

Activity:

Using the following website: (http://www.onhealth.com/probiotics/article.htm#probiotics), please answer the following questions.

1. What are probiotics?

   _____

   _____

   _____

   _____

2. Please list the different types of probiotics.

   _____

   _____

   _____

   _____

3. Please list the different health benefits of probiotics.

   _____

   _____

   _____

   _____

4. Why do you think probiotics would be a good treatment option while a patient is taking antibiotics?

   _____

   _____

   _____

   _____

Student Name: _____

Lab Partner: _____

Grade/Comments: _____

_____

_____

Student Comments: _____

_____

_____

CHAPTER 27
The Musculoskeletal System

After completing Chapter 27 from the textbook, you should be able to:	Related Activity in the Workbook/Lab Manual
1. List, identify, and diagram the basic anatomical structure and parts of the muscles and bones.	Review Questions, PTCB Exam Practice Questions, Activity 27-1
2. Describe the functions of the muscles and bones and their physiology.	Review Questions, PTCB Exam Practice Questions, Activity 27-1
3. List and define common diseases affecting the muscles and bones and demonstrate an understanding of the causes, symptoms, and pharmaceutical treatments associated with each disease.	Review Questions, PTCB Exam Practice Questions, Activity 27-2, Activity 27-3, Activity 27-4, Lab 27-1, Lab 27-2
4. Describe the mechanisms and the complications of the following musculoskeletal diseases and comprehend how each class of drugs works: osteomyelitis, osteoarthritis, gout, inflammation, multiple sclerosis, and cerebral palsy.	Review Questions, PTCB Exam Practice Questions, Activity 27-2, Activity 27-3, Activity 27-4, Lab 27-1, Lab 27-2
5. List the indications for use and mechanisms of action of ASA, NSAIDs, COX-2 inhibitors, antigout agents, calcitonin, bisphosphonates, SERMs, and skeletal muscle relaxants.	Review Questions, PTCB Exam Practice Questions, Activity 27-2, Activity 27-3, Activity 27-4, Lab 27-2

INTRODUCTION

The musculoskeletal system, which consists of bones and skeletal muscles, provides the body with both form and movement. Its four main functions are to provide a framework or shape for the body, protect the internal organs, allow body movement, and provide storage for essential minerals. The musculoskeletal system is affected by numerous disorders, some of which cause only discomfort and pain, and some of which cause complete disability. Osteoporosis, the most prevalent bone disorder in the United States, affects approximately 20 million Americans and is a major cause of bone fractures. Osteoarthritis, a progressive disease of the joints, affects up to 40 million Americans.

A wide range of pharmaceuticals is used for the treatment of diseases of the musculoskeletal system, although many provide only symptomatic relief. However, as a result of intensive research, new products aimed at the prevention or retardation of disease, particularly osteoporosis and osteoarthritis, may provide hope for the millions of Americans afflicted with these debilitating diseases. As a pharmacy technician, you should be aware of the most common musculoskeletal disorders that require pharmacological treatment, including conditions treated with OTC drugs.

REVIEW QUESTIONS

Match the following.

1. _____ bones
2. _____ marrow
3. _____ cartilage
4. _____ hematopoiesis
5. _____ joints
6. _____ ligaments
7. _____ muscle
8. _____ myocyte
9. _____ sarcomere
10. _____ synovial fluid
11. _____ tendons

a. soft tissues that line every joint and give shape to the ears and nose

b. the location or position where bones are connected to each other

c. specialized tissue that contracts when stimulated

d. one of the segments into which a fibril of striated muscle is divided

e. strong fibrous bands of connective tissue that hold bones together

f. specialized form of dense connective tissue consisting of calcified intercellular substance that provides the shape and support for the body

g. a muscle cell

h. cords of connective tissue that attach muscle to bone

i. spongy type of tissue found inside most bones

j. liquid that fills the space between the cartilage of each bone; provides smooth movement by lubricating the cartilage

k. formation and development of blood cells

Choose the best answer.

12. Smooth muscles comprise or line all of the following *except*:
    a. stomach.
    b. lungs.
    c. neck.
    d. intestines.

13. Chemical and _____ interactions between actin and myosin cause muscles to react.
    a. electrical
    b. physical
    c. enzymatic
    d. synovial

14. Cranial and rib bones are classified as:
    a. long bones.
    b. short bones.
    c. flat bones.
    d. sesamoid bones.

15. An example of a bisphosphonate is:
    a. alendronate.
    b. celecoxib.
    c. calcitonin.
    d. tiludronate.

Match the following.

16. _____ osteoporosis
17. _____ bursitis
18. _____ myalgia
19. _____ anemia
20. _____ leukemia
21. _____ osteoarthritis
22. _____ rheumatoid arthritis
23. _____ gout
24. _____ osteomyelitis
25. _____ Paget's disease

a. a progressive form of arthritis that has devastating effects on the joints, body organs, and general health

b. when one or more white blood cells experience DNA loss or damage

c. bone brittleness due to lack of calcium

d. a progressive disease characterized by the breakdown of joint cartilage

e. changes the normal process of bone growth: Bone breaks down more quickly and then grows back softer than normal bone

f. failure of bone marrow to produce the components of the red blood cell

g. is an inflammation of the bursae, which are the small, fluid-filled pouches between bones and ligaments, or between bones and muscles, that serve as cushions

h. caused by an excess or overproduction of uric acid or by the inability of the kidneys to adequately excrete uric acid from the body

i. muscle pain

j. bacterial infection inside the bone that destroys bone tissue

Match the following drugs with their classifications or indications.

26. _____ Dantrium
27. _____ phenytoin
28. _____ Ridaura
29. _____ colchicine
30. _____ Dolobid
31. _____ diclofenac
32. _____ Zomig

a. gout
b. salicylate
c. direct skeletal muscle relaxant
d. seizures
e. NSAID
f. antirheumatic agent
g. spasticity

PHARMACY CALCULATION PROBLEMS

Calculate the following.

1. If an employee gets paid $100/day and has to miss an average of 12 work days each year because of fibromyalgia, how much income is the employee losing each year due to illness?

2. Calculate the monthly medical (traditional and nontraditional) expenses for this fibromyalgia patient:

   medical insurance—$150/month

   medications—$89

   chiropractic and acupuncture—$119

   massage therapy—$45

   physician co-payments—$15

3. If an insurance company pays 60% of the retail price for medications, how much is the customer's co-pay if the total retail price is $223?

4. A patient comes in with a prescription for 30 leflunomide 20 mg tablets with the directions stated as 1 tab po qd. While checking the lab to see if this drug is in your inventory, you realize that you only have the 10 mg strength in stock. The pharmacist calls the physician to change the order and the physician is in compliance with changing the strength. What will the new directions be, and how many tablets will be dispensed to the patient?

5. 6 g of active ingredient is in 120 g of a compounded ointment. What is the concentration (w/w)?

PTCB EXAM PRACTICE QUESTIONS

1. An example of an NSAID is:
   a. carisoprodol.
   b. piroxicam.
   c. baclofen.
   d. aspirin.

2. Gout is a disorder involving the deposit of which of the following compounds in the joints and soft tissues, resulting in significant pain?
   a. potassium chloride
   b. hydrochloric acid
   c. uric acid
   d. calcium chloride

3. All of the following drugs are skeletal muscle relaxants *except*:
   a. Valium.
   b. Flexeril.
   c. Robaxin.
   d. Celebrex.

4. NSAIDs are a class of drugs used to treat:
   a. infection.
   b. inflammation.
   c. muscle weakness.
   d. bone loss.

5. A combination of salicylate and an antibiotic used to treat RA is:
   a. penicillamine.
   b. SMZ/TMP.
   c. sulfasalazine.
   d. hydroxychloroquine sulfate.

ACTIVITY 27-1: Anatomy Worksheet

Types of Muscle

Label the following illustration of the different types of muscle.

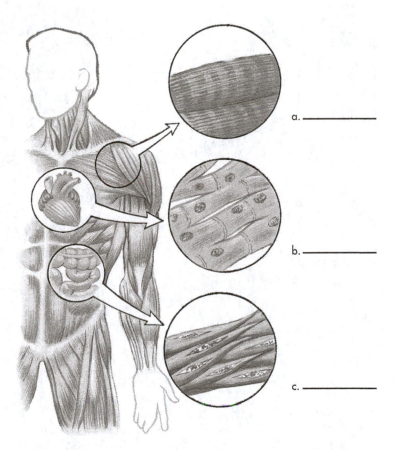

a. _____

b. _____

c. _____

The Long Bone

Label the following illustration of the long bone.

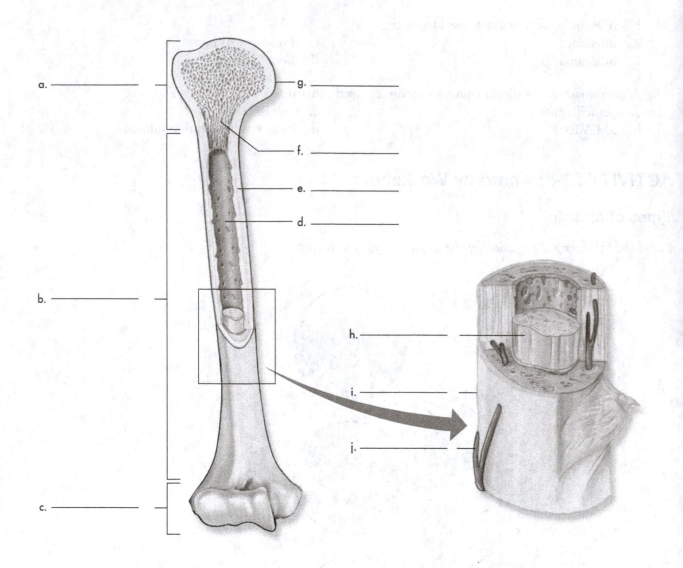

The Skeletal System

Label the following illustration of the skeletal system.

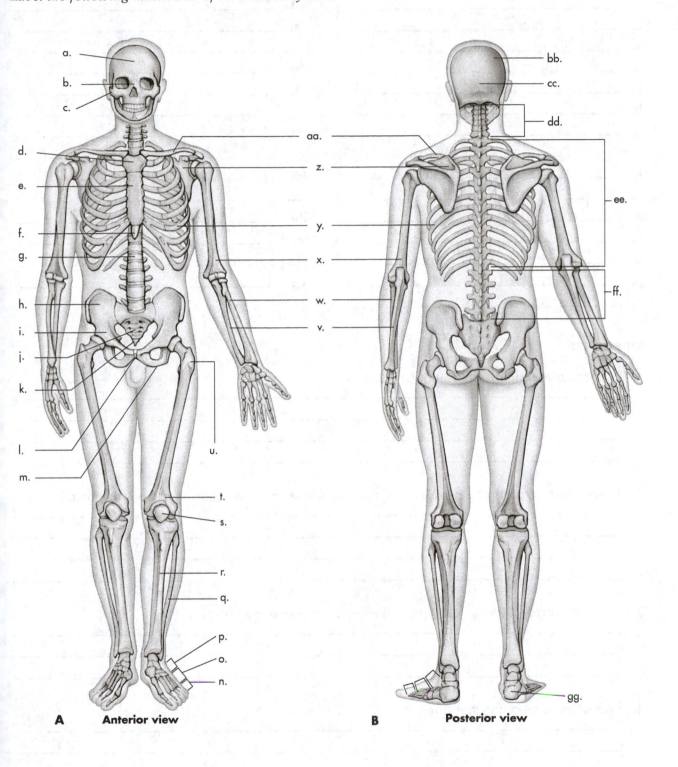

A   **Anterior view**

B   **Posterior view**

a. _____   r. _____
b. _____   s. _____
c. _____   t. _____
d. _____   u. _____
e. _____   v. _____
f. _____   w. _____
g. _____   x. _____
h. _____   y. _____
i. _____   z. _____
j. _____   aa. _____
k. _____   bb. _____
l. _____   cc. _____
m. _____   dd. _____
n. _____   ee. _____
o. _____   ff. _____
p. _____   gg. _____
q. _____

Questions:

1. Name four functions of the muscles.

_____

_____

_____

_____

2. Describe which parts of a muscle are responsible for its action and how they work together.

_____

_____

_____

_____

3. Name the three major muscle types and give an example of each.

_____

_____

_____

4. Name five or more functions of bones.

_____

_____

_____

_____

_____

5. Name the two types of bone marrow and the functions of each.

_____

_____

_____

_____

6. Research the changes that occur in the skeleton as we age. Start with an infant and end with an elderly adult. Create a timeline to track your findings.

ACTIVITY 27-2: Case Study—Arthritis and Inflammation

Instructions: Read the following scenario and then answer the critical thinking questions.

Arthur is a 57-year-old obese farmer who eats as much meat as he raises. He frequently experiences joint pain and inflammation and has for years. As the years go on, he finds it harder and harder each day to do simple things such as hitch a rope or even drive his tractor. Eventually he sees a doctor and is diagnosed with arthritis in both hands. He is prescribed NSAIDs, wears a copper bracelet, and seems to have the condition under control for now.

Early one morning, a constant throbbing pain on his hand awakens Arthur. He discovers a nodule that is red, swollen, and tender to the touch. When Arthur presses on it for relief, it moves around slightly, but it still is painful. Stubborn as he is and aware of his arthritis, he takes an NSAID and tries to go about his day. The NSAID does not work and the pain is too much, so Arthur heads in to see the doctor. For him, this is another day's work on the farm that he is losing. The doctor orders a blood and urine uric acid test but no X-ray of the bones.

1. What is this nodule on Arthur's hand? Is it arthritis?

_____

_____

2. What causes this condition in Arthur?

_____

_____

_____

_____

3. Based on the information given in the scenario, what might have contributed to this condition?

_____

_____

_____

_____

4. Initially, treatment includes timely pain relief, but how can Arthur help prevent this from happening again?

_____

_____

_____

_____

ACTIVITY 27-3: Case Study—Long Hours

Instructions: Read the following scenario and then answer the critical thinking questions.

All the pharmacy technicians at the pharmacy benefit management (PBM) company where you work put in long hours processing claims, including yourself. The scheduled hours were extended after the organization added two more employer groups. The office team and you have all been working at this pace for over a year. Luckily, everyone in the office gets along well, and everyone fulfills his or her own workload demands. The majority of the work you all perform is by using a computer and a telephone. What was once an eight-hour day has turned into 12–14 hour days that also includes going into the office on scheduled Saturdays. There is a good amount of compensation, but you are feeling as if the trade-off with less family time is not worth the extra hours.

Every so often, your hands become tired and they tingle a bit. You take a 10-minute scheduled break, go to visit the restroom, and by the time you come back, your hands do not tingle any more. One day, you are working at your computer and you find it difficult to ignore the tingling as the tingling has radiated toward your wrists as well. You remember that when you were in bed last night you could hardly sleep because your hands were numb and burning at the same time.

You take your 10-minute break as usual, hoping that the sensation will go away, but when you return to your computer you experience sharp, sudden, and piercing pains from your wrists that now radiates up toward your arms. As you are experiencing this pain, you express to your coworker that you are in a great deal of pain in both of your arms. Your coworker tells you that he or she has been having the same problem and takes about 400–800 mg of ibuprofen to reduce the pain. The coworker recommends that you do the same for the pain you are experiencing. Your coworker offers you two 200 mg ibuprofen tablets.

1. Should you follow your coworker's recommendation and take the ibuprofen he or she is offering?
   _____
   _____
   _____
   _____

2. What is the likely condition/diagnosis in this particular case?
   _____
   _____
   _____
   _____

3. Drawing from the scenario, what factors strongly contributed to your assessed diagnosis?
   _____
   _____
   _____
   _____

4. Do you believe the coworker has the same diagnosis as you do? If not, what diagnosis could the coworker have?
   _____
   _____
   _____
   _____

5. What precautions can be taken by you in order to prevent this condition from happening in your place of business?

_____

_____

_____

ACTIVITY 27-4: Case Study—Posture Changes

Instructions: Read the following scenario and then answer the critical thinking questions.

Mrs. Sweet is a 68-year-old postmenopausal woman with hypothyroidism and experiences frequent heartburn and constipation.

Mrs. Sweet is extremely proud of the roses in her garden. She spends a good amount of time tending to them daily, pruning them, and always planting new species. On Saturdays mornings, she also teaches adults and children how to grow roses at the community center in her town.

Mrs. Sweet has noticed that over the years her posture has changed. Her physician also notices the change as she is now hunched slightly forward when she goes to see him for her yearly checkup. The physician asks a few questions about her posture and if she has been noticing any pain related to her change in posture. Mrs. Sweet does state to her physician that she has been experiencing lower back pain for a few months. The physician next orders a bone mineral density assessment and an X-ray of Mrs. Sweet's spine.

1. What do you think that the physician has assessed and is contributing to Mrs. Sweet's pain?

_____

_____

2. What are the factors in this case that would contribute to Mrs. Sweet's condition?

_____

_____

_____

_____

3. What treatment and prevention options are available for Mrs. Sweet's condition?

_____

_____

_____

_____

4. What are the precautions that Mrs. Sweet should be aware of with supplements that her physician has ordered?

_____

_____

_____

_____

5. Will Mrs. Sweet have to give up her favorite activities in order to control her condition?

_____

_____

_____

_____

LAB 27-1: Treating Arthritis

Objective:

Familiarize yourself with the medications commonly prescribed and recommended for arthritis.

Pre-Lab Information:

• Review Chapter 27 in the textbook.

Explanation:

In our current market, there are many commonly prescribed medications that are used to effectively treat arthritis.

Activity:

Visit www.arthritis.org to locate the various treatment options that a patient may consider for his or her arthritis. Please answer all of the questions below and be sure to view the lists of drugs from each chart.

1. What are the nine classes of medications currently listed in the Drug Lookup section that are used to treat arthritis?

   • _____

   • _____

   • _____

   • _____

   • _____

   • _____

   • _____

   • _____

   • _____

2. Which class of medications has listed controlled substances that are used to treat arthritis?

   _____

   _____

   _____

   _____

3. What does the acronym DMARDs mean, and how are these medications effective in arthritis treatment?

   _____

   _____

   _____

   _____

   _____

4. Please provide the brand and generic names of the biologic response modifiers that are effective for arthritis.

Brand   Generic

_____   _____

_____   _____

_____   _____

_____   _____

_____   _____

5. Please provide the brand and/or generic manes of the corticosteroids that are effective for arthritis.

Brand   Generic

_____   _____

_____   _____

_____   _____

_____   _____

_____   _____

_____   _____

_____   _____

Student Name: _____

Lab Partner: _____

Grade/Comments: _____

_____

_____

Student Comments: _____

_____

_____

LAB 27-2: Treating Inflammation

Objective:

Familiarize yourself with the medications commonly prescribed and recommended for acute and chronic inflammation.

Pre-Lab Information:

• Review Chapter 27 in the textbook.

Explanation:

In our current market, there are many commonly prescribed medications that are used to effectively treat inflammation of the musculoskeletal system.

Activity:

Using the lists below, please match up the brand and generic names as well as the classes of the commonly prescribed and recommended medications that are used to effectively treat inflammation of the musculo-skeletal system.

Brand	Generic	Class
_____	_____	_____
_____	_____	_____
_____	_____	_____
_____	_____	_____
_____	_____	_____
_____	_____	_____
_____	_____	_____
_____	_____	_____
_____	_____	_____
_____	_____	_____

Brand	Generic	Class
Celebrex	meloxicam	COX-II Inhibitor
Cortef	tramadol	NSAID
Medrol	prednisolone	Corticosteroid
Motrin	hydrocodone/IBU	
Ultram	ibuprofen	
Tylenol	celecoxib	
Mobic	methylprednisolone	
Feldene	hydrocortisone	
Vicoprofen	piroxicam	
Prednisone	acetaminophen	

Student Name: _____

Lab Partner: _____

Grade/Comments: _____

_____

Student Comments: _____

_____

CHAPTER 28
The Respiratory System

After completing Chapter 28 from the textbook, you should be able to:	Related Activity in the Workbook/Lab Manual
1. Identify and list the basic anatomical and structural parts of the respiratory tract.	Review Questions, PTCB Exam Practice Questions, Activity 28-1
2. Describe the function or physiology of the individual parts of the respiratory system and the external exchange of oxygen and waste.	Review Questions, PTCB Exam Practice Questions, Activity 28-1
3. List and define common diseases affecting the respiratory tract and understand the causes, symptoms, and pharmaceutical treatment associated with each disease.	Review Questions, PTCB Exam Practice Questions, Activity 28-2, Activity 28-3, Activity 28-4, Lab 28-1, Lab 28-2, Lab 28-3
4. List the trade and generic names and identify the classification of various drugs used in treatment of diseases and conditions of the respiratory tract.	Review Questions, PTCB Exam Practice Questions, Activity 28-2, Activity 28-3, Activity 28-4, Lab 28-2, Lab 28-3

INTRODUCTION

The respiratory system is responsible for providing all cells of the body with the oxygen necessary to perform their specific functions. It is the system involved in the intake of oxygen through inhalation and the excretion of carbon dioxide through exhalation. The respiratory system is divided into two parts, the upper and lower respiratory tracts. The upper respiratory tract includes the nasal cavity, paranasal sinuses, pharynx, and larynx. The lower respiratory tract includes the trachea, two lungs, two main bronchi, secondary and tertiary bronchi, bronchioles, alveolar ducts, and alveoli.

The most common disease of the respiratory system is the common cold. Uncomplicated common colds are generally treated with over-the-counter (OTC) medications, including antihistamines, decongestants, cough suppressants, analgesics, antipyretics, and anti-inflammatories. The aim in treatment is to provide relief of symptoms. Naturally, the respiratory system is also prone to more serious diseases and conditions, such as asthma, which affect more than 15 million people and are responsible for as many as 1.5 million emergency room visits and 500,000 hospitalizations every year. If left uncontrolled, asthma can cause a long-term decline in lung function. Because many respiratory diseases are treated with some form of inhalation therapy, it is important for you, as a pharmacy technician, to be able to assist the pharmacist in educating clients as to the proper, safe use of inhalation products. You should also be aware of the most common respiratory disorders that require pharmacological treatment, including conditions treated with OTC drugs.

REVIEW QUESTIONS

Match the following.

1. _____ allergen
2. _____ allergy
3. _____ cilia
4. _____ COPD
5. _____ epiglottis
6. _____ larynx
7. _____ pharynx
8. _____ rhinitis
9. _____ trachea

a. the result of the immune system's reaction to a foreign substance
b. inflammation of the nasal passages
c. tiny hair-like organelles in the nose and bronchial passageways
d. the windpipe
e. a substance capable of causing a hypersensitivity reaction
f. a condition resulting from continual blockage of oxygen external exchange in the lungs
g. the voice box
h. small, leaf-shaped cartilage attached to the tongue that prevents substances other than air from entering the trachea
i. part of the throat from the back of the nasal cavity to the larynx

Choose the best answer.

10. The primary function of the respiratory system is to:
    a. transport air to and from the lungs.
    b. supply oxygen to the blood.
    c. exchange oxygen for carbon dioxide.
    d. keep the brain alive.

11. The two purposes of the respiratory system are:
    a. to prevent allergens coming into the airways and filter out contaminants.
    b. transport of air (gases) to and from the lungs and exchange of oxygen for carbon dioxide.
    c. exhaling and inhaling.
    d. maintaining an adequate supply of oxygen to the brain and exhaling carbon dioxide.

12. The exchange of gases between blood and cells is called:
    a. pulmonary ventilation.
    b. internal respiration.
    c. external respiration.
    d. cellular respiration.

13. Which does not belong to the conducting portion of the respiratory system?
    a. alveoli
    b. bronchioles
    c. nose
    d. pharynx

14. A common lay term for the larynx is:
    a. Bob's apple.
    b. Adam's apple.
    c. Adam's orange.
    d. Eve's apple.

15. The exchange of gases occurs in the:
    a. trachea.
    b. bronchioles.
    c. alveoli.
    d. bronchus.

16. The volume of air that can be exhaled after normal exhalation is the:
    a. tidal volume.
    b. residual volume.
    c. inspiratory reserve volume.
    d. expiratory reserve volume.

17. The volume of air in a normal breath is called:
    a. total lung capacity.
    b. vital capacity.
    c. tidal volume.
    d. residual volume.

18. Gas exchange in the lungs is done by the process of:
    a. osmosis.
    b. diffusion.
    c. exocytosis.
    d. active transport.

19. The first line of immunity defense is:
    a. a rise in histamine levels.
    b. a rise in white blood cell count.
    c. mucus produced by the lungs.
    d. mucus produced in the nose and throat.

20. The primary chemical stimulus for breathing is the concentration of:
    a. carbon monoxide in the blood.
    b. carbon dioxide in the blood.
    c. oxygen in the blood.
    d. carbonic acid in the blood.

21. Asthma is a disorder that can be:
    a. cured with proper medication.
    b. treated with proper medication, but not cured.
    c. neither effectively treated nor cured.
    d. cured with antibiotics.

22. A bacterial infection most commonly found in the lungs and can spread to other parts of the body is:
    a. influenza.
    b. tuberculosis.
    c. pneumonia.
    d. pertussis.

For questions 23–27, correctly order the structures of the respiratory passageways through which air moves as it enters the body.

23. _____ pharynx

24. _____ trachea

25. _____ larynx

26. _____ bronchi

27. _____ bronchiole

Fill in the blanks.

28. _____ is the mechanism through which gases are exchanged.

29. _____ supports respiration by maintaining fluids, providing immunity, and removing inhaled solid materials and microorganisms.

30. Pneumonia is an illness of the _____ respiratory system.

PHARMACY CALCULATION PROBLEMS

Calculate the following.

1. If an inhaler contains 120 metered doses, how many days will the inhaler last if the patient is using 2 puffs qid prn?

2. A patient is using one levalbuterol 0.63 mg nebule in her home nebulizer tid. If levalbuterol comes in a box of 24 nebules, how many boxes will she need for a 24-day supply?

3. A patient is using an albuterol-ipratropium inhaler. The patient is using 2 puffs qid and prn, max 12 puffs/day. The inhaler contains 200 metered doses, calculate the day supply for this patient.

4. How many theophylline 200 mg tablets will be needed for a 30-day supply if the patient takes 1 po tid?

5. A five-year old female patient is prescribed albuterol syrup 0.2 mg/kg tid. The patient weighs 35 lbs. and the dosage is not to exceed 12 mg/day. Is the dose prescribed safe for this patient to take?

PTCB EXAM PRACTICE QUESTIONS

1. During respiration, the body inhales _____ and exhales _____.
   a. nitrogen, carbon dioxide
   b. oxygen, nitrogen
   c. oxygen, carbon dioxide
   d. carbon dioxide, oxygen

2. The common cold should *not* be treated with which medication?
   a. an analgesic
   b. an antibiotic
   c. a mucolytic
   d. a decongestant

3. Which of the following is *not* a respiratory disease?
   a. asthma
   b. GERD
   c. COPD
   d. emphysema

4. The Combat Methamphetamine Epidemic Act of 2005 requires nonprescription products to be sold from behind the pharmacy counter if they contain any of the following ingredients *except*:
   a. dextromethorphan.
   b. ephedrine.
   c. pseudoephedrine.
   d. phenylpropanolamine.

5. Which of the following drugs would be considered the most appropriate for an acute asthma attack?
   a. albuterol
   b. Singulair
   c. amoxicillin
   d. Flagyl

ACTIVITY 28-1: Anatomy Worksheet

The Upper Respiratory Tract

Label the following illustration of the upper respiratory tract.

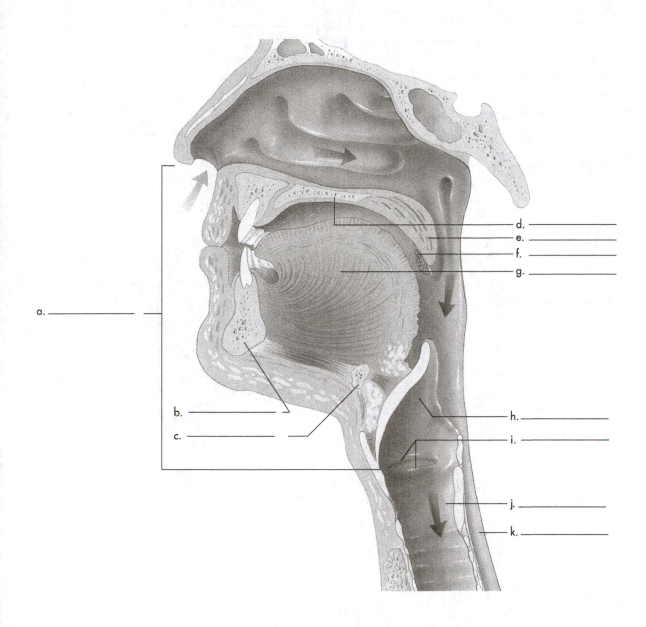

The Lower Respiratory Tract

Label the following illustration of the lower respiratory tract.

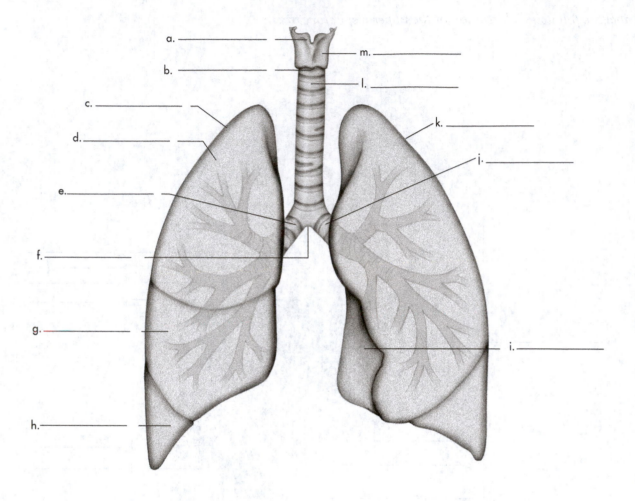

a. _____

b. _____

c. _____

d. _____

e. _____

f. _____

g. _____

h. _____

m. _____

l. _____

k. _____

j. _____

i. _____

The Lungs

Label the following illustration of the lungs.

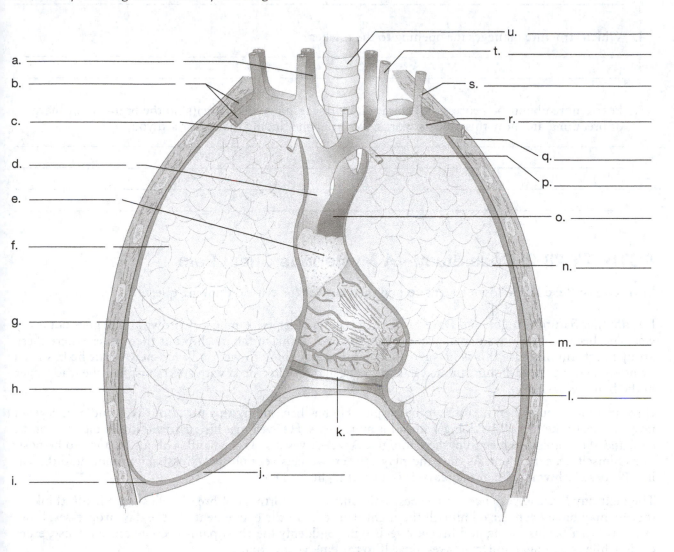

a. _____

b. _____

c. _____

d. _____

e. _____

f. _____

g. _____

h. _____

i. _____

j. _____

k. _____

l. _____

m. _____

n. _____

o. _____

p. _____

q. _____

r. _____

s. _____

t. _____

u. _____

Questions

1. Describe the two main functions of the respiratory system.

   _____

   _____

   _____

   _____

2. What occurs if a part of the body does not receive enough oxygen? What is the medical term for this?

   _____

   _____

   _____

   _____

CHAPTER 28 *The Respiratory System*   **421**

3. Which muscle is responsible for breathing?

_____

_____

4. Which structure manages the opening to the trachea?

_____

_____

5. Learn more about the process of respiration by researching which area(s) in the brain are in charge of breathing and how this process works. Describe one finding that surprised you.

_____

_____

_____

_____

ACTIVITY 28-2: Case Study—A Mysterious Chest Pain

Instructions: Read the following scenario and then answer the critical thinking questions.

It is another Saturday night, and Dave's favorite punk band is performing downtown. Dave goes out every weekend because he enjoys dancing and getting thrown about in the mosh pit at the venues where these groups perform. Because this is his favorite band, Dave is going to wear a brand-new outfit he has been dying to debut: printed T-shirt, printed flat sneakers, and a jacket laced with spikes just like the lead singer in the band wears.

Dave is no amateur when it comes to mosh pits. He has been doing this for about two and a half years now and feels like he will be doing it for a lot more years. He even met his girlfriend in the pit six months ago, and she is going to meet him there tonight. Dave arrives just as the band is about to start, so he positions himself near the front. As the band plays, the crowd gets very physical, tossing, jumping, and thrashing. Bodies clash while the music plays. It is a great night for Dave.

The next day Dave experiences some chest pain and some shortness of breath. He shrugs it off, thinking that he may have overexerted himself the night before in all the excitement. As the day progresses, however, his heart begins racing and his chest feels tight. Suddenly the chest pains become more intense, especially while coughing, and Dave takes himself to the emergency room.

At the emergency room, they initially think Dave is having a heart attack, because he is gripping his chest. They listen to his chest and are unable to find breathing sounds in the left lung. An X-ray is ordered so that the physicians can see if air is outside the lung. While Dave has his shirt off in the X-ray department, the technician notices a puncture wound in his back. The results of the X-ray are positive for air outside the lung.

1. What is Dave's condition?

_____

_____

2. Based on the scenario, what likely led Dave to acquire this condition?

_____

_____

_____

_____

3. What is the treatment for this condition?

_____

_____

_____

_____

4. How do you think this experience will affect his favorite mosh pit activity?

_____

_____

_____

_____

ACTIVITY 28-3: Case Study—A New Baby

Instructions: Read the following scenario and then answer the critical thinking questions.

Mr. and Mrs. Kent have successfully delivered a baby girl. Mrs. Kent is taking the next three months off from work to care for her newborn baby.

A short time after they take the baby home, they notice that the baby's stool is greasy and has a strong, pungent odor. Being first-time parents, they believe that this is normal. Shortly after this discovery, though, they notice that the baby coughs a lot and the Kent's feel that the cough is excessive. As both Mr. and Mrs. Kent are in excellent health, the Kent's bring the baby to the pediatrician.

The baby does present with a consistent, productive, and strong cough. A stool sample is ordered when Mrs. Kent explains to the pediatrician of the smelly stool situation. The baby's diaper is also full of diarrhea. The doctor orders an examination of the sputum, blood tests, as well as a sweat test.

1. What condition or disease does the pediatrician suspect might be causing these symptoms?

_____

_____

_____

2. Why does the pediatrician order a sweat test and examination of the sputum? What will the results of the exams and tests prove to the pediatrician and to the Kent's?

_____

_____

_____

_____

3. What is the average life span of a person with this disease? What complication will a patient diagnosed with the disease usually die from?

_____

_____

_____

_____

4. How can the baby have this disease when neither parent has symptoms of this disease?

_____

_____

_____

_____

5. How do you think that the baby's recent diagnosis of her disease might now change the family's lifestyle choices?

_____

_____

_____

_____

ACTIVITY 28-4: Case Study—Multi-Ingredient Products

Instructions: Read the following scenario and then answer the critical thinking questions.

The Hendersen family is home sick with a cold. Dad, Mom, 16-year-old Shari, 11-year-old Dan, and 18-month-old Brandy all have severe nasal congestion and coughs. As awful as Mrs. Hendersen is feeling, she has made several trips to the local grocery-pharmacy chain store to purchase different cold remedies for her family members. Mrs. Hendersen has purchased the remedies in the dosage forms of capsules, gelcaps, disintegrating tablets, and powders that are mixed into liquids.

At first, Mrs. Hendersen chose the OTC product that she recalled seeing advertised in the magazines she has read. As time moved on while herself and the family have not gotten any relief from the first product, Mrs. Hendersen started making product choices based on the attractive packaging as well as the many ingredients that were in the formulation, believing that if there is more it should work better for her and her family.

Frustrated by all of her attempts to find an OTC product that would work, Mrs. Hendersen decides to stop by the pharmacy on her next visit to the grocery-pharmacy chain. She then asks the pharmacist for a recommendation of the most effective OTC product that would help her and her family. The pharmacist asks if she or her family members have any other symptoms aside from the nasal congestion. Mrs. Hendersen then replies no. The pharmacist provides Mrs. Hendersen with the standard information about drinking plenty of fluids, chicken soup, and using saline nasal drops. The pharmacist then suggests to Mrs. Hendersen that she should take a decongestant; however, there is one family member who will not be able to take the decongestant.

1. Based on the information in the scenario, what was Mrs. Kent doing or not doing successfully by selecting the different medications she had purchased?

_____

_____

_____

_____

2. What way is the common cold commonly contracted?

_____

_____

_____

_____

3. What can be done to avoid spreading the common cold to individuals?

_____

_____

_____

_____

4. Which family member was the pharmacist referring to as the one family member who could not use the decongestant? Why?

_____

_____

_____

_____

5. What other medicines might negatively interact with OTC decongestants?

_____

_____

_____

_____

LAB 28-1: Proper Usage and Maintenance of a Nebulizer Machine

Objectives:

Demonstrate the proper use and maintenance of a nebulizer machine.

Demonstrate ability to teach patients how to set up, use, and clean a nebulizer.

Pre-Lab Information:

Gather the materials needed:

- nebulizer machine
- nebulizer kit assembly, including:
  - nebulizer cup unit
  - tubing
  - mouthpiece or mask
  - tee adapter
  - training respiratory treatment or normal saline ampule
  - nebulizer filter
  - warm water
  - mild detergent solution
  - vinegar

Explanation:

If you work as a pharmacy technician in a retail pharmacy setting, you will need to assist patients who require prescribed nebulizer treatments. Many patients do not learn from their physicians how to set up, use, and clean the nebulizer properly; this means that your skilled assistance is critical to them and ensures proper medication compliance.

Activity:

Part 1

Procedure: Operating a Nebulizer Machine

1. Open the nebulizer cup unit by turning it counterclockwise. Pour the medication (3 mL training respiratory treatment or normal saline) into the bottom portion of the unit.
2. Close the nebulizer by turning the cup unit clockwise.
3. Connect one end of the tubing to the air outlet located on the nebulizer machine and the other end of the tubing to the nebulizer cup unit.
4. Attach the tee adapter to the top of the nebulizer cup unit.
5. Attach the mouthpiece or mask to one end of the tee adapter, leaving the opposite end open.
6. Connect the nebulizer machine to a power outlet and turn on the machine using the ON/OFF switch. It is normal for the machine to make a loud vibrating sound and to emit a smoking mist from both ends of the tee adapter.
7. The patient should insert the mouthpiece into the mouth, or have a mask secured over the nose and mouth and then breathe normally until the treatment is complete.
8. Upon completion of the treatment, turn the nebulizer machine off and remove the nebulizer kit assembly for proper cleaning.

Part 2

Procedure: Cleaning/Maintenance of a Nebulizer Kit Assembly

1. After each use, the nebulizer kit assembly should be cleaned to avoid possible infection.
2. Clean each component of the nebulizer kit assembly, excluding the tubing, with warm water and a mild detergent solution.
3. Rinse the components with warm water for 30 seconds to remove the detergent.
4. Soak all the parts in a mixture of 3 parts warm water to 1 part vinegar for 30 minutes.
5. Rinse the components with warm water and allow them to air-dry on clean paper towels.
6. The nebulizer filter should be changed every six months or as soon as it turns a gray color.

Discussion Questions:

1. Why is it important for pharmacy technicians to be knowledgeable about the operation and maintenance of nebulizer machines?

   _____

   _____

   _____

   _____

2. Which patient categories would benefit from using a face mask for administration, as opposed to a mouthpiece?

   _____

   _____

   _____

   _____

3. Why is it important that the nebulizer components be cleaned following each treatment?

   _____

   _____

   _____

   _____

Student Name: _____

Lab Partner: _____

Grade/Comments: _____

_____

_____

Student Comments: _____

_____

_____

LAB 28-2: Treating Allergies

Objective:

To understand the different treatment options that allergic reaction and/or allergic condition from seasonal or yearly allergies are treated both pre and post reaction or condition.

Pre-Lab Information:

- Review Chapter 28 in the textbook.

Explanation:

Many consumers and patients, during the course of their lives, may experience the unfortunate effects and symptoms of an allergic reaction and/or allergic condition from seasonal or yearly allergies. There are many treatment options for these consumers and patients to consider and also to take precautions with so that their allergic reaction and/or allergic condition may not be bothersome and/or potentially fatal for them.

Activity:

Match the following allergic reaction and/or allergic condition to the class and medications from the following lists.

Hint: Different OTC medications might be used by a consumer for an allergic condition or reaction.

Allergic Condition/Allergic Reaction

Poison Ivy _____

Allergic rhinitis _____

Sneezing _____

Foods _____

Runny nose _____

Antibiotics _____

Bee sting _____

Urticaria _____

Seasonal allergies _____

Poison oak _____

Watery eyes _____

Class/Medication

a) Nasal corticosteroids/beclomethasone, flunisolide, fluticasone, triamcinolone

b) H-1 antagonist/cetirizine, diphenhydramine, fexofenadine, hydroxyzine, loratadine

c) Topical antihistamine/diphenhydramine, fexofenadine

d) Topical corticosteroid/hydrocortisone

e) Vasopressor/sympathomimetic/epinephrine

f) Oral decongestant/phenylephrine

Student Name: _____

Lab Partner: _____

Grade/Comments: _____

_____

_____

Student Comments: _____

_____

_____

LAB 28-3: Treating Asthma

Objective:

To understand asthma and the different treatment options for patients who are diagnosed with asthma.

Pre-Lab Information:

- Review Chapter 28 in the textbook.
- Visit the website www.asthma.com

Explanation:

To date, there are more than 15 million individuals who have been diagnosed with asthma. There are many different classes of medications and medications within those classes that are prescribed for patients who are affected by this disease.

Activity:

While visiting the website www.asthma.com, take a few minutes to visit the toolbox and take the "DO I HAVE ASTHMA?" questionnaire, as well as take the "TEST YOUR ASTHMA CONTROL" "FOR ADULTS" questionnaire. Even if you do not have asthma, answering these questions may assist you with enhancing your customer service skills while working with the patients you know have asthma.

Next explore the MANAGE tab at the website. Please answer the following questions below.

1. What is a peak flow meter?
   _____
   _____
   _____

2. Peak flow readings can help a health care provider to determine:
   - _____
   - _____
   - _____

3. What is spirometry test? Is this test a common or uncommon test to diagnose asthma?
   _____
   _____
   _____

4. What is the class of medication within the "QUICK-RELIEF" tab?
   _____

5. What are the classes of medications within the "LONG-TERM" tab?
   _____
   _____
   _____
   _____

6. What is the class of medication within the "COMBINATION" tab?

_____

7. What are the classes of medications within the "OTHER" tab?

_____

_____

8. What are the four types of "DELIVERY DEVICES" that a patient might use to effectively treat his or her asthma?

_____

_____

_____

9. What are the "OTHER THERAPIES" that patients might consider to manage their asthma?

_____

_____

_____

_____

10. While visiting the "ASTHMA BASICS FOR PARENTS," what is the 2010 statistic of people with asthma who are children? _____

11. What should a parent do to help their child manage his or her asthma?

_____

_____

_____

_____

12. If a child is old enough to participate with managing his or her asthma, what should the parent do to help the child understand?

_____

_____

_____

_____

Student Name: _____

Lab Partner: _____

Grade/Comments: _____

_____

_____

Student Comments: _____

_____

_____

CHAPTER 29

The Cardiovascular, Circulatory, and Lymph Systems

After completing Chapter 29 from the textbook, you should be able to:	Related Activity in the Workbook/Lab Manual
1. List, identify, and diagram the basic anatomical structure and parts of the heart.	Review Questions, PTCB Exam Practice Questions, Activity 29-1
2. Explain the function of the heart and the circulation of the blood within the body.	Review Questions, PTCB Exam Practice Questions, Activity 29-1
3. List and define common diseases affecting the heart, including the causes, symptoms, and pharmaceutical treatment associated with each disease.	Review Questions, PTCB Exam Practice Questions, Activity 29-2, Activity 29-3, Activity 29-4, Activity 29-5, Lab 29-1, Lab 29-2
4. Explain how each class of drugs works to mitigate symptoms of heart diseases.	Review Questions, PTCB Exam Practice Questions, Lab 29-1, Lab 29-2
5. Describe the mechanism of action of anticoagulants, indications for use, and antidotes for overdose.	Review Questions
6. List a variety of drugs intended to affect the cardiovascular system, their classifications, and the average adult dose.	Review Questions, PTCB Exam Practice Questions
7. List the total cholesterol, LDL, HDL, and triglyceride ranges for an average adult, and describe the differences between HDL, LDL, and triglycerides.	Review Questions, Activity 29-5, Lab 29-1, Lab 29-2
8. Describe the structure and main functions of the lymphatic system, and explain its relationship to the cardiovascular system.	Review Questions, PTCB Exam Practice Questions, Activity 29-1

INTRODUCTION

The cardiovascular system, or circulatory system, is responsible for transporting blood to all parts of the body. It includes the heart, arteries, arterioles, veins, venules, and capillaries. The arteries are responsible for carrying oxygen-rich blood to the cells, while the veins carry the deoxygenated blood back to the heart and lungs. The lungs and respiratory system work in tandem with the cardiovascular system to sustain life. To accomplish its primary purpose as a pumping mechanism that circulates blood to all parts of the body, the heart relies on a conduction system comprised of nodes and nodal tissues that regulate the various aspects of the heartbeat. In addition, the nervous system plays a vital role in regulating heart rate. The lymphatic system and circulatory system also work closely together as blood and lymph fluid move through the same capillary system. Lymph fluid removes wastes and debris from the body and supports the immune system by filtering out pathogens and draining excess fluid from the body.

The two common diseases affecting the cardiovascular system are congestive heart failure (CHF) and coronary artery disease (CAD). CHF occurs when the heart pumps out less blood than it receives, resulting in a weakened and enlarged heart, and in less blood being pumped to feed the other organs. CAD is a condition characterized by insufficient blood flow to the heart. Hypertension, or high blood pressure, and hyperlipidemia, or high blood cholesterol, are two additional conditions that affect the cardiovascular system. Often, both hypertension and hyperlipidemia go undetected, as these conditions do not cause substantial symptoms. As a pharmacy technician, you should also be aware of the most common cardiovascular disorders that require pharmacological treatment, including conditions treated with over-the-counter (OTC) drugs.

REVIEW QUESTIONS

Match the following.

1. _____ arterioles
2. _____ atrioventricular valves
3. _____ contractility
4. _____ DOC
5. _____ DVT
6. _____ dyscrasia
7. _____ hematuria
8. _____ hyperlipidemia
9. _____ leukocyte
10. _____ venules
11. _____ plaque
12. _____ pulmonary edema
13. _____ hematuria
14. _____ semilunar valves
15. _____ thrombophlebitis

a. the smallest veins
b. the smallest arteries
c. high concentrations of lipids in the blood
d. large quantities of protein in the urine
e. include the tricuspid and mitral valves of the heart
f. inflammation of a vein with a thrombus
g. the drug preferred for treatment of a particular condition or disease
h. the ability to contract; also, the degree of contraction
i. a blood clot in one of the veins of the legs or other deep veins
j. a white blood cell
k. abnormal condition of the body, especially a blood imbalance
l. include the aortic and pulmonary valves of the heart
m. blood in the urine
n. fluid collection in the pulmonary vessels or lungs
o. fatty deposits that are high in cholesterol

Choose the best answer.

16. The human body contains _____ of blood.
    a. 4,300 gallons
    b. 15.6 L
    c. 5.6 L
    d. none of the above

17. The heart muscle pumps _____ of blood daily.
    a. 4,300 gallons
    b. 16.6 L
    c. 5.6 L
    d. none of the above

18. The _____, a double layer of serous and fibrous tissue, is a fluid-filled sac that surrounds and protects the heart. It also permits free movement of the heart during contraction.
   a. endocardium
   b. myocardium
   c. septum
   d. pericardium

19. The two top chambers of the heart are called:
   a. ventricles.
   b. valves.
   c. atria.
   d. arteries.

20. The two bottom chambers of the heart are called:
   a. ventricles.
   b. valves.
   c. atria.
   d. arteries.

21. Which of the following is not a risk factor for high blood pressure?
   a. genetics
   b. stress
   c. race
   d. heart size

Match each medication with its classification.

22. _____ flecainide
23. _____ propranolol
24. _____ sotalol
25. _____ spironolactone
26. _____ hydrochlorothiazide
27. _____ bumetanide
28. _____ methazolamide
29. _____ hydralazine
30. _____ nitroglycerin
31. _____ captopril
32. _____ irbesartan
33. _____ pindolol
34. _____ atenolol
35. _____ clonidine
36. _____ clopidogrel
37. _____ warfarin
38. _____ atorvastatin
39. _____ gemfibrozil
40. _____ nicotinic acid

a. angiotensin II receptor blocker
b. antiplatelet agent
c. coronary vasodilator
d. selective beta-adrenergic blocker
e. Class II antiarrhythmic
f. anticoagulant
g. water-soluble vitamin
h. nonselective beta-adrenergic blocker
i. carbonic anhydrase inhibitor
j. HMG CoA reductase inhibitor
k. thiazide diuretic
l. Class I antiarrhythmic
m. ACE inhibitor
n. Class III antiarrhythmic
o. potassium-sparing diuretic
p. lipid-regulating agent
q. peripheral vasodilator
r. loop diuretic
s. antiadrenergic agent

PHARMACY CALCULATION PROBLEMS

Calculate the following.

1. A patient is to receive lidocaine 2 g/250 mL IV that will run at 2 mg/min. What is the infusion rate in milliliters per hour?

2. If an amiodarone drip is to run at 33 mL/hr for six hours, how many milligrams of drug will be infused in that time if the bottle contains 500 mg/250 mL?

3. A patient weighing 240 lbs. is receiving dopamine 5 mcg/kg/min IV. The concentration of the dopamine bag is 400 mg/250 mL. What is the infusion rate in milliliters per hour?

4. An infant patient has been prescribed heparin 10 units q6–8h. On stock you have 100 units/mL. How many milliliters will you prepare to cover 24 hours?

5. What concentration (v/v) would be obtained when 20 mL of alcohol is combined with 60 mL of SWFI?

PTCB EXAM PRACTICE QUESTIONS

1. What is the American Heart Association's recommendation for healthy blood pressure levels?
   a. 80/120
   b. 140/90
   c. 120/80
   d. 90/140

2. Which of the following drugs is *not* used to treat hyperlipidemia?
   a. Toprol
   b. Questran
   c. Zocor
   d. Tricor

3. Which of the following is used as the antidote for a heparin overdose?
   a. vitamin K
   b. protamine sulfate
   c. enoxaparin
   d. warfarin

4. In the cardiovascular system, _____ carries oxygenated blood to the cells and _____ carries deoxygenated blood back to the heart and lungs.
   a. arteries, veins
   b. veins, arteries
   c. arterioles, veins
   d. capillaries, veins

5. INR as it relates to blood coagulation stands for:
   a. independent normalized ratio.
   b. international nominal ratio.
   c. international normalized ratio.
   d. international normalized rations.

ACTIVITY 29-1: Anatomy Worksheet

The Heart

Label the following illustration of the heart.

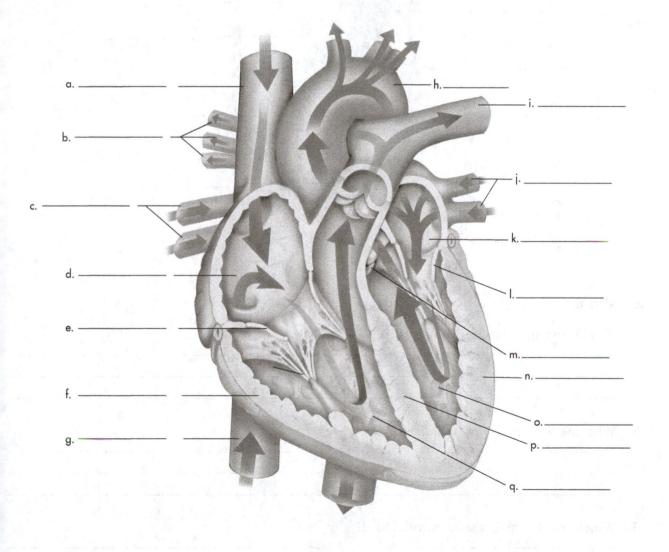

a. _____

b. _____

c. _____

d. _____

e. _____

f. _____

g. _____

h. _____

i. _____

j. _____

k. _____

l. _____

m. _____

n. _____

o. _____

p. _____

q. _____

Pulmonary Circulation

Label the following illustration showing pulmonary circulation.

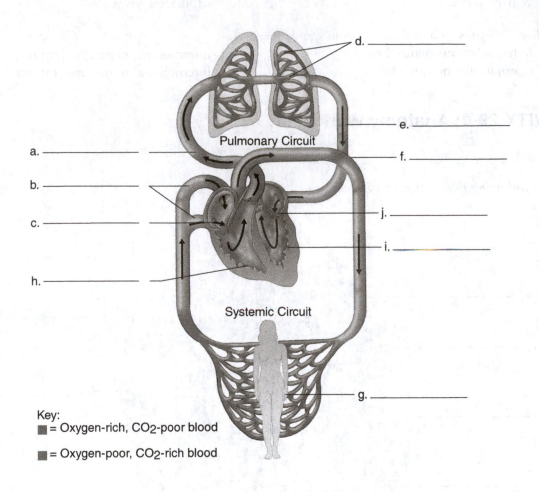

Key:
■ = Oxygen-rich, CO2-poor blood

■ = Oxygen-poor, CO2-rich blood

Questions:

1. What is the main function of the heart?
    _____
    _____
    _____

2. What are three functions of blood?
    _____
    _____
    _____

3. Which vessels supply the heart with blood?
    _____
    _____
    _____

4. Describe the process of pulmonary circulation in your own words. Use your textbook or other medical resources to help you.

_____

_____

_____

_____

_____

_____

5. Describe the cardiac cycle in your own words. Use your textbook or other medical resources to help you.

_____

_____

_____

_____

_____

6. How is lymph circulated throughout the body?

_____

_____

_____

_____

ACTIVITY 29-2: Case Study—Leg Pain

Instructions: Read the following scenario and then answer the critical thinking questions.

Eleanor Stark is an active and healthy 62-year-old woman who volunteers at the community food bank up to four days a week. Other than docusate sodium for constipation and an occasional acetaminophen for pain, the maintenance medication she takes consistently is estrogen. Eleanor recently returned from a visit to her sister's home, 10 states away, where she traveled by bus for three days.

Eleanor is now presenting with pain and tenderness in one leg. She says that it feels hot, and it is red-hot as the leg is swelling up a bit more each day. She makes an appointment with her physician when she can no longer tolerate the pain in her leg. Eleanor is sent to the hospital by her physician and is admitted there to treat her condition.

1. What condition does Eleanor have?

_____

_____

2. Based on the facts presented to you about Eleanor, what is the cofactor that has placed her in a high-risk category for this condition?

_____

_____

3. What treatment option or therapy is first-line protocol for Eleanor's condition?

_____

4. What is the goal of the therapy for Eleanor's condition?

_____

_____

5. Because Eleanor is a very active lady and does not desire being in the hospital for her current therapy, is there an alternative therapy option for her and her physician to agree with?

_____

_____

ACTIVITY 29-3: Case Study—A Medical Emergency

Instructions: Read the following scenario and then answer the critical thinking questions.

An ambulance is dispatched to an apartment complex about 45 minutes away from the nearest hospital. Mr. Jones' neighbor has called 911, stating she heard a suspicious thump and that he did not respond to her knocking on his door. The ambulance and fire truck arrives to Mr. Jones' door at 6:30 a.m. as the firemen pound on the door of Mr. Jones' apartment. They hear a whimper from inside the apartment and the firemen pry open the door. They find a man, about 50 years old, hunched over a chair clenching his fist against the center of his chest.

Mr. Jones states that his chest is tight and it has been feeling that way for almost an hour. He states that he does not have pain anywhere else. The paramedics ask him about his medical history as Mr. Jones reveals that he has high blood pressure and has been prescribed nitroglycerin for chest pain. Mr. Jones also states that because of the sudden onset of his chest pain, he could not get to it in the bathroom medicine cabinet.

On the way to the hospital, Mr. Jones has been administered three doses of nitroglycerin 0.4 mg sublingual that provides him no relief. The paramedics provide oxygen therapy to Mr. Jones as well as, administer him an IV push of morphine. Within minutes, the pain is subsiding. Upon arrival to the emergency department, a nurse begins an IV of nitroglycerin.

1. What does a clenched fist mean to emergency personnel?

_____

_____

2. How does nitroglycerin work in the body? How does it provide relief for Mr. Jones?

_____

_____

3. What safety precaution, in relation to a patient's blood pressure, must be considered when using nitroglycerin?

_____

_____

4. Why is the morphine subsiding Mr. Jones's pain?

_____

_____

ACTIVITY 29-4: Case Study—A Bad Headache

Instructions: Read the following scenario and then answer the critical thinking questions.

Carmen is a 54-year-old, diabetic, overweight mother of six children who range in age from 32 to 7. She has always been a model housewife and mother, preparing all family meals, keeping the house tidy, and helping the children with schoolwork. In addition to taking care of her children, she is also raising two grandchildren, ages 7 and 9. Carmen's medical history includes diabetes, asthma, periodic constipation, heartburn, and mild depression at times.

One evening, Carmen develops a mild headache and takes some acetaminophen before retiring to sleep after another long day. By morning, her headache is so bad that her head is throbbing, she is sensitive to light, her ears are ringing, and she sees spots before her eyes. She cannot get out of bed because moving intensifies the headache.

1. What do you suspect is going on with Carmen?

   _____

   _____

2. What tests might be conducted to confirm this diagnosis?

   _____

   _____

3. What lifestyle changes could Carmen make that would make a difference in her health condition?

   _____

   _____

ACTIVITY 29-5: Analyzing Cholesterol Screening Test Results

In Chapter 29 of the textbook, you learned about the role cholesterol plays in causing heart disease, stroke, and other health conditions. Physicians screen their patients to determine their lipid levels: total cholesterol, LDL, HDL, and triglycerides. They then compare these levels against acceptable ranges to determine if a patient may be at risk for developing a heart attack or stroke. They then use this information to decide if the patient requires medication, lifestyle and/or behavioral changes, or a combination of both.

As a pharmacy technician, it is important for you to understand how the cholesterol screening tests work and to be familiar with the different ranges. Your place of employment may also offer free screenings to patients or customers.

Part One

Review the information on cholesterol in Chapter 29 of your textbook. Then, visit the American Heart Association website and locate the information sheet called "What Do My Cholesterol Levels Mean?" (http://www.americanheart.org/presenter.jhtml?identifier=3004817). Now, answer the following questions.

1. What does the abbreviation *HDL* mean?
   _____

2. Why is HDL considered "good" cholesterol?
   _____
   _____

3. What is the normal range, for both women and men, for HDL cholesterol?
   _____
   _____

4. What does the abbreviation *LDL* mean?
   _____

5. Why is this considered "bad" cholesterol?
   _____
   _____

6. What is the normal range for LDL cholesterol? What is an optimal range for a person at risk of heart attack or death from heart attack? What is an optimal range for a person with heart disease or diabetes?
   _____
   _____

7. What are triglycerides, and how are they related to heart disease?
   _____
   _____

8. What is a normal range for triglycerides?
   _____
   _____

Part Two

Now you will review some cholesterol screening test results for three fictitious patients. Review the results, then go to http://www.americanheart.org/presenter.jhtml?identifier=183 to determine the ranges for each patient and answer the related questions.

Patient 1

Mary Smathers, age 53, had her annual physical checkup last week. Here are the results of her cholesterol screening.

Lipid Screen	Result	What is the range for this patient?
Total cholesterol	181	
Triglycerides	56	
HDL cholesterol	74	
LDL cholesterol	96	

1. Based on these ranges, does Mary Smathers appear to be at risk for developing coronary heart disease?

_____

2. How about her risk of having a heart attack or stroke?

_____

Patient 2

John Price, age 83, just received the results of his cholesterol screening.

Lipid Screen	Result	What is the range for this patient?
Total cholesterol	242	
Triglycerides	163	
HDL cholesterol	32	
LDL cholesterol	140	

1. Based on these ranges, does John Price appear to be at risk for developing coronary heart disease?

_____

2. How about his risk of having a heart attack or stroke?

_____

3. Name five things John can do to improve his lipid result numbers.

_____

_____

_____

_____

_____

4. What are some risk factors for coronary heart disease?

_____

_____

_____

_____

Patient 3

Manny Lewis, an overweight smoker in his 50s, also received the results of his cholesterol screening.

Lipid Screen	Result	What is the range for this patient?
Total cholesterol	198	
Triglycerides	153	
HDL cholesterol	37	
LDL cholesterol	119	

1. Based on his levels, what condition is Manny at risk of developing?

_____

_____

2. What specific lifestyle changes should Manny adopt immediately to improve his numbers?

_____

_____

LAB 29-1: Treating High Blood Pressure

Objectives:

To understand the different treatment options for high blood pressure.

Pre-Lab Information:

• Review Chapter 29 in the textbook.

Explanation:

Many patients have been diagnosed with hypertension or high blood pressure. The American Heart Association has designated hypertension into the three categories of:

1. Prehypertension   120–139   or   80–89
2. High blood pressure (hypertension) Stage 1   140–159   or   90–99
3. High blood pressure (hypertension) Stage 2   160 or higher or 100 or higher

Whichever category their consistent blood pressure readings are, patients who require either lifestyle changes or prescribed regimens of medications to treat their hypertension can choose a course of action under the direction of a physician to produce a successful outcome.

Activity:

Using the website www.heart.org, please answer the following questions.

1. What are the eight ways that a person can control his or her blood pressure?

   • _____

   • _____

   • _____

   • _____

   • _____

   • _____

   • _____

   • _____

2. When a patient adopts a heart-healthy lifestyle, he or she can:

   • _____

   • _____

   • _____

   • _____

3. OTC decongestants that may raise a person's blood pressure are:

- _____
- _____
- _____
- _____
- _____
- _____
- _____
- _____
- _____
- _____

4. Is the sodium content in OTC medications important for patients with hypertension to consider? If so, why?

_____

_____

_____

5. According to the American Heart Association, how many classes of blood pressure medications are there?

_____

6. What is the generic suffix associated with the ACE inhibitor class?

_____

7. What is the generic suffix most associated with the beta-blocker class?

_____

8. What is the generic suffix associated with the alpha-blocker class?

_____

9. The medication minoxidil is listed as a vasodilator. What is the another indication that minoxidil is approved for?

_____

10. What are the cardiovascular risks associated with drinking alcohol?

_____

Student Name: _____

Lab Partner: _____

Grade/Comments: _____

_____

_____

Student Comments: _____

_____

_____

LAB 29-2: Treating Cholesterol

Objectives:

To understand the different treatment options for cholesterol.

Pre-Lab Information:

• Review Chapter 29 in the textbook.

Explanation:

Many patients have been diagnosed with hyperlipidemia or high cholesterol. As the optimal range for most adults is 200 mg/dL or lower, the American Heart Association has suggestions to improve borderline and high cholesterol levels as well as the prevention of hyperlipidemia.

Activity:

Using the website www.heart.org, please answer the following questions.

1. What is the female sex hormone that contributes to raising HDL cholesterol?
   _____

2. What are the recommendations for a female with high LDL cholesterol?
   _____

3. What are the symptoms of high cholesterol?
   _____

4. How is cholesterol tested?
   _____

5. What three lifestyle changes can an individual make in order to affect his or her cholesterol levels?
   • _____
   • _____
   • _____

6. What are three cooking tips to help lower cholesterol suggested by the American Heart Association?
   • _____
   • _____
   • _____

7. What are the four classes of cholesterol medications currently available for patients with high cholesterol to consider?
   _____

8. What is the generic suffix most associated with HMG CoA reductase inhibitors?
   _____

9. How often should cholesterol be checked?
_____

10. What situations might apply to an individual to where their cholesterol levels will have to be checked more often?

- _____
- _____
- _____
- _____

Student Name: _____

Lab Partner: _____

Grade/Comments: _____

_____

Student Comments: _____

_____

_____

CHAPTER 30
The Immune System

After completing Chapter 30 from the textbook, you should be able to:	Related Activity in the Workbook/Lab Manual
1. Explain how the body's nonspecific and specific defense mechanisms work to keep the body safe from disease-causing microorganisms.	Review Questions, Activity 30-1
2. Understand the basic relationships between the immune system and the various body systems.	Review Questions, Activity 30-1, Activity 30-4, Lab 30-2
3. List and describe the different types of infectious organisms.	Review Questions, PTCB Exam Practice Questions, Activity 30-1, Lab 30-1
4. List the five stages of progression of HIV to AIDS.	Review Questions
5. Explain how the different classes of HIV drugs work.	Review Questions
6. Describe autoimmune disease and identify various types.	Review Questions, PTCB Exam Practice Questions
7. Understand how drug resistance develops and what steps can be taken to stop it.	Review Questions, Lab 30-1
8. List and define common anti-infective drug classifications, their mechanisms of action, and their side effects.	Review Questions, PTCB Exam Practice Questions, Activity 30-3, Lab 30-1
9. Describe both tuberculosis and malaria and their causes, treatments, and prevention.	Review Questions, Activity 30-3
10. Identify the different types and uses of vaccines and how they work in the body.	Review Questions

INTRODUCTION

The immune system protects the body from foreign invaders that would otherwise destroy it, or parts of it, via infection or cancer. The immune system uses numerous kinds of responses to attacks from these foreign invaders and is amazingly effective most of the time. Its defensive barriers and mechanisms include nonspecific mechanisms such as the skin, mucus, and cilia in the linings of the respiratory and digestive passageways, and the blood clotting process. It also includes specific defense mechanisms such as the white blood cells, thymus gland, lymph nodes, antibodies, and lymphocytes (B-cells and T-cells).

Many different classes of medications affect the immune system. These include drugs for the treatment of HIV/AIDS, tuberculosis, and malaria, as well as for many other conditions and diseases of the immune system. Pharmacotherapeutic treatment of pathogens includes antibacterials, anti-infectives, and antifungals, to name a few. As a pharmacy technician, it is important for you to have a clear understanding of what these drugs are and how they work to protect the body.

In addition to fighting foreign invaders, sometimes the immune system is called upon to help defend against the autoimmune process in cases of autoimmune diseases, such as lupus erythematosus or rheumatoid arthritis, in which a person's immune system mistakenly attacks itself. The end result of this defense is often inflammation. These autoimmune diseases are treated both pharmacologically and nonpharmacologically. The pharmacotherapeutic goal of treatment is to reduce inflammation, or to stop or suppress the inflammatory process.

REVIEW QUESTIONS

Match the following.

1. _____ aerobic
2. _____ anaerobic
3. _____ antibodies
4. _____ antigens
5. _____ complement
6. _____ DNA
7. _____ epitopes
8. _____ cytoplasm
9. _____ hematopoietic
10. _____ genome
11. _____ lysis
12. _____ macrophage
13. _____ pathogen
14. _____ phagocytes
15. _____ RNA

a. a fluid where cell respiration takes place; usually contains RNA (a nucleic acid that enables protein synthesis)

b. the destruction of cells

c. specific molecules that trigger an immune response

d. blood-forming

e. a nucleic acid that carries genetic information and is capable of self-replication and synthesis of RNA

f. a nucleic acid needed for the metabolic processes of protein synthesis

g. a large group of proteins that is activated in sequence when cells are exposed to a foreign substance; activation eventually results in the death or destruction of the substance

h. white blood cell, found primarily in connective tissue and the bloodstream

i. region on the surface of an antibody that is capable of producing an immune response

j. specialized cells that engulf and ingest other cells

k. a disease-causing organism

l. requires oxygen for life

m. the complete hereditary material or code of an organism

n. does not require oxygen for life

o. proteins that specifically seek and bind to the surface of pathogens or antigens.

Choose the best answer.

16. Which of the following is not a defense against infection?
    a. mucus
    b. bone marrow
    c. vertebral column
    d. skin

17. Viruses are difficult to cure because:
    a. a capsid protects their DNA/RNA.
    b. they are resistant to antibiotics.
    c. they mutate constantly.
    d. a and c

18. What type of pathogen is TB?
    a. viral
    b. parasitic
    c. bacterial
    d. fungal

19. Which are protozoa that most often consume algae and bacteria?
    a. sporozoans
    b. zooflagellates
    c. ciliates
    d. amoeboids

20. Which have a specialized opening in the outer edge to capture their prey?
    a. sporozoans
    b. zooflagellates
    c. ciliates
    d. amoeboids

21. Which are parasites that live inside a host and often cause disease to the host by robbing the host of nutrients?
    a. sporozoans
    b. zooflagellates
    c. ciliates
    d. amoeboids

22. Which of the following is not a solution to resistance?
    a. Avoid using antibiotics unnecessarily.
    b. Complete each antibacterial regimen; do not have leftover pills.
    c. Use the widest spectrum antibiotic possible.
    d. Use the common antibiotics first.

True or False?

23. *Candida albicans* is also known as athlete's foot.

    T   F

24. Currently in the market, there are three generations of cephalosporin antibiotics that are available for use.

    T   F

25. About 20% of nosocomial bacterial infections (often acquired in hospitals) are resistant to at least one of the most commonly prescribed antibiotics.

    T   F

26. Some organisms are resistant to all FDA-approved antibiotics and can be treated only with experimental and potentially toxic drugs.

    T   F

Match the following.

27. _____ Stage 1
28. _____ hormonal treatment
29. _____ Stage 2
30. _____ chemotherapy
31. _____ Stage 3
32. _____ radiation
33. _____ Stage 4
34. _____ specific inhibitors
35. _____ Stage 5
36. _____ surgery

a. AIDS opportunistic infections begin; CD4 cell count or level at or below 200 per cubic millimeter of blood

b. usually the first line of treatment for solid tumors

c. final stage of wasting and infections; ends in death

d. may be used in conjunction with surgery and/or drug treatments

e. signs and symptoms of HIV begin to appear

f. uses cytotoxic agents—a wide array of drugs—to kill cancer cells

g. infection without presentation of signs or symptoms (may last 10 or more years)

h. prevent cancer cells from receiving the signals necessary for continued growth and division

i. initial transmission and infection with HIV

j. a relatively new class of drugs that works by targeting specific proteins and processes used by cancer cells

PHARMACY CALCULATION PROBLEMS

Calculate the following.

1. If cefuroxime 750 mg IV is administered to a patient tid × 3 days, how many grams will the patient receive over the entire course?

2. A patient has a prescription for acyclovir 200 mg capsules. If the script reads, "Take one capsule five times daily for 10 days," how many milligrams will the patient take during the entire course of treatment?

3. A patient who weighs 159 lbs. and is 5'8" is coming into the infusion center for his or her weekly dose of chemotherapy. What is the body surface area for this patient?

4. Your pharmacy marks up all herbal medication 40% above cost. If a bottle of Echinacea costs the pharmacy $3.25, what is the retail price?

5. Conversion: 180 lbs = _____ kg

PTCB EXAM PRACTICE QUESTIONS

1. All of the following are types of infectious organisms *except*:
   a. yeasts.
   b. bacteria.
   c. viruses.
   d. lipids.

2. How many different strains of HIV are in existence?
   a. one
   b. two
   c. three
   d. four

3. Ciprofloxacin (Cipro) belongs to what class of antibiotics?
   a. quinolone
   b. sulfa
   c. cephalosporin
   d. aminoglycoside

4. All of the following are considered to be autoimmune diseases *except*:
   a. cystic fibrosis.
   b. Crohn's disease.
   c. lupus.
   d. multiple sclerosis.

5. Which of the following antibiotics is a macrolide?
   a. amoxicillin
   b. tetracycline
   c. azithromycin
   d. clindamycin

ACTIVITY 30-1: Anatomy Worksheet

A Lymph Node

Label the following illustration of a lymph node.

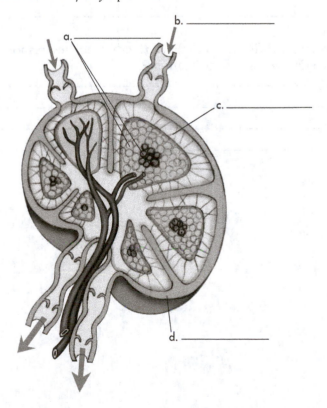

A Virus

Label the following illustration of a virus.

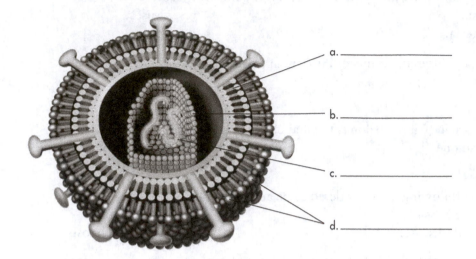

a. _____

b. _____

c. _____

d. _____

Questions:

1. What are nonspecific defense mechanisms? Give five examples and discuss how each one functions.

   _____
   _____
   _____
   _____
   _____

2. How is the cell-mediated response different from the antibody-mediated response? Which type of response plays a role in the effectiveness of vaccinations?

   _____
   _____
   _____
   _____

3. How does the immune system affect or assist the other systems within the body? Match each immune system effect with the correct body system.

Match the following.

1. _____ Provides antibodies found in skin (IgA, IgG, etc.) to assist in immune function of protection.

2. _____ Lymph vessels carry absorbed lipids to the bloodstream.

3. _____ Assists in repair after injuries. Assists in repair of bone. Macrophages (phagocytes) fuse to make bone cells.

4. _____ Tonsils, which are lymphoid tissue, protect against infection at the entrance to the respiratory tract. Lungs remove inhaled and deposited solid material and microorganisms. Plays a supportive role in maintaining and eliminating fluids.

5. _____ Fights blood vessel infections. Returns interstitial tissue fluid to circulation via veins.

6. _____ Fights bladder and kidney infections.

7. _____ Thymus gland secretes thymosin.

8. _____ Produces antibodies to assist in immune system function. Through cytokine- and interleukin-mediated pathways, regulates this system by inducing the release of gonadotropins (luteinizing hormone and follicle-stimulating hormone).

9. _____ Produces *cytokines*, immune hormones that affect the production of other hormones by the hypothalamus.

a. nervous
b. circulatory
c. endocrine
d. renal
e. respiratory
f. musculoskeletal
g. integumentary
h. reproductive
i. digestive

4. Name six kinds of infectious organisms.

_____

_____

_____

_____

_____

_____

ACTIVITY 30-2: Case Study—A Severe Cold

Instructions: Read the following scenario and then answer the critical thinking questions.

Mrs. Tindle has been coming into your retail pharmacy quite frequently during the past four days. She has purchased two over-the-counter multi-ingredient cough/cold remedies. She looks miserable and appears to have a resistant cold. She returns two days later for a different over-the-counter product and states to you that her son has also been sick and that her husband is beginning to show the initial symptoms of the cold as well. She further tells you that her son was the first one in the family to get sick.

Mrs. Tindle finally takes herself and her 16-year-old son to the physician's office after six days of suffering with their symptoms. She presents with sore throat, chills, diarrhea, and vomiting that has worsened over time. Occasionally, she has a fever and has been taking 1,000 mg bid of acetaminophen. Her son presents with symptoms of thick and yellow to green nasal discharge as well as a productive cough. He has been taking an over-the-counter cough syrup with dextromethorphan and guaifenesin. You know that her son has been volunteering at the local food bank on the weekends.

Mrs. Tindle explains to her physician that they have tried "everything" over the counter, including multiple popular cough/cold preparations. They want to know if they can both have a prescription for an antibiotic.

1. What could the doctor do to see if this is a bacterial infection that can be treated with antibiotics?

   _____

   _____

   _____

2. What are the diagnoses for Mrs. Tindle and her son?

   _____

   _____

   _____

3. What are the treatment options for Mrs. Tindle and her son?

   _____

   _____

   _____

4. What is the most appropriate course of action for Mrs. Tindle to take for her specific diagnosis?

   _____

   _____

   _____

5. As Mrs. Tindle's son has an antibiotic for his condition and Mrs. Tindle does not, should the prescription be moved up to the front of the line? There are four other prescriptions in line waiting to be filled by the other pharmacy technician and the pharmacist.

   _____

   _____

   _____

ACTIVITY 30-3: Case Study—TB

Instructions: Read the following scenario and then answer the critical thinking questions.

A 49-year-old Jamaican male moved to the United States about 10 years ago. His medical history includes a diagnosis of rheumatoid arthritis, for which he is prescribed prednisone 20 mg, methotrexate, and Humira.

The patient has just returned from Jamaica, where he visited family members, and noticed within days that he was having increasing difficulty breathing, accompanied by a cough. He did not recall being around anyone sick while in Jamaica. The patient becomes very sick with fever and chills and stops taking the Humira. He visits the doctor, who finds nothing wrong and tells him that the symptoms will disappear in a few days.

A few months later, he visits Jamaica again. Within days of returning, he has a bad cough that produces blood and shortly he ends up in the emergency room. TB is suspected, and he is placed into a negative-pressure room. The TB skin test comes up negative, but another type of lung biopsy comes back positive for TB.

1. What are the symptoms of an active TB infection?

_____

_____

_____

2. Given the facts provided in the case study, what fact may have contributed to the TB infection?

_____

_____

_____

3. Knowing that TB is a communicable disease, what are the public exposure concerns for this scenario?

_____

_____

_____

4. What are some of the side effects for Humira?

_____

_____

_____

5. What is the first line of treatment for TB? How many medications are listed as first-line therapy?

_____

_____

_____

ACTIVITY 30-4: Case Study—Birthday Party Emergency

Instructions: Read the following scenario and then answer the critical thinking questions.

Tommy is an eight-year-old, precocious little boy who is quite a handful for his teachers in school. To his teachers, it seems that Tommy cannot sit still for a minute, and he is always getting into something. Because Tommy is constantly jumping around and unable to focus his attention, the teachers think he might have ADHD. The school convinces Tommy's mother to seek medication for this condition. Tommy also suffers from headaches, asthma, and constant stomach pain that has lasted ever since his mother can remember. At her wit's end, Tommy's mother makes an appointment for him the following week.

Over the weekend, Tommy attends his cousin's birthday party, where all the children are playing and running around. All of a sudden, Tommy is on the floor with what appears to be an anaphylactic reaction to something. As people scramble to call an ambulance, Tommy's mother frantically tries to find out from the other children what happened to Tommy. One of the other little boys says that the last thing he saw was Tommy eating a Snickers candy bar in the kitchen.

1. Drawing from the facts in this scenario, what is the most likely cause of Tommy's anaphylactic reaction?

   _____

   _____

   _____

2. What is an anaphylactic reaction?

   _____

   _____

   _____

3. Tommy has eaten Snickers bars before, so why did he not have this reaction then?

   _____

   _____

   _____

4. What is the treatment for this condition?

   _____

   _____

   _____

LAB 30-1: Treating an Infection

Objectives:

To understand the different treatment options for methicillin-resistant staphylococcus aureus (MRSA).

Pre-Lab Information:

• Review Chapter 30 in the textbook.

Explanation:

The bacterial strain of MRSA has become very prevalent in our current fight toward combating dangerous microorganisms. As the arsenal of existing antibiotics has been proven to be ineffective against *Staphylococcus aureus*, which because of their overuse have assisted with evolving staphylococcus aureus into MRSA, new therapeutic approaches have been fostered and old ones have been modified to help slow down this microorganism's dangerous and sometimes fatal effects.

Activity:

Using the websites http://www.webmd.com/skin-problems-and-treatments/understanding-mrsa-methicillin-resistant-staphylococcus-aureus and http://www.webmd.com/skin-problems-and-treatments/understanding-mrsa-detection-treatment, please answer the following questions.

1. What areas or parts of the body system can MRSA infect?

   _____

   _____

   _____

   _____

2. What is MRSA sometimes called?

   _____

3. What four antibiotics are MRSA resistant to?

   • _____

   • _____

   • _____

   • _____

4. What is the term for MRSA that is showing up in healthy people who have not been hospitalized?

   _____

5. How is MRSA diagnosed?

   _____

   _____

   _____

6. What are the first two antibiotics used for an MRSA infection?

_____

_____

7. What are the other six antibiotics that are used optionally for an MRSA infection?

_____

_____

_____

8. Are antibiotics always necessary for an MRSA infection of the skin? If not, what other option might a physician choose for a skin boil?

_____

_____

_____

9. Why is it important for a patient to finish all of an antibiotic for an MRSA infection?

_____

_____

Research:

Use the Internet to find out more about the global problem of drug resistance. Visit the World Health Organization (WHO) website (http://www.who.int) to find out more on this topic. What options for action does the WHO propose? What can you, as a pharmacy professional, do to in relation to this global problem?

Student Name: _____

Lab Partner: _____

Grade/Comments: _____

_____

_____

Student Comments: _____

_____

_____

LAB 30-2: Treating Human Immunodeficiency Virus (HIV)

Objective:

To understand the different treatment options for the human immunodeficiency virus (HIV).

Pre-Lab Information:

• Review Chapter 30 in the textbook.

Explanation:

Ever since its modern-day discovery in the early 1980s, HIV has been on the forefront of the minds of our own government, the Centers for Disease Control, and the WHO. Ever since the first medication was approved for HIV/AIDS in 1990, the medication known as Retrovir or AZT, the discovery of the pipeline of medications used to treat HIV/AIDS has been of great importance during the last 30 years. These medications enable HIV positive patients to live a successful quality of life. Individuals, who are living with HIV and on the combination therapy regimen known as highly active antiretroviral therapy (HAART), will most likely to live their full life expectancy age.

Activity:

Using the website www.thebody.com, please answer the following questions below.

1. As of this writing, what are the names of the five current classifications of HIV medications?

   • _____

   • _____

   • _____

   • _____

   • _____

2. What is the goal of the design for the five classifications of HIV medications?

   _____

   _____

3. As there are many different HIV medications within each classification, currently there are eight medications that contain more than one medication in a single tablet. Please list those eight medications below.

   Brand Name   **Generic Name(s)**

   _____   _____

   _____   _____

   _____   _____

   _____   _____

   _____   _____

   _____   _____

   _____   _____

4. Why are the above-listed eight combination medications that are used to treat HIV developed this way?

_____

5. What are some of the side effects of the medication Sustiva? What schedule I substance might a patient test positive for while taking Sustiva?

_____
_____
_____
_____

6. Why is the adult single dose of the medication Viramune one 200 mg tablet (once a day) for 14 days rather than one 200 mg tablet (twice a day)?

_____
_____
_____

7. What is the overall goal of HAART?

_____
_____
_____

8. Is an HIV positive individual more likely or less likely to pass on his or her HIV if he or she is taking HAART? Why?

_____
_____
_____

9. A new controversial therapy has been discovered for the treatment of leukemia, please discuss and notate this controversial therapy below.

_____
_____

10. What are some treatment options for individuals to consider for both pre and post exposure to HIV?

_____
_____
_____

Student Name: _____

Lab Partner: _____

Grade/Comments: _____
_____
_____

Student Comments: _____
_____
_____

CHAPTER 31
The Renal System

After completing Chapter 31 from the textbook, you should be able to:	Related Activity in the Workbook/Lab Manual
1. List, identify, and diagram the basic parts of the renal system.	Review Questions, PTCB Exam Practice Questions, Activity 31-1
2. Explain the functions of the nephron, kidney, and bladder.	Review Questions, PTCB Exam Practice Questions, Activity 31-1
3. List and define common diseases and conditions affecting the renal system, and explain the mechanisms of action of each class of drugs used to treat each disease.	Review Questions, PTCB Exam Practice Questions, Activity 31-2, Activity 31-3, Activity 31-4
4. Explain how homeostasis of fluid and electrolytes affects the body.	Review Questions, PTCB Exam Practice Questions, Activity 31-3

INTRODUCTION

The renal system, or urinary system, is a fairly simple system with few components; however, its condition has a grave impact on many parts of the body. Genitourinary tract infections, poor kidney filtration, and water imbalance can indicate or cause diabetes, high blood pressure, or dehydration. The proper functioning of the kidneys is essential to maintain life. The drugs most commonly used to treat diseases of the renal system are anti-infectives and diuretics. The use of strong diuretics that help to remove excess water may also cause a loss of potassium, which may lead to muscle and heart problems. A delicate balance of electrolytes, kidney function, filtration, and waste removal must be maintained at all times during illnesses and while taking medications that affect or treat the urinary tract. As a pharmacy technician, you should be aware of the most common urinary system disorders that require pharmacological treatment, including conditions treated with OTC drugs.

REVIEW QUESTIONS

Match the following.

1. _____ acidosis
2. _____ bilirubin
3. _____ dialysis
4. _____ Kegel exercises
5. _____ ketone
6. _____ palliative
7. _____ pH
8. _____ specific gravity
9. _____ urobilinogen
10. _____ void

a. pelvic muscle training and toning exercises
b. empty the bladder
c. a by-product of fat metabolism
d. a measure of the density of a substance as compared to water
e. medical procedure that removes waste from the blood of patients with renal failure
f. substance produced by the breakdown of bilirubin
g. substance produced by the breakdown of hemoglobin
h. excessive acid in the body fluids
i. the measure of acidity or alkalinity of a solution
j. reducing the severity of symptoms

Choose the best answer.

11. The specific gravity of water is:
    a. 1.
    b. 2.
    c. 3.
    d. 4.

12. Microscopic kidney cells are known as:
    a. michrons.
    b. nephrons.
    c. nephews.
    d. microns.

13. What is the filter station of the kidney called?
    a. loop of Henle
    b. glomerulus
    c. distal convoluted tubule
    d. none of these

14. Phenazopyridine may cause the urine to be colored:
    a. red.
    b. orange.
    c. green/blue-green.
    d. brown/black.

15. Approximately how much urine collects in the bladder prior to signals being sent to the brain for voidance?
    a. 100–200 mL
    b. 300–400 mL
    c. 50–100 mL
    d. 200–300 mL

True or False?

16. Bilirubin is normally detected in the urine.

    T   F

17. Obesity is not a cause of incontinence.

    T   F

18. Pyelonephritis is an infection of the bladder and the lower urinary tract.

    T   F

19. Cranberry juice is effective for a urinary tract infection (UTI) because it makes the urine more acidic.

    T   F

20. Kidney damage can lead to diabetes.

    T   F

PHARMACY CALCULATION PROBLEMS

Calculate the following.

1. If a patient needs phenazopyridine 200 mg 1 po tid prn × 4 days, how many tablets should you dispense?

2. A new prescription has been dropped off for oxybutynin po, 10 mg bid. If the pharmacy carries only 5 mg tablets, how many tablets will be needed for a 30-day supply?

3. A woman is to receive a trimethoprim/sulfamethoxazole IV for a complicated UTI. Her dose is 200 mg based on the trimethoprim content. Trimethoprim (TMP)/sulfamethoxazole (SMZ) IV comes as TMP 80 mg/SMZ 400 mg per 5 mL vial. How many milliliters should be drawn up for the IV?

4. A patient took one hydrocodone/APAP tablet po qid × 5 days for pain from kidney stones. How many grams of hydrocodone would the patient be consuming for the full course of therapy, if each tablet contained 5 mg of hydrocodone and 500 mg of acetaminophen?

5. What is the day supply if the directions for a prescription for ciprofloxacin 500 mg are 2 tabs po STAT?

PTCB EXAM PRACTICE QUESTIONS

1. If the renal system does not maintain water and electrolyte balance then the body will not be in:
   a. stasis.
   b. homeostasis.
   c. homeopathic.
   d. homo sapiens.

2. What is the medical term for difficult or painful urination?
   a. dysuria
   b. hematuria
   c. pyuria
   d. anuria

3. The renal system is responsible for all of the following functions *except*:
   a. filtration of waste from the blood.
   b. maintenance of electrolyte balance.
   c. oxygen transport.
   d. maintenance of acid–base balance.

4. Diabetic kidney disease is also known as:
   a. diabetic nephropathy.
   b. diabetic ketoacidosis.
   c. peripheral neuropathy.
   d. end-stage renal disease.

5. All of the following are used to treat urinary incontinence *except*:
   a. Diovan.
   b. Ditropan.
   c. Detrol.
   d. Urispas.

ACTIVITY 31-1: Anatomy Worksheet

The Urinary System

Label the following illustration of the urinary system.

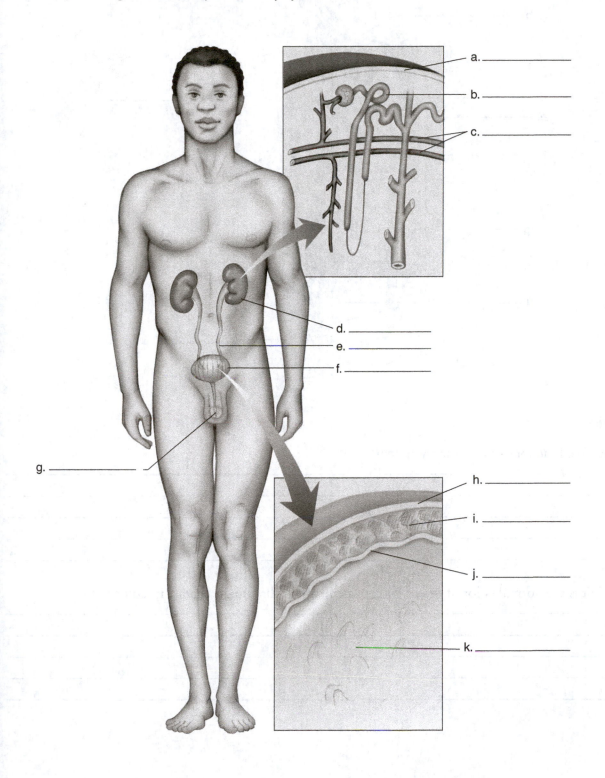

a. _____

b. _____

c. _____

d. _____

e. _____

f. _____

g. _____

h. _____

i. _____

j. _____

k. _____

The Nephron

Label the following illustration of the nephron.

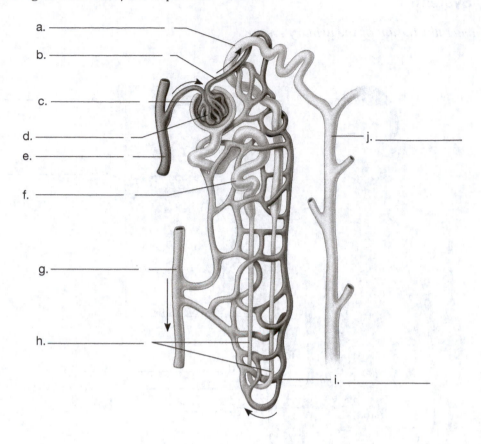

a. _____

b. _____

c. _____

d. _____

e. _____

f. _____

g. _____

h. _____

i. _____

j. _____

Questions:

1. List five functions of the urinary system.

   _____

   _____

   _____

   _____

   _____

2. What is the normal color of urine? Discuss some things that might change its color.

   _____

   _____

   _____

   _____

   _____

3. Use your textbook or other medical reference to learn more about the process of urine formation; then describe it in your own words.

_____

_____

_____

_____

ACTIVITY 31-2: Case Study—UTI

Instructions: Read the following scenario and then answer the critical thinking questions.

Ms. Andelo, a healthy 24-year-old woman, is a periodic customer at the retail pharmacy where you work. She shares the good news that she has been dating a nice young man for about a month and it seems serious. She also lets you know that they have a very physical relationship as well.

Today she is here to pick up some medicine for some symptoms she has been experiencing. Ms. Andelo just came from her doctor's office, where she complained that she is repeatedly experiencing the urge to urinate. However, when she attempts to urinate, it is painful and accompanied by a burning sensation. She is very skittish about the pain and has refrained as much as possible from urinating because of fear. She had hoped it would stop by now. The last time she was able to urinate, she had a spotting of blood but nothing substantial. This has been going on for about four days.

1. What other symptoms would present if this were a lower UTI?

_____

_____

_____

2. What could be prescribed for a patient such as Ms. Andelo for a UTI, and for how long?

_____

_____

_____

3. Are any popular alternative methods available for UTI prevention?

_____

_____

_____

4. Based on the information given in the scenario, what is the probable cause of the UTI?

_____

_____

_____

ACTIVITY 31-3: Case Study—Dialysis

Instructions: Read the following scenario and then answer the critical thinking questions.

Mr. Sanders is a frequent patient of the dialysis center where you work as a clinical pharmacy technician. He comes to the hospital for dialysis treatments three times a week on an outpatient basis. Generally, his treatment days can be very long. By the time he checks in to the center, begins his dialysis treatment, and completes his cycle, several hours pass. He is used to being tired for a good amount of time, but lately it seems that he is even more tired than usual. An example is when he occasionally lifts a phone book, he becomes very fatigued. Mr. Sanders is also experiencing shortness of breath and an increasing loss of memory. He questions if these recent stressors are progressing due to the dialysis procedures.

Mr. Sanders's list of current medications includes diphenhydramine, warfarin, docusate sodium, calcium, and PhosLo.

1. Based on the information in this case study, what condition could Mr. Sanders be experiencing in addition to his chronic renal failure?

   _____

   _____

   _____

2. What are the treatment options available for Mr. Sander's newly diagnosed condition?

   _____

   _____

   _____

3. What are the reasons that Mr. Sanders is prescribed the current medications on his list?

   _____

   _____

   _____

ACTIVITY 31-4: Case Study—Incontinence

Instructions: Read the following scenario and then answer the critical thinking questions.

Maryellen Montell is a 42-year-old-woman who recently had a total hysterectomy. Three weeks after this surgery, she is still unable to control urinary leakage, and it occurs at the most inopportune times. She presents with leakage any time she coughs or laughs and sometimes when she climbs stairs.

She comes to the ostomy supply pharmacy where you work, on a very busy day, to pick up some incontinence products, including undergarments. Your coworker takes in her prescription for the undergarments and begins to process it. He or she questions Maryellen about sizing. Maryellen replies in a soft voice. Your coworker tells Maryellen that her insurance will not pay for that size or the brand of "diapers" she needs and starts to rattle off the list of undergarments your pharmacy does have available. It seems like a lengthy conversation to Maryellen, who just says, "Never mind," and leaves the pharmacy counter in a huff without the prescription. You look at your coworker, who shakes his or her head and says, "What was her problem?"

1. According to the description in this scenario, Maryellen exhibits symptoms of which of the four types of incontinence?

   _____

   _____

   _____

   _____

   _____

   _____

   _____

   _____

2. What happens within the body with this type of incontinence?

   _____

   _____

   _____

   _____

   _____

   _____

   _____

3. Is this condition treatable with or without medicine?

   _____

   _____

   _____

   _____

   _____

   _____

   _____

   _____

4. Given the description of this scenario, why do you think Maryellen left the pharmacy the way she did?

_____

_____

_____

_____

_____

_____

_____

5. If you had taken in the prescription, how would you have handled the transaction differently to help prevent Maryellen from leaving?

_____

_____

_____

_____

_____

_____

LAB 31-1: Treating Prostatitis

Objective:

To understand about the pathology and treatment options for prostatitis.

Pre-Lab Information:

• Review Chapter 31 in the textbook.

Explanation:

Prostatitis can affect every male at a specific point in his lifetime. The condition may be either acute or chronic. The treatment options for a male to consider with his individual case may vary depending on the cause and severity of the inflammation of the prostate.

Activity:

Using the website (http://www.mayoclinic.com/health/prostatitis/DS00341), please answer the following questions.

1. Besides a bacterial infection, what are the three other causes of prostatitis?

_____

_____

_____

2. What are the 10 risk factors for prostatitis?

_____

_____

_____

_____

_____

3. What are the four complications of prostatitis?

_____

_____

_____

_____

4. What four preparations should a patient take prior to his appointment?

_____

_____

_____

_____

5. What six tests might lead to a diagnosis of prostatitis?

_____
_____
_____

6. What are the five treatment options for prostatitis?

_____
_____
_____

7. What are the home remedies and lifestyle changes that a male with prostatitis can do to lessen some of his prostatitis symptoms?

_____
_____
_____
_____

8. What are alternative therapies that the patient may choose to reduce his symptoms of prostatitis?

_____
_____

Student Name: _____

Lab Partner: _____

Grade/Comments: _____
_____
_____

Student Comments: _____
_____
_____

LAB 31-2: Treating Urinary Tract Infections (UTI)

Objective:

To understand the different treatment options for a UTI.

Pre-Lab Information:

• Review Chapter 31 in the textbook.

Explanation:

As of this writing, there are currently 20 different antibiotics and other medications that are approved and indicated for the treatment of a UTI.

Activity:

Match up the 20 antibiotics and other medications according to brand name, the generic counterpart, and the classification that the antibiotic or medication belongs to.

Generic	Brand	Classification
amoxicillin	_____	_____
amoxicillin/clavulanate	_____	_____
cefaclor	_____	_____
cefadroxil	_____	_____
cefpodoxime	_____	_____
ceftriaxone	_____	_____
cefuroxime	_____	_____
cephalexin	_____	_____
demeclocycline	_____	_____
doxycycline	_____	_____
flavoxate	_____	_____
fosfomycin	_____	_____
methenamine	_____	_____
minocycline	_____	_____
nitrofurantoin	_____	_____
norfloxacin	_____	_____
ofloxacin	_____	_____
phenazopyridine	_____	_____
sulfamethoxazole/ trimethoprim	_____	_____
tetracycline	_____	_____

Brand Names:

Vibramycin	Ceclor	Noroxin	Rocephin	Duricef
Bactrim, Bactrim DS	Sumycin	Urispas	Pyridium	Ceftin
Declomycin	Keflex	Augmentin	Macrobid, Macrodantin	Vantin
Urised, Urex	Floxin	Minocin	Amoxil, Trimox	Monurol

Classifications:

Cephalosporin (1st, 2nd, or 3rd generation)	Penicillin	Tetracycline
Urinary anti-infective	Analgesic	Sulfonamide
Nitrofuran antimicrobial agent	Broad-spectrum antibiotic	

Student Name: _____

Lab Partner: _____

Grade/Comments: _____

_____

_____

Student Comments: _____

_____

_____

CHAPTER 32
The Endocrine System

After completing Chapter 32 from the textbook, you should be able to:	Related Activity in the Workbook/Lab Manual
1. Identify and describe the glands of the endocrine system.	Review Questions, PTCB Exam Practice Questions, Activity 32-1
2. Describe the functions of the hypothalamus and pituitary gland, and list other body parts that are affected by these glands.	Review Questions, PTCB Exam Practice Questions, Activity 32-1
3. List and define the hormones of the endocrine system and know which gland or organ secretes each hormone.	Review Questions, PTCB Exam Practice Questions, Activity 32-1, Activity 32-2, Activity 32-3
4. Describe male and female hormones and some products used for replacement in cases of deficiency of these hormones.	Review Questions, PTCB Exam Practice Questions, Activity 32-2, Activity 32-3
5. Identify and describe the major diseases and conditions that affect the endocrine system.	Review Questions, PTCB Exam Practice Questions, Activity 32-4, Lab 32-1, Lab 32-2, Lab 32-3, Lab 32-4
6. Compare and contrast diabetes mellitus and diabetes insipidus.	Review Questions, Activity 32-4, Lab 32-1, Lab 32-2
7. Understand the effects of anabolic steroid use.	Review Questions, Activity 32-2

INTRODUCTION

The endocrine system is a collection of glands that produce hormones, substances that help regulate the body's growth, metabolism, and sexual development and function. The hormones, which are released into the bloodstream and transported to tissues and organs throughout the body, influence every cell in some way. The glands of the endocrine system are ductless. The hormones secreted from the endocrine glands are thus released directly into the bloodstream and travel in the body to specific target organs where they exert their effect.

The driving forces of the endocrine system are the hypothalamus, located in the brainstem, and the pituitary gland, which is attached to the base of the hypothalamus. The hypothalamus directs the pituitary gland, which, in turn, controls the thyroid, parathyroid, pancreas, adrenal glands, and the gonads. A complete review of these glands, their secretions, and their effects on body systems illustrates how important the endocrine system is to the proper functioning of the body. For example, every cell in the body depends on thyroid hormones for regulating metabolism.

Some diseases of the endocrine system, such as diabetes, are very familiar to most people; others, such as Graves' disease or Cushing's syndrome, are less common. As a pharmacy technician, you should be aware of the most common endocrine system disorders that require pharmacological treatment, including conditions treated with OTC drugs.

REVIEW QUESTIONS

Match the following.

1. _____ corticosteroid
2. _____ gonads
3. _____ homeostasis
4. _____ hormone
5. _____ isotonic
6. _____ negative feedback
7. _____ polydipsia
8. _____ polyphagia
9. _____ polyuria
10. _____ priapism

a. a chemical substance, produced by an organ or gland, that travels through the bloodstream to regulate certain bodily functions and/or the activity of other organs or glands

b. the process by which the body returns to homeostasis

c. painful, extended-duration erection

d. excessive hunger or eating

e. excessive urination

f. a stable and constant environment

g. steroidal hormones produced in the adrenal cortex

h. testes and ovaries

i. having the same salt concentration as that of blood

j. ingestion of abnormally large amounts of fluid

Fill in the blanks.

11. _____ is the study of the chemical communication system that provides the means to control a large number of physiologic processes.

12. The _____ is often referred to as the "master gland," because it controls many of the other _____.

13. Thyroid cells combine iodine and the _____ to make T3 and T4.

14. The _____ _____ are located on the upper part of each kidney.

15. The adrenal cortex secretes two types of corticosteroids or hormones: _____ and _____.

Match each drug to its classification.

16. _____ glucocorticoid
17. _____ mineralocorticoid
18. _____ lab-modified estrogen
19. _____ plant-derived estrogen
20. _____ natural hormone
21. _____ secreted hormone
22. _____ androgen
23. _____ brain hormone
24. _____ synthetic form of somatostatin
25. _____ synthetic long-acting somatostatin

a. testosterone
b. somatostatin
c. estradiol
d. octreotide
e. fludrocortisone
f. lanreotide
g. estropipate
h. Premarin
i. prednisone
j. cortisol

Choose the best answer.

26. Anabolic steroids belong to which schedule of controlled substances?
    a. Schedule I
    b. Schedule II
    c. Schedule III
    d. Schedule IV

27. Which of the following is not an irreversible effect of steroids?
    a. body hair
    b. clitoris enlargement
    c. chills
    d. breast shrinkage

28. Which of the following endocrine glands main function is to keep the body in homeostasis?
    a. pituitary
    b. adrenal
    c. hypothalamus
    d. thyroid

29. Gestational diabetes affects about what percentage of all pregnant women in the United States each year?
    a. 14%
    b. 34%
    c. 40%
    d. 4%

30. Which type of insulin is the only insulin that can be injected IV?
    a. Humulin N
    b. R
    c. Lantus
    d. lente

PHARMACY CALCULATION PROBLEMS

Calculate the following.

1. If the directions for conjugated estrogen cream read, "Apply 0.5 g PV qd," how long will a 60 g tube last?

2. A diabetic patient gives himself 20 units of insulin tid with meals. How many vials will the patient need for a 30-day supply? The vial contains 10 mL and has a concentration of 100 units/mL.

3. A patient requires a tapering prescription for methylprednisolone 4 mg tablets for a severe allergic reaction. It normally is stocked in a convenience pack, but that form is currently back-ordered. The patient agreed that he or she could take the tablets in a bottle as long as all the directions are included. The directions read:

   Day 1: Take six tablets (at once or in divided doses)

   Day 2: Take five tablets (at once or in divided doses)

   Day 3: Take four tablets (at once or in divided doses)

   Day 4: Take three tablets (at once or in divided doses)

   Day 5: Take two tablets (at once or in divided doses)

   Day 6: Take one tablet

   How many tablets will you dispense?

4. A patient brings in a prescription for 0.75 mg of levothyroxine. How many micrograms would the patient take for a 30-day supply if the directions are 1 tab qd?

5. You just received a prescription for desiccated thyroid 180 mg tablets. The computer system only lists the product in grains. How many grains are in one tablet?

PTCB EXAM PRACTICE QUESTIONS

1. Which gland in the endocrine system is responsible for the regulation of calcium in the body?
   a. thymus
   b. thyroid
   c. pituitary
   d. parathyroid

2. Which disease is characterized by the body's failure to produce insulin?
   a. type 1 diabetes
   b. type 2 diabetes
   c. gestational diabetes
   d. pre-diabetes

3. Insulin delivery technology has developed the following innovations *except* for:
   a. pens.
   b. oral tablets.
   c. external pumps.
   d. oral spray.

4. Glucotrol is to glipizide as Glucophage is to:
   a. acarbose.
   b. metformin.
   c. glyburide.
   d. glimepiride.

5. Male sex hormones are also referred to as:
   a. estrogens.
   b. progestins.
   c. insulins.
   d. androgens.

ACTIVITY 32-1: Anatomy Worksheet

The Endocrine Glands

Label the following illustration of the endocrine glands.

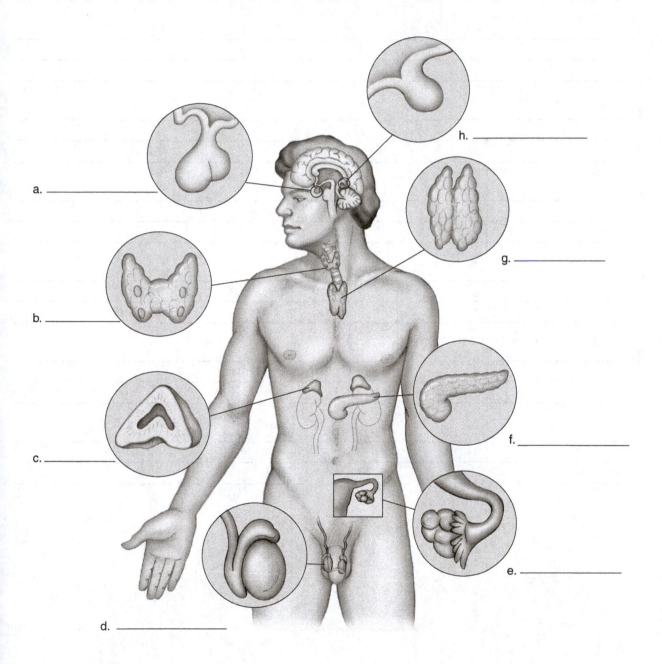

a. _____

b. _____

c. _____

d. _____

e. _____

f. _____

g. _____

h. _____

Now that you have labeled the endocrine glands in the figure, use the following spaces to describe the hormone(s) each gland produces and each hormone's function within the body.

1. _____
   _____
   _____

2. _____
   _____
   _____

3. _____
   _____
   _____

4. _____
   _____
   _____

5. _____
   _____
   _____

6. _____
   _____
   _____

7. _____
   _____
   _____

8. _____
   _____
   _____

ACTIVITY 32-2: Case Study—Anabolic Steroid Use

Instructions: Read the following scenario and then answer the critical thinking questions.

Rob is a 17-year-old male who finally was selected as a defensive tackle for his high school football team. It turns out that Rob is one of the smallest players on the team, but his coach has encouraged him to work out more often and eat certain foods to help him increase his body size and strength. Rob feels the need to be popular with the rest of the high school football team and goes to great lengths to fit in. For example, he works out daily in the well-equipped school gym long after the rest of the team goes home.

Rob is not gaining muscle or strength as fast as he would like, so he resorts to using anabolic steroids to bulk up. Everyone at school is aware of Rob's steroid use, and the athletes typically accept steroid use among themselves.

One day, Rob is randomly tested after he assaults another player. During questioning, he is asked to reveal who supplies the steroids that are in his system. Rob brags that he volunteers at a hospital picking up trash, and while in the pharmacy area he walks over to the shelf, out of camera range, and places the capsules in his pocket. He states that he has been doing this the entire time and has no other source.

1. What key component(s) in the story reveal that Rob is lying about obtaining the steroids from the pharmacy?

   _____

   _____

   _____

   _____

2. What are some signs of steroid use in a case such as this?

   _____

   _____

   _____

   _____

3. How much pressure (psychologically or otherwise) do you think teenagers like Rob are under to use steroids to meet athletic goals and fit in socially?

   _____

   _____

   _____

   _____

4. What discipline (legal or otherwise) should be applied here, and to whom?

   _____

   _____

   _____

   _____

ACTIVITY 32-3: Case Study—Hormone Replacement Therapy for Men

Instructions: Read the following scenario and then answer the critical thinking questions.

Fifty-year-old Ron has been not felling so well mentally. Ron has been on hormonal replacement therapy for approximately nine months as things were going well for him. Ron presents to his physician with new issues of a developed severe case of acne and he is also gaining weight. Ron feels certain that these new issues are due to his hormone replacement therapy. Also, within the past few weeks Ron has been perspiring more heavily than usual and he finds that his perspiration has a foul odor. Ron also noticed that he is losing more hair than usual from his scalp.

All of these unfavorable symptoms have Ron wondering if the hormone replacement therapy is worth the trouble correlating to these new issues. The physician tells Ron that these symptoms are normal with this kind of therapy, and the physician adjusts the dose. As Ron continues his hormone replacement therapy, some symptoms persist while others are subsiding.

1. What kind of hormone replacement therapy do you think that Ron has been prescribed?

   _____

   _____

   _____

   _____

2. What are some other issues or symptoms, aside from the ones that Ron is currently experiencing, that he may experience in the near future?

   _____

   _____

   _____

   _____

3. What psychological effects do you think that Ron might be experiencing with his body and appearance changes?

   _____

   _____

   _____

   _____

ACTIVITY 32-4: Case Study—Insulin

Instructions: Read the following scenario and then answer the critical thinking questions.

Mrs. Kendall has been coming to the community pharmacy for years. You always look forward to seeing her. She is a very proactive patient who knows exactly what kind of medicine she is taking and for what reason. Your prescription profile shows that Mrs. Kendall is currently taking three medications for maintenance therapy, as she is in good health.

Today Mrs. Kendall comes into the pharmacy a little distraught. She has been crying and is quite upset. Mrs. Kendall tells you in a sullen voice that the physician has just prescribed a few new medications and that she is there to pick them up. You view her profile and now notice that she has been prescribed devices, equipment, and medications for type 1 diabetes, including a glucose meter, test strips, other testing supplies, insulin, and syringes.

Even though she appeared to be in good health, Mrs. Kendall reveals to you that she has been taking oral diabetes medication for six months and has ordered her medication through a mail order pharmacy. She was certain that she could arrest her diabetes and that she would not require insulin therapy. She feels as if her body has betrayed her and her health. Although Mrs. Kendall is a bit scared and upset with the changes of her diabetes management and therapy, she feels confident in your abilities to help her to understand the devices and equipment, as well as the pharmacist to help educate her with self-injecting her insulin therapy.

1. As a pharmacy technician, are you able to assist Mrs. Kendall with educating her as to how she can use her new glucose meter?

2. How can you further assist Mrs. Kendall's changes in her diabetes management?

3. If Mrs. Kendall's disease progresses, what other products might she possibly require from the pharmacy?

_____

_____

_____

_____

_____

_____

_____

LAB 32-1: Using a Blood Glucose Meter

Objectives:

Demonstrate the procedure for testing blood glucose levels.

Learn what supplies are required to perform blood glucose monitoring.

Pre-Lab Information:

- Review Chapter 32 in your textbook to learn more about diabetes.
- Visit the American Diabetes Association website: www.diabetes.org
- Gather the following materials:
  - blood glucose meter
  - blood glucose meter test strip
  - lancing device
  - lancet
  - control solution (optional)

Explanation:

Approximately 6.6% of the U.S. population has diabetes, but about one-third of that group is unaware of their serious medical condition. Diabetes is a disease in which the body does not produce or properly use insulin, a hormone that is needed to convert sugar, starches, and other food into the energy necessary for daily life. The cause of diabetes is not certain, but both genetics and environmental factors (such as obesity and lack of exercise) appear to play roles.

As a pharmacy technician, you need to understand how diabetic patients monitor their blood glucose levels using a blood glucose meter. This knowledge will help you assist customers who have questions about equipment and supplies.

Activity:

In this activity, you will test your own blood glucose levels.

Blood Testing Procedure

1. Wash hands with warm, soapy water.
2. Insert a new lancet into the lancing device.
3. Adjust the lancing device to the appropriate depth to collect a proper sample.
4. Turn on the blood glucose meter and ensure that it is properly coded for the test strips, if necessary. (Follow the specific manufacturer's instructions.)
5. Remove a test strip from the vial and recap the remaining test strips immediately.
6. Insert the test strip into the blood glucose meter.
7. Lance your finger and allow an ample blood drop to form.
8. Place the sample tip/section of the test strip next to the blood drop and hold it there until the blood glucose meter confirms that the blood sample was adequate for testing.
9. Remove the finger from the test strip and wait for the blood glucose meter to display the test results.
10. Discard the used lancet and test strip in a biohazard waste container.

Note: Control solution can be used in place of an actual blood sample for training purposes. For step 7, squeeze a drop of control solution onto the fingertip.

Note: Due to the variety of blood glucose monitors, you should thoroughly read the instructions provided by the manufacturer to ensure that the proper procedures are being followed.

Discussion Questions:

1. What was your blood glucose level? Is your result low, normal, or high?
   _____
   _____

2. How often should type 2 diabetics test their blood sugar?
   _____
   _____

3. Why is it important that used lancets and test strips be thrown away in a biohazard waste container?
   _____
   _____
   _____
   _____

Student Name: _____

Lab Partner: _____

Grade/Comments: _____

_____

_____

Student Comments: _____

_____

_____

LAB 32-2: Simulated Insulin Injection

Objective:
Become familiar with the procedure for giving an insulin injection.

Pre-Lab Information:
Gather the following materials:

- insulin syringe
- vial of normal saline or sterile water
- alcohol swab
- biohazard waste container

Explanation:
Some patients who have type 1 diabetes require daily insulin injections. Giving yourself a daily injection can be emotionally and psychologically difficult, as well as physically demanding.

Activity:
In this exercise, you will experience the process of giving yourself an insulin injection, using saline or sterile water as your "mock" insulin.

Procedure

1. Using a new, unopened vial of normal saline or sterile water, label it as U-100 insulin, 100 units/mL.
2. Calculate the proper dosage in milliliters needed for 10 units.
3. Select the appropriate-size insulin syringe (U-100) to use for injection.
4. Remove the vial cap, and swab the rubber diaphragm with an alcohol swab.
5. Pull back the plunger on the syringe to the calculated dosage for adding air into the syringe.
6. Insert the needle into the vial. Push the plunger in to transfer the air from the syringe to the vial, then invert the vial and pull back on the plunger to draw up the needed volume of solution.
7. Using your thumb and index finger, gently pinch up a section of skin on the side of your abdomen.
8. Insert the needle into the pinched skin. Push the plunger to inject the solution and then remove the syringe.
9. Dispose of the syringe in a biohazard waste container.

Note: Normal saline is the preferred solution for training use, as its pH is close to that of the human body.

Discussion Questions:

1. How did you feel, emotionally, preparing to inject yourself?

_____

_____

_____

_____

2. How did you feel, physically, as you administered the injection?

_____

_____

_____

_____

3. In what ways will this exercise help you to provide better patient care?

_____

_____

_____

_____

Student Name: _____

Lab Partner: _____

Grade/Comments: _____

_____

_____

Student Comments: _____

_____

_____

LAB 32-3: Treating Diabetes

Objective:
To become familiar with the management of diabetes.

Pre-Lab Information:

• Visit the website http://www.diabetes.org/

Explanation:
Depending on his or her type of diabetes that a patient is managing, many diabetics are prescribed a therapy regimen that will help control their glucose levels.

Activity:
Using the website www.diabetes.org, please answer the following questions.

1. When monitoring blood glucose levels, what is vital for a patient to do so that a provider can help the patient with a good care plan?

   _____

2. If a patient has type-2 diabetes, what therapy option is prescribed to him or her to manage his or her diabetes?

   _____

3. What are the six oral therapy classifications of diabetes medications currently available?

   _____

   _____

   _____

4. How many types of insulin are sold in the United States?

   _____

5. What are the four types of insulin?

   _____

   _____

   _____

6. If there are 100 units of insulin per 1 mL, how many milliliters are in 50 units of insulin?

   _____

7. According to "Site Rotation 101," what is the preferred infusion site for proper insulin delivery? What are the other alternate sites that a patient may consider?

   _____

   _____

   _____

   _____

Student Name: _____

Lab Partner: _____

Grade/Comments: _____

_____

_____

Student Comments: _____

_____

_____

LAB 32-4: Treating Menopause

Objective:

To become familiar with the management of menopause.

Pre-Lab Information:

• Review Chapter 32 in your textbook to learn more about menopause.

Explanation:

Estrogen replacement therapy is the primary resource for females who are experiencing menopause. The decline in a female's estrogen levels during this time in their lives presents both challenges and rewards with the proper use of hormone replacement therapy.

Activity:

Using your textbook as a resource, match up the following hormone replacement therapy medications with their brand name counterpart. Also notate the method of the delivery systems/dosage forms for each of the medications.

Generic	Brand Name(s)	Delivery System/ Dosage Form(s)
conjugated animal estrogen	_____	_____
estradiol	_____	_____
progesterone	_____	_____
conjugated plant estrogens	_____	_____
estrone estropipate	_____	_____
esterified estrogens	_____	_____
norethindrone acetate	_____	_____
medroxyprogesterone acetate	_____	_____
synthetic progesterone and animal estrogens	_____	_____
estradiol/norethindrone acetate	_____	_____

Student Name: _____

Lab Partner: _____

Grade/Comments: _____

_____

_____

Student Comments: _____

_____

_____

The Reproductive System

After completing Chapter 33 from the textbook, you should be able to:	Related Activity in the Workbook/Lab Manual
1. List, identify, and diagram the basic anatomical structures and parts of the male and female reproductive systems.	Review Questions, PTCB Exam Practice Questions, Activity 33-1
2. Describe the functions and physiology of the male and female reproductive systems and the hormones that govern them.	Review Questions, PTCB Exam Practice Questions, Activity 33-1
3. List and define common diseases affecting the male and female reproductive systems and understand the causes, symptoms, and pharmaceutical treatments associated with each disease or condition.	Review Questions, PTCB Exam Practice Questions, Activity 33-2, Activity 33-3, Activity 33-4, Lab 33-1, Lab 33-2, Lab 33-3
4. Describe the indications for use and mechanisms of action of various contraceptives.	Review Questions, PTCB Exam Practice Questions, Activity 33-2

INTRODUCTION

The reproductive system is made up of internal reproductive organs, associated ducts, and external genitalia. Its primary function is the reproductive process. Sex hormones are produced in the gonads: in males, in the testes; and in females, in the ovaries.

Although many diseases can affect the reproductive system, a pharmacy technician will most frequently encounter conditions involving contraception, infertility, sexually transmitted diseases (STDs), and benign prostatic hyperplasia (BPH). As a pharmacy technician, it is important for you to be well informed regarding the different types of contraceptives, as well as their side effects and contraindications, and to be familiar with common conditions and disorders of the reproductive system.

REVIEW QUESTIONS

Match the following. Some answers may be used more than once.

1. _____ contraception
2. _____ endometrium
3. _____ hyperplasia
4. _____ oocyte
5. _____ ovaries
6. _____ ovulation
7. _____ ovum
8. _____ STD
9. _____ STI
10. _____ testes

a. the reproduction of cells within an organ at an increased rate
b. female reproductive organs that produce eggs
c. process in which the ovarian follicle ruptures and releases the egg
d. a sexually transmitted disease
e. the male reproductive organs that produce sperm
f. a disease caused by a pathogen (virus, bacterium, parasite, or fungus) that spreads from person to person through sexual contact
g. birth control
h. the lining of the uterus
i. a mature egg
j. an immature egg

Choose the best answer.

11. The most abundant and active of the estrogens is:
    a. estrace.
    b. estropipate.
    c. estrodil.
    d. estradiol.

12. Federal law requires that all drugs containing estrogen:
    a. be dispensed with a patient package insert.
    b. also contain progesterone.
    c. be clearly labeled "do not take if pregnant."
    d. be redispensed for 28 days only.

13. Which of the following will not interact with oral contraception?
    a. antibiotics
    b. antipyretics
    c. antifungals
    d. antiepileptics

14. During the fourth or fifth month of gestation, the pituitary gland secretes:
    a. colostrum.
    b. oxytocin.
    c. prolactin.
    d. all of the above.

15. Endometriosis is a condition characterized by:
    a. fragments of the uterine lining found in other parts of the pelvic cavity.
    b. vaginal odor and discharge.
    c. sterility.
    d. increased fertility.

16. A latex or silicon cervical barrier form of birth control is a:
    a. cervical cap.
    b. diaphragm.
    c. condom.
    d. intrauterine device.

True or False?

17. Activities that increase a male's risk for infertility include bicycling.

    T   F

18. Oxidants negatively affect DNA in the sperm.

    T   F

19. Syphilis and gonorrhea infection can cause a female to develop pelvic inflammatory disease (PID).

    T   F

20. Oral contraception medications can prevent a person from contracting HIV.

    T   F

PHARMACY CALCULATION PROBLEMS

Calculate the following.

1. A female patient is prescribed Depo-Provera 150 mg IM for three months. What is the total day supply until this prescription can be refilled again?

2. A prescription for clomiphene 50 mg tablets is being processed for a quantity of 30 tablets. The insurance company will only adjudicate a five-day supply for every 30 days. How many refills will you have to add to the prescription?

3. A man has brought in a prescription for prazosin 5 mg capsules. The prescription indicates that he is to take 10 mg bid. How many capsules would you need to dispense for a 90-day supply?

4. For latent syphilis, the recommended treatment is penicillin g benzathine (long-acting), 7.2 million units, divided into three weekly intramuscular injections. How many milligrams will the patient receive per dose?

5. A man is receiving 50 mg of testosterone cypionate IM every two weeks for hormone replacement therapy. If the clinic pharmacy stocks testosterone cypionate 100 mg/mL, how many milliliters of drug will the patient receive over the course of eight weeks?

PTCB EXAM PRACTICE QUESTIONS

1. Women who are experiencing premenstrual dysphoric disorder (PMDD) may be treated with all of the following *except*:
   a. antidepressants.
   b. NSAIDs.
   c. testosterone.
   d. oral contraceptives.

2. Which class of medications is first prescribed for BPH?
   a. antihypertensives
   b. alpha-adrenergic blockers
   c. 5-alpha reductase inhibitors
   d. beta blockers

3. Which of the following medical terms describes the most common cause of male infertility?
   a. oligospermia
   b. azoospermia
   c. dysspermia
   d. aspermia

4. Which of the following drugs is *not* used to treat erectile dysfunction (ED)?
   a. vardenafil
   b. tadalafil
   c. sildenafil
   d. triavil

5. Which of the following is the generic name for Flomax?
   a. terazosin
   b. prazosin
   c. tamsulosin
   d. alfuzosin

ACTIVITY 33-1: Anatomy Worksheet

The Female Reproductive System

Label the following illustration of the female reproductive system.

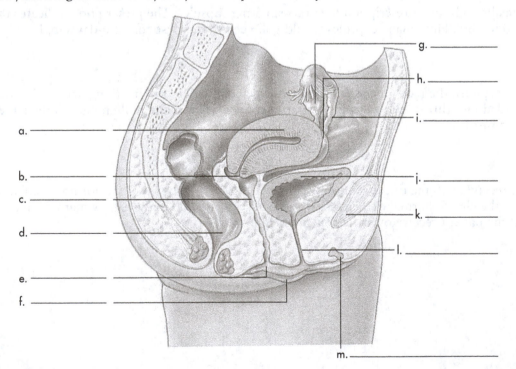

The Male Reproductive System

Label the following illustration of the male reproductive system.

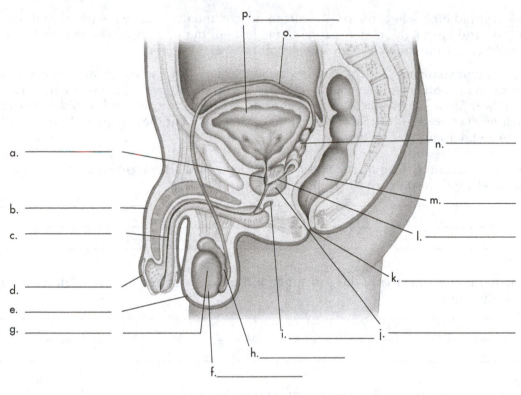

p. _____
o. _____
a. _____
b. _____
c. _____
d. _____
e. _____
g. _____
f. _____
h. _____
i. _____
j. _____
k. _____
l. _____
m. _____
n. _____

Questions:

1. Name the four hormones that are responsible for the female menstrual cycle. Where are these hormones produced within the body?

   _____

   _____

   _____

   _____

2. What is the main hormone that is responsible for male secondary sexual characteristics? Where is it produced within the body?

   _____

   _____

   _____

   _____

3. Name three different forms of contraception, explain how each method works, and give examples of each.

   _____

   _____

   _____

   _____

ACTIVITY 33-2: Case Study—Gonorrhea

Instructions: Read the following scenario and then answer the critical thinking questions.

Anna, a 17-year-old high school senior, presents to the community clinic with a vaginal discharge accompanied by pain and burning during urination. Anna just got out of a physically abusive relationship with an 18-year-old male from the same high school after two years of dating.

Anna is scared that something is very wrong with her because of these symptoms and comes to the clinic to get a checkup in confidence. The doctor who sees her orders lab tests that eventually lead to a diagnosis of gonorrhea. Anna is prescribed some medication for the gonorrhea and is told to notify her sexual partner that he may need to be treated as well. Anna is terrified at the prospect of notifying her abusive ex-boyfriend and does not know what to do.

1. Does Anna have an obligation to tell her ex-boyfriend (and his current partner, if he is involved with someone else)? Can someone else contact him?

   _____

   _____

   _____

2. What are the consequences of this condition for Anna and her past partner if left untreated? How does it affect health?

   _____

   _____

   _____

3. What can Anna do to avoid contracting an STD in the future?

   _____

   _____

   _____

ACTIVITY 33-3: Case Study—Erectile Dysfunction

Instructions: Read the following scenario and then answer the critical thinking questions.

Gary, a 52-year-old hardware store owner, has battled with BPH for four months. He also has other medical conditions, including high blood pressure, which is being treated with an oral antihypertensive medication. He feels that he is too young to be experiencing this condition.

Originally, Gary tried to control his BPH by limiting fluids in the evening, moderating his caffeine consumption, and scheduling his void times. He even tried a popular herbal supplement that stated that it would help with subsiding BPH symptoms. When these options proved to be unsuccessful for Gary, he was prescribed an alpha-adrenergic blocker. Unfortunately, the therapy did not work either, and he had to have a transurethral resection of the prostate (TURP) procedure.

After this procedure, Gary then experienced ED. His physician prescribed Viagra to treat the ED. Gary has arrived at the pharmacy today to pick up his first order of Viagra. Normally when Gary visits at the pharmacy, he is in a good mood. Today Gary is not in a good mood.

1. What popular herbal supplement did Gary use for his BPH? Please provide three names of these supplements.

   _____

   _____

   _____

2. Based on the information in the case study, is Gary's ED due to his high blood pressure or the TURP procedure?

   _____

   _____

   _____

3. What do you think you can do to help Gary with his current mood?

   _____

   _____

4. Which alpha-adrenergic blockers may have been appropriately prescribed early on for the pharmaceutical management of Gary's BPH plan?

   _____

   _____

   _____

ACTIVITY 33-4: Case Study—Oxytocin

Instructions: Read the following scenario and then answer the critical thinking questions.

Thirty-two-year-old Amanda is two weeks overdue with delivering her second baby. She finds it both challenging and uncomfortable to move. Today her water has broken, and she then calls her OB/GYN who instructs her to be driven to the hospital.

When Amanda arrives at the emergency department, she is quickly taken to labor and delivery as the OB/GYN team begins to monitor her condition. Amanda's blood pressure is slightly elevated, but the contractions are so mild that she cannot feel them. She has dilated to only 3 cm.

Six hours later, Amanda has dilated to 5 cm and her contractions are becoming stronger; however, she remains at this stage for the next four hours. Eventually, Amanda's physician decides to induce labor in order to move the delivery further along. Amanda is given oxytocin both pre and post the delivery of the baby.

1. Why is oxytocin generally used for predelivery of a baby?

   _____

   _____

   _____

2. Why is oxytocin generally used for postdelivery of a baby?

   _____

   _____

   _____

3. In what dosage form and route of administration will a pharmacy technician prepare oxytocin doses for obstetric patients?

   _____

   _____

   _____

4. Oxytocin has an approved yet controversial indication to help abort the fetus in cases of incomplete abortion or miscarriage. What is your perspective and viewpoint about this controversy?

   _____

   _____

   _____

LAB 33-1: Treating Infertility

Objective:

To become familiar with the infertility treatment options for parents who are unable to conceive an infant naturally.

Pre-Lab Information:

- Visit the website http://www.webmd.com/infertility-and-reproduction/guide /infertility-reproduction-treatment-care.
- Review Chapter 33 in your textbook about infertility.

Explanation:

Many individuals who are unable to conceive an infant, for one reason or another, can now choose from various treatment options to help assist in the process of conception.

Activity:

Using the website (http://www.webmd.com/infertility-and-reproduction/guide/infertility-reproduction-treatment-care), please answer the questions below.

1. What are the eight assisted reproduction options that partners may choose from?

   _____

   _____

   _____

   _____

2. What is tubal ligation more commonly referred to as? What is a tubal ligation reversal?

   _____

   _____

   _____

3. How many medications are currently available for infertility treatment?

   _____

4. What are the six injectable medication names (brand and generic) for infertility treatment?

   _____

   _____

   _____

   _____

   _____

5. What is artificial insemination?

   _____

   _____

6. What is in vitro fertilization?

_____

_____

7. What is a surrogate? What two kinds of surrogate mothers are there?

_____

_____

_____

Student Name: _____

Lab Partner: _____

Grade/Comments: _____

_____

_____

Student Comments: _____

_____

_____

LAB 33-2: Treating Erectile Dysfunction

Objective:

To become familiar with treatment options for male patients who have been diagnosed with ED.

Pre-Lab Information:

• Review Chapter 33 in your textbook about ED.

Explanation:

Many male patients who are unable to achieve an erection due to either inorganic or organic conditions can now choose from various treatment options to help assist them in the process of achieving a prolonged and successful erection.

Activity:

Match up the following generic medications to their brand-name counterparts.

Generic	Brand
yohimbine	_____
sildenafil	_____
alprostadil	_____
tadalafil	_____
vardenafil	_____

Brand Names:

Viagra	Muse	Aphrodyne	Levitra
Caverject	Cialis		

Student Name: _____

Lab Partner: _____

Grade/Comments: _____

_____

_____

Student Comments: _____

_____

_____

LAB 33-3: Understanding Pregnancy Categories

Objective:

To understand the importance of caution when pregnant women use prescription drugs.

Pre-Lab Information:

- Review Chapter 33 in your textbook.
- Visit the following U.S. Department of Health and Human Services website: http://www.womenshealth .gov/publications/our-publications/fact-sheet/pregnancy-medicines.pdf

Explanation:

Pregnancy categories are determined on the basis of the potential harm a drug may cause to the fetus. The five pregnancy categories are A, B, C, D, and X, with A being the lowest risk and X being the highest. As a pharmacy technician, it is important for you to understand the concept of risk versus benefit—especially as it applies to drugs taken during pregnancy.

Activity:

Visit the following U.S. Department of Health and Human Services website and use the information there to answer the questions related to drugs used in pregnancy: http://www.womenshealth.gov/publications /our-publications/fact-sheet/pregnancy-medicines.pdf

1. Write the definition of Pregnancy Category A as it applies to human studies only.

   _____

   _____

   _____

2. Write the definition of Pregnancy Category B as it applies to *human studies* only.

   _____

   _____

   _____

3. Write the definition of Pregnancy Category C as it applies to *human studies* only.

   _____

   _____

   _____

4. Write the definition of Pregnancy Category D as it applies to *human studies* only.

   _____

   _____

   _____

5. Write the definition of Pregnancy Category X as it applies to *human studies* only.

   _____

   _____

   _____

6. To which pregnancy category does the drug phenytoin (Dilantin) belong?

   _____

7. To which pregnancy category does the drug isotretinoin (Accutane) belong?

   _____

8. To which pregnancy category does the drug fluconazole (Diflucan) belong?

   _____

9. To which pregnancy category does the drug levothyroxine (Synthroid) belong?

   _____

10. To which pregnancy category does the drug ondansetron (Zofran) belong?

   _____

Student Name: _____

Lab Partner: _____

Grade/Comments: _____

_____

_____

Student Comments: _____

_____

_____

CHAPTER 34
The Nervous System

After completing Chapter 34 from the textbook, you should be able to:	Related Activity in the Workbook/Lab Manual
1. Explain the functions of the nervous system and its division into the central and peripheral nervous systems.	Review Questions, PTCB Exam Practice Questions, Activity 34-1
2. Compare and contrast the sympathetic and parasympathetic nervous systems.	Review Questions, PTCB Exam Practice Questions, Activity 34-1
3. Describe the function or physiology of neurons and nerve transmission and the various neurotransmitters.	Review Questions, Activity 34-1
4. Explain the relationship of the nervous system to the other body systems.	Review Questions, Activity 34-1, Activity 34-2, Activity 34-3, Activity 34-4, Lab 34-1
5. Explain the functions of the blood–brain barrier and describe what types of substances will and will not cross it.	Review Questions, Activity 34-1
6. List and define common diseases affecting the nervous system and discuss the causes, symptoms, and pharmaceutical treatment associated with each disease.	Review Questions, PTCB Exam Practice Questions, Activity 34-2, Activity 34-3, Activity 34-4, Lab 34-1, Lab 34-2
7. Identify the common drugs used to treat diseases and conditions of the nervous system.	Review Questions, PTCB Exam Practice Questions, Activity 34-2, Activity 34-3, Activity 34-4, Lab 34-1, Lab 34-2

INTRODUCTION

The nervous system is a very complex system that interacts with every other system in the body to ensure homeostasis and regulate the body's responses to internal and external stimuli. The nervous system communicates with all cells in the body through nerve impulses that are conducted from one part of the body to another via the transmission of chemicals called *neurotransmitters*.

The nervous system is divided into two parts, the central nervous system (CNS) and the peripheral nervous system (PNS). The CNS includes the brain, the spinal column, and their nerves. The PNS is also divided into two parts: the somatic nervous system, which controls voluntary movement of the body through muscles; and the autonomic nervous system, which controls involuntary motor functions and affects such things as heart rate and digestion.

Diseases and conditions affecting the nervous system include anxiety, depression, bipolar disorder, Parkinson's disease, alcohol addiction, and seizures. Pain due to injury or cancer also affects the nervous system. *Neuropharmacology*, or pharmacology related to the nervous system, is one of the most diverse and complicated areas of pharmacology. As a pharmacy technician, you must have a solid understanding of the common diseases affecting the nervous system and the pharmaceutical treatments associated with these diseases.

REVIEW QUESTIONS

Match the following.

1. _____ adjuvant
2. _____ afferent
3. _____ anxiety
4. _____ anxiolytic
5. _____ CNS
6. _____ cerebrospinal fluid
7. _____ EEG
8. _____ efferent
9. _____ gray matter
10. _____ hypotension
11. _____ PNS
12. _____ narcolepsy
13. _____ white matter

a. condition characterized by frequent and uncontrolled periods of deep sleep

b. all parts of the nervous system excluding the brain and spinal cord

c. component of myelinated nerve tissue in the CNS

d. low blood pressure

e. helping or assisting

f. a drug used in the treatment of anxiety

g. the part of the nervous system made up of the brain and spinal cord

h. an uncomfortable emotional state of apprehension, worry, and fearfulness

i. sending impulses away from the CNS

j. the fluid surrounding brain and spinal cord

k. a major component of the nervous system, composed of nonmyelinated nerve tissue with a gray-brown color

l. sending an impulse toward the CNS

m. a graphic record of the electrical activity of the brain

Choose the best answer.

14. Afferent impulses are said to be:
  a. sensory.   c. motor.
  b. integrative.   d. perceived.

15. The changes in the environment that set off the nerve impulse to communicate with another neuron are called:
  a. simuli.   c. stimulus.
  b. stimulation.   d. stimuli.

16. The sympathetic nervous system is governed by the neurotransmitter:
  a. acetylcholine.   c. cytoplasm.
  b. synapse.   d. norepinephrine.

17. The _____ is concerned with higher intellect or reasoning, problem solving, parts of speech, movement, and emotion.
  a. occipital lobe   c. frontal lobe
  b. parietal lobe   d. temporal lobe

18. Which of the following is not a general property of the blood–brain barrier (BBB)?
  a. Water-soluble or low-lipid/low-fat-soluble molecules do not penetrate.
  b. Infectious agents cannot open up the BBB.
  c. Large molecules do not easily pass through the BBB.
  d. Highly electrically charged molecules are slowed down.

19. Which of these drugs bind to the GABA-A receptors and increase the actions of GABA?
  a. β-adrenergic blockers   c. benzodiazepines
  b. SSRIs   d. MAOIs

Match the following drugs with their categories or treatment uses.

20. _____ imipramine   **a.** nonbenzodiazepine
21. _____ selegiline   **b.** atypical antidepressant
22. _____ haloperidol   **c.** tetracyclic
23. _____ propranolol   **d.** TCA
24. _____ gabapentin   **e.** SSRI
25. _____ duloxetine   **f.** β-adrenergic blocker
26. _____ dextroamphetamine   **g.** benzodiazepine
27. _____ citalopram   **h.** MAOI
28. _____ zolpidem   **i.** anticonvulsant
29. _____ alprazolam   **j.** antipsychotic
30. _____ mirtazapine   **k.** CNS stimulant
31. _____ divalproex   **l.** narcotic used for pain
32. _____ carbidopa/levodopa   **m.** migraine treatment
33. _____ methysergide   **n.** Alzheimer's
34. _____ morphine sulfate   **o.** Parkinson's
35. _____ tacrine   **p.** delays sodium influx

PHARMACY CALCULATION PROBLEMS

Calculate the following.

1. If chlorpromazine 25 mg/100 mL IV is to run over 30 minutes, what is the infusion rate in milliliters per hour?

2. A patient is to receive 37.5 mg of risperidone long-acting injection. The pharmacy only has 50 mg/2 mL in stock. How many milliliters are needed for the dose?

3. You need to fill a prescription for duloxetine 30 mg. The directions read "3 caps po qd." The patient only wants a 14-day supply. How many capsules will you need to fill the prescription?

4. If a patient is receiving 1 mg of alprazolam bid for 15 days, how many milligrams is the patient receiving each day? How much will the patient receive for the course of therapy?

5. If a patient weighs 132 lbs., what is his or her weight in kilograms?

PTCB EXAM PRACTICE QUESTIONS

1. The drugs Prozac, Zoloft, and Paxil are examples of drugs that selectively inhibit the reuptake of which of the following neurotransmitters?
   a. troponin
   b. GABA
   c. serotonin
   d. nortriptyline

2. Which of the following drugs is indicated for the treatment of bipolar disorder?
   a. lithium
   b. Librium
   c. Lasix
   d. Lyrica

3. What class of drugs does Clozaril belong to?
   a. anticonvulsant
   b. antidepressant
   c. antipsychotic
   d. anti-anxiety

4. Which of the following drugs would *not* be used to treat status epilepticus?
   a. Cerebyx
   b. Ativan
   c. Celebrex
   d. Valium

5. Benzodiazepines belong to which schedule of controlled substances?
   a. Schedule I
   b. Schedule II
   c. Schedule III
   d. Schedule IV

ACTIVITY 34-1: Anatomy Worksheet

The Nervous System

Label the following illustration of the nervous system.

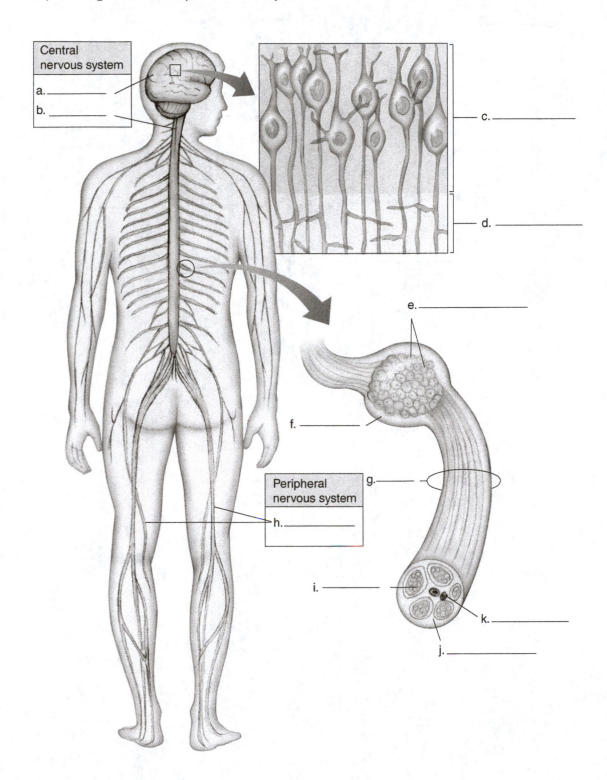

Central
nervous system

a. _____

b. _____

c. _____

d. _____

e. _____

f. _____

g. _____

Peripheral
nervous system

h. _____

i. _____

j. _____

k. _____

The Neuron

Label the following illustration of the neuron.

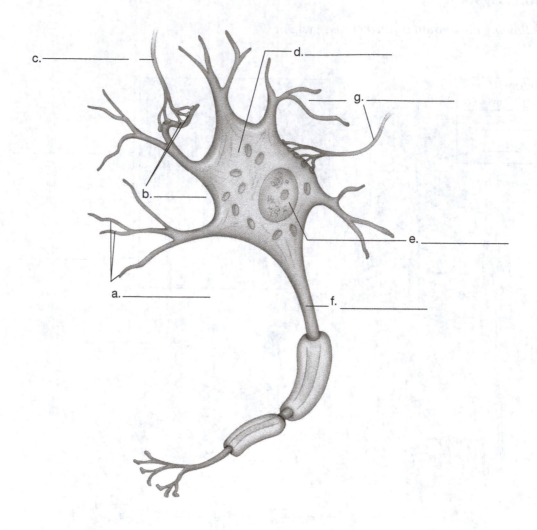

The Brain

Label the following illustration of the brain.

a. _____

b. _____

c. _____

d. _____

e. _____

f. _____

g. _____

h. _____

i. _____

j. _____

k. _____

l. _____

m. _____

n. _____

o. _____

p. _____

q. _____

r. _____

s. _____

t. _____

u. _____

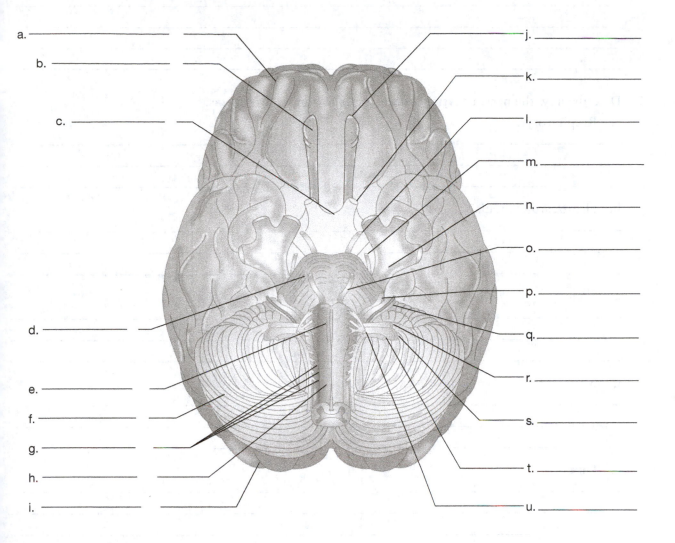

Questions:

1. What are the functions of the nervous system?

   _____
   _____
   _____
   _____

2. Describe how the nervous system affects the following body systems:
   a. Respiratory

   _____
   _____
   _____

   b. Heart/cardiovascular

   _____
   _____
   _____

   c. Skeletal

   _____
   _____
   _____

   d. Muscular

   _____
   _____
   _____

   e. Digestive

   _____
   _____
   _____

   f. Endocrine

   _____
   _____
   _____

   g. Lymphatic/immune

   _____
   _____
   _____

h. Renal (urinary)

_____

_____

_____

i. Integumentary

_____

_____

_____

3. Compare and contrast the sympathetic and parasympathetic nervous systems.

_____

_____

_____

_____

4. What are the functions of the neurons? Discuss the process of neurotransmission.

_____

_____

_____

_____

5. What are the functions of the BBB? What are some disease states or physical changes that can compromise its integrity?

_____

_____

_____

_____

ACTIVITY 34-2: Case Study—A Change in a Friend

Instructions: Read the following scenario and then answer the critical thinking questions.

About eight months ago, you used to consistently play racquetball twice a week with your neighbor Mrs. Vanderbank. However, she has no longer been able to meet with you for your games. At first, she would miss a game here and there, and then one day she plainly stated to you that she hated racquetball and never wanted to play again. Her recent change in behavior also happened around the same time she stopped taking phone calls from her mother, to whom she had always been close. The reasons she gave to you for not playing racquetball with you included a lack of sleep and a decrease in her energy.

As Mrs. Vanderbank comes in to pick up her prescriptions, you notice that she has lost a lot of weight. You mention to her that you did not realize that she was dieting. She sternly replies to you that she is not dieting and that she is truly never hungry. You are aware that Mrs. Vanderbank weighed 135 lbs. a few months ago and has lost weight since then. She also seems quieter than usual. As a friend, you ask her if she is alright and then you offer to go out with her to lunch tomorrow, but she tells you everything is alright and declines your lunch invitation.

She is picking up a prescription for fluoxetine. You remember that she was taking sertraline a short time ago. Another prescription that she is also picking up is for trazodone to help combat her insomnia. She states to you that the trazodone is not working, just like the sertraline that did not work. You tell her that the pharmacist would like to counsel her about the medications but she declines.

1. What condition do you believe that Mrs. Vanderbank is experiencing?

   _____

   _____

   _____

2. What class of drugs do fluoxetine and sertraline belong to?

   _____

   _____

   _____

3. As you are Mrs. Vanderbank's friend, do you believe that there is a conflict of interest with asking Mrs. Vanderbank personal questions while you are at work?

   _____

   _____

   _____

ACTIVITY 34-3: Case Study—The Blue Dog

Instructions: Read the following scenario and then answer the critical thinking questions.

Mr. Ogdahl is a regular at your outpatient pharmacy. At times, he exhibits some behaviors that seem rather silly to a lot of folks in other areas where you work. Occasionally, he seems comfortable enough to have light conversation with you while he waits for his medications.

At times, he talks about cartoons that come on in the mornings, specifically the one with the "blue dog." As his visits become more frequent, he seems to talk about the blue dog more and more in a personal sense. He tells you that before he can watch the blue dog each and every morning, he first has to clear off his favorite chair, fold his favorite blanket, scrub his hands until they almost hurt, and pour a cup of orange juice—only orange juice—into a blue cup that matches the blue dog. One time you ask, "Have you ever had apple juice?" and he seems to become upset and rigid, reinforcing that only orange juice will do.

The medicine he has refilled every month like clockwork is oxazepam. One day he tells you that he was prescribed this medicine after cognitive behavior therapy failed.

1. To what class of drugs does oxazepam belong?

   _____

   _____

   _____

2. Based on the short description in the scenario, what seems to be Mr. Ogdahl's condition?

   _____

   _____

   _____

3. In what mental disorder category does this condition fall?

   _____

   _____

   _____

4. How can you explain to other people that Mr. Ogdahl's thoughts are not silly?

   _____

   _____

   _____

ACTIVITY 34-4: Case Study—Pain Relief for Cancer

Instructions: Read the following scenario and then answer the critical thinking questions.

Mrs. Eddleton is a 37-year-old housewife with cancer who asks to speak to a pharmacist for a recommendation. She explains that some days her pain from cancer is debilitating. The pain used to subside after she took her tablet and not return until just before the next dose was due; now, though, the pain is constant. Mrs. Eddleton reads extensively about her condition, hoping to discover a pain medication that will work.

She has regular follow-up visits at the pain management clinic, where they have been prescribing oral morphine three times a day for pain over the last year. She has tried several other pain medications before the morphine. Lately, even the morphine has not brought relief. She asks the pharmacist if there is an option where she would not have to take the medicine three times a day and might control the pain a little better. She has read that an opioid patch is available to help with pain like hers.

1. To what patch could Mrs. Eddleton be referring?
   _____
   _____
   _____

2. How is the patch used by the patient, and for what type of pain?
   _____
   _____
   _____

3. Do you know of anything Mrs. Eddleton could do, outside of or in conjunction with taking medication, to ease the pain?
   _____
   _____
   _____

4. Do you think it is acceptable for patients to be proactive in their own medication therapy in ways such as research?
   _____
   _____
   _____

LAB 34-1: Treating Attention Deficit Hyperactivity Disorder (ADHD)

Objective:

To understand about the different treatment options for attention deficit hyperactivity disorder (ADHD).

Pre-Lab Information:

Review Chapter 34 in your textbook to learn more about ADHD.

Explanation:

ADHD is prevalent in the preadolescent to adolescent age ranges as well as in some adults. There are a few treatment options for parents and adults to consider; after proper assessment, observation can be made for a diagnosis of ADHD.

Activity:

Using your textbook as a resource, match up the following medications that are commonly used as a treatment option for ADHD. Please match the generic medications with their brand-name counterpart. Also notate if the medication is a controlled substance and what schedule it belongs to.

Generic	Brand Name(s)	Controlled Substance Schedule
atomoxetine	_____	_____
dextroamphetamine	_____	_____
dextroamphetamine sulfate, dextroamphetamine saccharate, amphetamine aspartate, amphetamine sulphate	_____	_____
methylphenidate	_____	_____
methylphenidate (once daily)	_____	_____

Student Name: _____

Lab Partner: _____

Grade/Comments: _____

_____

_____

Student Comments: _____

_____

_____

LAB 34-2: Treating Migraines

Objective:

To understand about the different treatment options for migraines.

Pre-Lab Information:

Review Chapter 34 in your textbook to learn more about migraines.

Explanation:

Migraines can be both debilitating and bring about many uncomfortable symptoms for the migraine sufferer. Currently, there are 11 different kinds of medications to help patients either abort a migraine after its sudden onset or there is a prophylactic treatment option to prevent a migraine.

Activity:

Using your textbook as a resource, match up the following migraine therapy medications with their brand-name counterpart. Also notate the method of the delivery systems/dosage forms for each of the medications.

Generic	Brand Name(s)	Delivery System/ Dosage Form(s)
almotriptan	_____	_____
amitriptyline	_____	_____
naratriptan	_____	_____
ergotamine + caffeine	_____	_____
frovatriptan	_____	_____
sumatriptan	_____	_____
propranolol	_____	_____
rizatriptan	_____	_____
eletriptan	_____	_____
methysergide	_____	_____
zolmitriptan	_____	_____

Brand Name:

Amerge	Elavil	Sansert	Frova
Axert	Maxalt	Relpax	Inderal LA
Imitrex	Zomig		

Student Name: _____

Lab Partner: _____

Grade/Comments: _____

_____

_____

Student Comments: _____

_____

_____

CHAPTER 35
Medication Errors

After completing Chapter 35 from the textbook, you should be able to:	Related Activity in the Workbook/Lab Manual
1. List and describe the five rights of medication administration.	Review Questions, PTCB Exam Practice Questions, Activity 35-1, Activity 35-2, Activity 35-3, Activity 35-4, Lab 35-1, Lab 35-2
2. Outline and define the various categories of medication errors.	Review Questions, PTCB Exam Practice Questions, Activity 35-1, Activity 35-2, Activity 35-3, Activity 35-4, Lab 35-1, Lab 35-2
3. Discuss key statistics related to medication errors and pharmacy practice.	Review Questions, PTCB Exam Practice Questions, Activity 35-1, Activity 35-2, Activity 35-3, Activity 35-4, Lab 35-1, Lab 35-2
4. Identify look-alike, sound-alike drugs and tall man lettering.	Review Questions, PTCB Exam Practice Questions, Activity 35-1, Activity 35-2, Activity 35-3, Activity 35-4, Lab 35-1, Lab 35-2
5. Review specific case studies of medication errors, and discuss the causes, outcomes, and recommended preventable solutions.	Review Questions, PTCB Exam Practice Questions, Activity 35-1, Activity 35-2, Activity 35-3, Activity 35-4, Lab 35-1, Lab 35-2
6. Outline and describe best practices for preventing medication errors.	Review Questions, PTCB Exam Practice Questions, Activity 35-1, Activity 35-2, Activity 35-3, Activity 35-4, Lab 35-1, Lab 35-2
7. List various agencies involved in the monitoring and reporting of medication errors and describe their role(s).	Review Questions, PTCB Exam Practice Questions, Activity 35-1, Activity 35-2, Activity 35-3, Activity 35-4, Lab 35-1, Lab 35-2

REVIEW QUESTIONS

Match the following.

1. _____ medication error
2. _____ right patient
3. _____ right drug
4. _____ right route
5. _____ right dose
6. _____ right time
7. _____ right technique
8. _____ right documentation

a. the patient must receive the right dose. A dose that is too high or too low is considered a medication error

b. correct documentation must be completed

c. the patient must receive the medication within the prescribed time frame

d. the drug must be given via the correct route of administration. If the correct drug and dose are given, but via the wrong route, a medication error has occurred

e. the right drug must always be chosen

f. correct technique must be used when preparing the drug

g. the drug must always go to the correct patient

h. any preventable event that may cause or lead to inappropriate medication use or patient harm while the medication is in the control of the health care professional, patient, or consumer

Fill in the blanks.

9. An _____ or _____ is defined as administration of a dose of medication that was never ordered for that patient.

10. An _____ is counted if a dose is given in excess of the total number of times ordered by the physician, such as a dose given on the basis of an expired order, after a drug has been discontinued, or after a drug has been put on hold.

11. If a patient fails to receive a dose of medication that was ordered, an _____ _____ is noted if no attempt was made to administer the dose.

12. A _____ occurs when any dose is given that contains the wrong number of preformed dosage units (such as tablets) or was, in the judgment of the observer, more than 17% greater or less than the correct dosage.

13. _____ are typically defined as those situations where a medication is administered to the patient using a different route than was ordered.

14. _____ are typically defined as the administration of a dose more than 30 minutes (or 60 minutes depending on the site) before or after the scheduled administration time, unless there is an acceptable reason for this time difference.

15. A _____ involves the administration of a dose form different from that ordered by the physician, provided the physician specified or implied a particular form.

Choose the best answer.

16. The recommended dosage of digoxin for a child who is 5–10 years is:
    a. 10–15 mcg.
    b. 35–60 mcg/kg.
    c. 20–35 mcg.
    d. 35–60 mcg/kg.

17. More people die each year from:
    a. AIDS.
    b. motor vehicle accidents.
    c. breast cancer.
    d. medical errors.

18. Which medication is associated with medication errors?
    a. propofol
    b. heparin
    c. levothyroxine
    d. magnesium sulfate

19. The ultimate tool in preventing medication errors will always be:
    a. education.
    b. training sessions.
    c. becoming nationally certified.
    d. all of the above.

20. What piece of technology is most likely to reduce medication errors?
    a. personal electronic devices
    b. e-prescribing
    c. automated dispensing units
    d. none of the above

PHARMACY CALCULATION PROBLEMS

Calculate the following

1. How many milligrams are in 0.75 mcg if the direction for the patient is 1 tab po bid?

2. The order for cefazolin is 1 g/500 mL IV q12h for two days. The pharmacy has just run out of the 500 mL bags but there are 500 mg/250 mL bags currently in stock. The flow rate for the infusion of the 500 mL bag was for 60 minutes. How many bags will the patient now receive for the duration of the therapy, and what will the infusion rate in mL/hr be for each 250 mL bag?

3. The oncologist has prescribed gemcitabine 1,000 mg/mL over 30 minutes once weekly for up to seven weeks followed by one week of rest for a patient with pancreatic cancer. The patient's current height and weight are 79.5 kg and 5'10", respectively. The direction for reconstitution is to add 25 mL of 0.9% Sodium chloride to make a solution 38 mg/mL. Shake to dissolve. How many milliliters will you prepare for this patient?

4. You have a stock vial of sodium bicarbonate 0.5 mEq/mL. How many milliliters are needed to provide 60 mEq?

5. You have a stock vial of potassium chloride 2 mEq/mL. How many milliliters are needed to provide 35 mEq?

1. An environmental factor that can deter or distract health care professionals from their tasks is:
   a. heat.
   b. screaming babies.
   c. pollution.
   d. dust.

2. An example of a cardiovascular medication is:
   a. HCTZ.
   b. GABA.
   c. AZT.
   d. ASA.

3. A prescription for an antibiotic eardrop is prescribed to a patient who has otitis media. The direction is 1gtt bid × 7 days. How should the directions be translated for the patient?
   a. Instill one drop into the left eye twice a day for seven days
   b. Instill one drop into the right eye twice a day for seven days
   c. Instill one drop into the left ear twice a day for seven days
   d. Instill one drop into both ears twice a day for seven days

4. The correct way to type or write out 500 mg after converting it to a grams weight is:
   a. .5 g.
   b. 5 g.
   c. 0.05 g.
   d. 0.5 g.

5. Coumadin is to warfarin as Xanax is to:
   a. lorazepam.
   b. temazepam.
   c. alprazolam.
   d. diazepam.

ACTIVITY 35-1: Case Study—Communicating a Medication Error

Instructions: Read the following scenario and then answer the critical thinking questions.

Your intrapersonal relationships and rapport with both the nursing team and the inpatient pharmacy team have been positive since you began your tenure at the hospital three months ago. You enjoy the work of an inpatient technician, and you feel that your communication skills are both effective and efficient along with the management of your daily activities and tasks. However, at certain times of the day, the central IV area can be quite noisy and it is challenging to hear dosage changes or changes in orders.

As you are currently and diligently compounding and processing five IV orders, one of the female nurses who you are familiar with from the ER department suddenly calls down to the pharmacy. An adult male has just been brought in to the ER with status epilepticus. The nurse is ordering diazepam 10 mg STAT IM to be given in five initial separate doses for this patient.

When the order is called out to you for immediate process, you recall that the usual adult dose for diazepam to treat the indication of status epilepticus is an initial maximum dose of 30 mg. Also for initial treatment with diazepam for status epilepticus, a 5 mg or a 10 mg dose may be repeated every 10–15 minutes.

1. What kind of medication error could happen if you process all five doses?
   _____
   _____

2. What will you do to successfully communicate this medication error to the pharmacy team?
   _____
   _____
   _____

3. Why should the pharmacy supervisor address this medication error with the nursing team?

_____

_____

_____

4. You also recall that this particular nurse has called in an overage of doses for a controlled substance before with two other ER cases. What can you do to address this finding with the pharmacy team?

_____

_____

_____

ACTIVITY 35-2: Case Study—Recognizing Dangerous Abbreviations

Please match up the following dangerous abbreviations with their intended meanings and the common errors from the lists below.

Abbreviation	Intended Meaning	Common Errors
U	_____	_____
		_____
μg	_____	_____
		_____
Q.D.	_____	_____
		_____
Q.O.D.	_____	_____
		_____
SC or SQ	_____	_____
TIW	_____	_____
D/C	_____	_____
		_____
		_____
HS	_____	_____
Cc	_____	_____
AU, AS, AD	_____	_____
		_____
		_____
IU	_____	_____
MS, MSO$_4$, MgSO$_4$	_____	_____

Units	International Unit	Half strength	Confused for one another
Three times a week	Every other day	Cubic centimeters	Subcutaneous
Discharge; also discontinue	Both ears; left ear; right ear	Every day	Micrograms

Mistaken for "mg" (milligrams), resulting in an overdose.

Misinterpreted as "QD" (daily) or "QID" (four times daily). If the "O" is poorly written, it looks like a period or "I."

Misinterpreted as "three times a day" or "twice a week."

Mistaken as "SL" (sublingual) when poorly written.

The period after the "Q" has sometimes been mistaken for an "I," and the drug has been given "QID" (four times daily) rather than daily.

Mistaken as "U" (units) when poorly written.

Mistaken as IV (intravenous) or 10 (ten).

Patient's medications have been prematurely discontinued when D/C (intended to mean "discharge") was misinterpreted as "discontinue," because it was followed by a list of drugs.

Misinterpreted as the Latin abbreviation "HS" (hour of sleep).

Misinterpreted as the Latin abbreviations "OU" (both eyes), "OS" (left eye), and "OD" (right eye).

Mistaken as IV (intravenous) or 10 (ten).

Can mean morphine sulfate or magnesium sulfate.

Mistaken as a zero or a four (4), resulting in an overdose. Also mistaken for "cc" (cubic centimeters) when poorly written.

ACTIVITY 35-3: Case Study—Wrong Drug, Wrong Patient

Instructions: Read the following scenario and then answer the critical thinking questions.

Mr. Price is a consistent patient at the retail pharmacy to where you are the lead technician. You have had a positive and strong rapport with Mr. Price, and you are also very familiar with his patient profile. His list of medications comprises of atorvastatin, timolol, and esomeprazole 20 mg. He has just phoned in his refill requests for the three medications to you, and he will pick them up later on in this afternoon.

Another consistent patient at your pharmacy, Ms. Prince, has been taking the medication omeprazole 20 mg for the past four months for GERD. She has also phoned in her refill request and will also be picking up her prescription this afternoon. A few minutes after you completed the call with Ms. Prince, four patients arrive at the drop-off counter with new orders for you and the pharmacy team to process. You successfully convey to the team that the expected wait time for each patient is now 15–30 minutes. To your knowledge, the four new orders as well as the refill requests have all been successfully processed.

Mr. Price comes into the pharmacy at 4:00 p.m., and Ms. Prince comes into the pharmacy a few minutes after Mr. Price does. Both Mr. Price and Ms. Prince pay for their prescriptions and thank you for your service. A half hour later, Ms. Price calls the pharmacy and asks to speak with the pharmacist. Soon after that, Mr. Price calls also asking to speak with the pharmacist. After the pharmacist has completed the calls with both patients, he asks to speak with you and the two other technician colleagues.

He explains to you all that both Ms. Prince and Mr. Price took the wrong prescription home with them. He further explains to you all that the major indicator for the two of them that they received the wrong medication was that the colorings of the capsules were different than what they have been receiving with their prior refills. Both patients are immediately returning to the pharmacy to exchange their prescriptions per the pharmacist's instruction. Fortunately, neither patient has taken any of his or her medication that was incorrectly dispensed.

1. What two medications were incorrectly dispensed to Ms. Prince and Mr. Price?
   _____
   _____

2. What type of medication error has occurred in this case?
   _____
   _____

3. What should have been done to prevent this medication error from happening?
   _____
   _____

4. What were the two factors that contributed to this medication error?
   _____
   _____

5. Is this type of medication error reportable by law? Why or why not?
   _____
   _____

6. Which team member is to blame for this error?
   _____
   _____

ACTIVITY 35-4: Case Study—Dispensing an Antibiotic Suspension

Instructions: Read the following scenario and then answer the critical thinking questions.

The morning at the retail pharmacy has been very busy. Along with five refill requests for five different patients, three new orders have been phoned in by physicians along with four new walk-in orders, one of those new walk-in orders has been brought in by Amy's grandmother. For the first time in her life, three-year-old Amy has been prescribed amoxicillin and clavulanate potassium suspension 125 mg/mL with the quantity as 100 mL after reconstitution.

One of the pharmacy clerks has called in sick for the day; therefore, you have been delegated to run the front counter and register as well as process all new walked-in prescription orders at the drop-off counter.

Amy's order is ready and her grandmother is eager to get home so that Amy can take the medication and feel better. You hurriedly ring the grandmother up while at the same time noticing that something feels different about the weight of the bag. The other prescriptions for the patients who have been waiting are also ready for pick-up as Amy's grandmother denies a consultation from the pharmacist. She figures that she can just read the directions on the label.

An hour goes by and Amy's grandmother calls the pharmacy in a panicked mode. She asks to speak with the pharmacist and tells the pharmacist that Amy has been crying loudly for the past 25 minutes since she gave her a teaspoonful of the powder. The pharmacist instructs Amy's grandmother to immediately call poison control and that the poison control team may tell Amy's grandmother to take Amy to the emergency room.

1. What type of medication error has occurred in this case?
   _____
   _____

2. What harm may come to Amy after she has been given 5 mL of the powder?
   _____
   _____

3. What should have been done to prevent this medication error from happening?
   _____
   _____

4. Is this type of medication error reportable by law? Why or why not?
   _____
   _____

5. Which team member is to blame for this error?
   _____
   _____

LAB 35-1: Preventing Errors

Objective:

To understand as a technician, how to prevent errors from happening inside and outside of the pharmacy.

Pre-Lab Information:

Review Chapter 35 in your textbook to learn more about preventing errors.

Explanation:

From the time a physician prescribes a medication to a patient until the time the patient starts and ends his or her medication therapy, there are 12 types of medication errors that could occur. The pharmacy technician is strongly relied upon to assist the health care team and the patient with preventing errors.

Activity:

Match up the following cases to strategies in order to be aware of and also to prevent errors.

Case	Strategy
1. AD, AS, AU, OD, OS, OU _____	A. Look for duplicate therapies and interactions
2. Celexa/Celebrex _____	B. Do not take shortcuts around technology safeguards
3. Patient is taking Alka-Seltzer PM and loratadine for a cold. She takes the Alka-Seltzer PM for her heartburn and the loratadine so that she does not fall asleep at work. _____	C. Recognize prescription look-alike/ sound-alike medications
4. Ketamine, propofol _____	D. Report errors to improve process
5. A geriatric patient has arthritis and is medication risking compliance. _____	E. Avoid abbreviations and nomenclature
6. Patient is taking two different brand-name drugs with the same generic ingredient. _____	F. Increase awareness of at-risk confusing her arthritis medication for the other populations
7. The patient talks with the pharmacist about the "5 Rights" for medication safety. _____	G. Control the environment
8. Pharmacist gives the technician initials to override alerts. _____	H. Educate the patient
9. The technician witnesses the pharmacist throwing away all evidence of an error. _____	I. Focus on high-alert medications
10. Lighting, shift changes, workload increases. _____	J. Beware of OTC family extensions and standardized labeling

Student Name: _____

Lab Partner: _____

Grade/Comments: _____

_____

_____

Student Comments: _____

_____

_____

LAB 35-2: Reporting an Error

Objective:

To understand how to report an error once it occurs.

Pre-Lab Information:

Review Chapter 35 in your textbook to learn more about reporting errors.

Explanation:

As the safety of a patient is imperative for pharmacy professionals to protect, the responsibility of a pharmacy technician to report any error, which may compromise the safety of the patient, is just as imperative.

Activity:

Using the website www.nccmerp.org, please follow the procedures and answer the following questions.

1. Click onto "Report a Medication Error."
2. Click "Go" for the ISMP Medication Errors Reporting Program (MERP).
3. What are the seven examples of medication and vaccine errors?

_____

_____

_____

_____

_____

_____

_____

_____

4. Which kind or types of submissions are reporters encouraged to provide to ISMP?

_____

_____

_____

5. Click on the "Healthcare Practitioners" tab.
6. Click on the "Report Medication Errors (ISMP MERP)" tab.
7. What content is needed to report a medication error? What other information is necessary to provide?

_____

_____

_____

_____

_____

_____

_____

_____

8. Is the information reported kept confidential? Why or why not?

_____

_____

Student Name: _____

Lab Partner: _____

Grade/Comments: _____

_____

_____

Student Comments: _____

_____

_____

CHAPTER 36
Workplace Safety and Infection Control

After completing Chapter 36 from the textbook, you should be able to:	Related Activity in the Workbook/Lab Manual
1. Define and describe the importance of workplace safety.	Review Questions, PTCB Exam Practice Questions, Activity 36-1, Activity 36-2, Activity 36-3, Activity 36-4, Lab 36-1, Lab 36-2
2. Explain the difference between an accident and an incident.	Review Questions, PTCB Exam Practice Questions, Activity 36-1, Activity 36-2, Activity 36-3, Activity 36-4, Lab 36-1, Lab 36-2
3. Outline the four key elements of workplace safety.	Review Questions, PTCB Exam Practice Questions, Activity 36-1, Activity 36-2, Activity 36-3, Activity 36-4, Lab 36-1, Lab 36-2
4. Identify specific workplace safety concerns related to pharmacy practice.	Review Questions, PTCB Exam Practice Questions, Activity 36-1, Activity 36-2, Activity 36-3, Activity 36-4, Lab 36-1, Lab 36-2
5. Outline the key requirements as prescribed by OSHA, state regulations, and institutional policies.	Review Questions, PTCB Exam Practice Questions, Activity 36-1, Activity 36-2, Activity 36-3, Activity 36-4, Lab 36-1, Lab 36-2
6. Define and describe infection control.	Review Questions, PTCB Exam Practice Questions, Activity 36-1, Activity 36-2, Activity 36-3, Activity 36-4, Lab 36-1, Lab 36-2

INTRODUCTION

The concerns of workplace safety and infection control are of great importance for pharmacy technicians. It is critical to understand that workplace safety is a must whether the technician is working in an institutional or community-based pharmacy practice setting. There are a variety of rules and best practices regarding workplace safety and infection control, for pharmacy professionals, based on the specific state, practice setting, and institution, in addition to federal regulations. In this chapter, we will review the major provisions of workplace safety and infection-control measures.

REVIEW QUESTIONS

Match the following.

1. _____ workplace safety
2. _____ infection control
3. _____ PPE
4. _____ HEP B, HIV
5. _____ TCJ
6. _____ OSHA

a. proper hand hygiene
b. blood-borne pathogens
c. the organization that provides protocols for the safe removal of different hazards and substances, chemicals, needles, body fluids, blood, fire safety and control, and emergency plans in case of a fire
d. formed to assist health care organizations and health care programs in improving quality health care standards, accreditation, and certification for better, safe, and effective workplaces for health care workers and patients
e. gloves, gowns, hair covers, and masks
f. prevention of injury and illness of employees, and volunteers, in the workplace

Fill in the blanks.

7. An _____ refers to a specific event that results in unintended harm or damage, whereas an _____ is an event that has the potential to result in unintended harm or damage.

8. An _____ of all workplace conditions should be performed on a regular and timely basis to identify or eliminate existing and potential hazards.

9. Workplace training sessions must be available to _____ in the pharmacy.

10. A _____ area for preparing dangerous chemicals and drugs, such as _____, should be designated along with safety posters and signs restricting access to only qualified personnel.

PHARMACY CALCULATION PROBLEMS

Calculate the following

1. The patient has been ordered clindamycin 450 mg IM STAT in both gluteal areas of the body while in the emergency room. Then upon the patient's admission to the hospital, the order will be 450 mg IV q8h for 48 hours. The patient will be discharged with an order to take clindamycin 150 mg po tid for 10 days. How much clindamycin has this patient been prescribed for the entire course of therapy?

2. A physician orders for a patient requiring anticoagulation therapy: 2 mg of warfarin for days Monday, Wednesday, Friday, and Sunday and 5 mg of warfarin for days Tuesday, Thursday, and Saturday for a 30-day supply. How many tablets of each strength will be dispensed?

3. A patient has been ordered prochlorperazine 25 mg suppositories for 10 days. The directions are 1 supp PR bid prn N/V. You currently have in stock prochlorperazine 25 mg suppositories that come in quantities of 12 per box. How many suppositories will you dispense to the patient?

4. 6 oz. = _____ mL

5. 1 oz. = _____ tsp.

PTCB EXAM PRACTICE QUESTIONS

1. Material Safety Data Sheets contain all of the following information except:
   a. trade name.
   b. date of manufacturing.
   c. synonyms for the chemical.
   d. manufacturers name.

2. OPIM stands for:
   a. other prevalent infectious materials.
   b. obvious prevalent infectious materials.
   c. other potentially infectious materials.
   d. obvious potentially infectious materials.

3. The CDC has stated that proper hand hygiene techniques include:
   a. decontaminating hands with an alcohol-based hand rub.
   b. washing the hands for at least 15 seconds.
   c. using disposable towels to thoroughly dry hand rub the hands.
   d. all of the above.

4. Chemotherapy medications/hazardous agents must be compounded in what type of airflow hood?
   a. horizontal laminar airflow hood
   b. compounding aseptic isolator
   c. vertical laminar airflow hood
   d. both b and c

5. An example of an OPIM is:
   a. vaginal secretions.
   b. plasma.
   c. sweat.
   d. athlete's foot.

ACTIVITY 36-1: Case Study—Experiencing a cytotoxic spill in the flow hood

Instructions: Read the following scenario and then answer the critical thinking questions.

Your first week in the central IV pharmacy at the hospital went great, as the pharmacy director made some really good observations about the consistency of your aseptic technique. For your second week, you have been delegated to work in the satellite oncology pharmacy as the technician in that pharmacy is on vacation for the week. On Thursday afternoon, you ask your former instructor if you can refresh your aseptic technique skills, as it applies to compounding hazardous medications, for a few hours during Friday and Saturday. Your instructor is able to accommodate you on both Friday and Saturday.

After a good amount of time refreshing your skill sets with USP <797> and compounding hazardous medications, you feel ready for the orders and tasks for the week. Monday goes well as you process 15 orders for different patients. During Tuesday afternoon, you are carefully attempting to withdraw 7 mL of a chemotherapy medication from a 10 mL ampule with a filter needle when you accidentally push into the ampule 5 mL of the drug and 4 mL more of air. The medication aspirates onto part of your glove as well as onto the surface of the workflow bench.

1. What should or will you do immediately after the spill?

   _____

   _____

   _____

2. Are you going to report this spill? Why?

   _____

   _____

   _____

3. Do you think that you will be reassigned to another pharmacy since this is your first spill? Why or why not?

   _____

   _____

   _____

ACTIVITY 36-2: Case Study—Hospital E-Tool Part 1—Working in a BSC

Instructions: Use the website https://www.osha.gov/SLTC/etools/hospital/pharmacy/pharmacy.html to follow the instructions and to also answer the following questions related to working in a biological safety cabinet.

1. Click on the "Biological Safety Cabinet" in the pharmacy and answer this question. What are some of the examples of antineoplastic drugs?

   _____

   _____

2. Exposure to hazardous drugs during preparation due to ineffective engineering/work practice controls and PPE are:

   _____

   _____

   _____

   _____

3. What should a BSC also contain?

   _____

   _____

4. When double gloving, how should the gloves be placed?

   _____

   _____

5. How often should gloves be changed?

   _____

   _____

6. Click on the box of "latex gloves" in the pharmacy. If any member of pharmacy personnel is allergic to latex, what is the possible solution that OSHA has developed as a part of the Blood Borne Pathogen standard?

   _____

   _____

   _____

   _____

ACTIVITY 36-3: Case Study—Hospital E-Tool Part 2—Ergonomics

Instructions: Use the website https://www.osha.gov/SLTC/etools/hospital/pharmacy/pharmacy.html to follow the instructions and to also answer the following questions about ergonomics.

1. Click on the "Ergonomics" tab. What are the potential hazards that pharmacy personnel may be exposed to?

    _____

    _____

    _____

    _____

2. What are the possible solutions that OSHA has developed in order to decrease these potential hazards?

    _____

    _____

    _____

    _____

    _____

    _____

ACTIVITY 36-4: Case Study Hospital E-Tool Part 3—Workplace Violence

Instructions: Use the website https://www.osha.gov/SLTC/etools/hospital/pharmacy/pharmacy.html to follow the instructions and to also answer the following questions about workplace violence.

1. Click on the "Workplace Violence" tab. What is the potential hazard that all pharmacy personnel may be exposed to while working in the pharmacy?

    _____

    _____

2. What are the possible solutions that OSHA has developed in order to decrease these potential hazards?

    _____

    _____

    _____

    _____

    _____

    _____

LAB 36-1: Handling Hazardous Waste

Objective:

To understand the importance of handling hazardous waste in the oncology pharmacy.

Pre-Lab Information:

Review Chapter 36 in your textbook to learn more about handling hazardous waste.

Use the website https://www.osha.gov/SLTC/etools/hospital/pharmacy/pharmacy.html to research information about handling hazardous waste.

Explanation:

Cytotoxic medication waste as well as radiopharmaceutical waste, when handled improperly, can cause harm to all pharmacy personnel. Following the proper procedures and standards for disposal of hazardous pharmaceutical waste will minimize the potential hazards to pharmacy personnel.

Activity:

After the successful completion of a mock intravenous chemotherapy admixture in the lab, be prepared to dispose of the "mock" hazardous waste and answer the following questions from your instructor.

1. What kind or type of sharp container will your needle, syringe, and vial of "hazardous" medication be carefully disposed in?

   _____

2. Should all hazardous waste be separated from the regular trash in a pharmacy? Why?

   _____

   _____

   _____

3. After you have properly disposed of your needle, syringe, and ampule or vials of "hazardous" medication, what kind or type of bag will your PPE be carefully placed into?

   _____

   _____

4. Why is it important for you to wash your hands after the proper disposal of hazardous waste?

   _____

   _____

   _____

Student Name: _____

Lab Partner: _____

Grade/Comments: _____

_____

_____

Student Comments: _____

_____

_____

LAB 36-2: Using an Eyewash Station

Objective:

To understand how to properly use an eyewash station.

Pre-Lab Information:

Review Chapter 36 in your textbook to learn more about an eyewash station.

Locate the eyewash station in your classroom laboratory.

Explanation:

An eyewash station is a permanent fixture in the pharmacy. Pharmacy technicians may come into contact with medications or OPIMs that may plash into their eyes.

Activity:

Use the eyewash station in the classroom laboratory to flush out your eyes for 30 seconds to one minute. The instructor and students will each take a turn at the eyewash station.

Note: If the eyewash station contains bottled eyewash solution(s), the instructor will demonstrate how to use a bottle of solution to wash the eye(s) without opening the bottle. Each student will take a turn demonstrating his or her competencies of using a bottle of eyewash solution.

Student Name: _____

Lab Partner: _____

Grade/Comments: _____

_____

_____

Student Comments: _____

_____

_____

CHAPTER 37
Special Considerations for Pediatric and Geriatric Patients

After completing Chapter 37 from the textbook, you should be able to:	Related Activity in the Workbook/Lab Manual
1. Discuss the physiological changes that occur in pediatric and geriatric patients.	Review Questions, PTCB Exam Practice Questions, Activity 37-2, Activity 37-3
2. Explain how the processes of pharmacokinetics in pediatric patients affect drug dosing.	Review Questions, PTCB Exam Practice Questions, Activity 37-1, Activity 37-2, Activity 37-5, Activity 37-6
3. Discuss pediatric drug administration and dosage adjustment considerations.	Review Questions, PTCB Exam Practice Questions
4. List two common childhood illnesses or diseases in pediatric patients.	Review Questions, PTCB Exam Practice Questions
5. Discuss the physiological changes that occur in geriatric patients.	Review Questions, PTCB Exam Practice Questions
6. List several factors that affect pharmacokinetic processes in geriatric patients.	Review Questions, PTCB Exam Practice Questions
7. Discuss polypharmacy and noncompliance in pediatric and geriatric medication therapy.	Review Questions, PTCB Exam Practice Questions, Activity 37-1, Activity 37-5, Activity 37-6
8. Discuss Medicare Part D and its effects on medication dispensing to the geriatric population.	Review Questions
9. Explain ways in which geriatric medication dispensing will change in the future, and how extended life expectancy will change pharmacy practice.	Review Questions, Activity 37-5, Activity 37-6

INTRODUCTION

Providing medical and pharmaceutical care for pediatric and older patients is a bit more challenging than caring for adults who need medications. Drug dosing is different for children than adults and carries the same responsibility for accuracy and attention to detail when filling prescriptions for this age group. For older adult patients, there is often more concern about side effects and how well the drug is tolerated by them. These two age groups need extra care and consideration when it comes to pharmaceutical services and care. As a pharmacy technician, you need to understand the unique factors involved in caring for pediatric and geriatric patients.

REVIEW QUESTIONS

Match the following.

1. _____ absorption
2. _____ adverse effects
3. _____ bioavailability
4. _____ distribution
5. _____ excretion
6. _____ geriatric
7. _____ half-life
8. _____ metabolism
9. _____ noncompliance
10. _____ OTC drugs
11. _____ polypharmacy
12. _____ side effects
13. _____ toxicity

a. drug poisoning; can be life-threatening or extremely harmful

b. chemical change of drugs or foreign compounds in and by the body

c. when a patient does not follow a prescribed drug regimen

d. amount of a drug that is available for absorption

e. amount of time it takes the body to break down and excrete one-half of a drug dosage

f. refers to persons over the age of 65

g. elimination of a drug from the body; usually occurs through urine, feces, or the respiratory system

h. undesirable and potentially harmful drug effects

i. the process by which a drug enters the bloodstream

j. drug effects other than the intended one; usually undesirable but not harmful

k. administration of more medications than clinically indicated

l. drugs that can be purchased without a prescription

m. the process by which a drug reaches the various organs and tissues of the body

Choose the best answer.

14. _____ are newborn babies from birth to one month of age; _____ are between the ages of one month and two years.
    a. neonates/toddlers
    b. infants/neonates
    c. infants/toddlers
    d. neonates/infants

15. Because the kidneys, liver, and brain are the organs that require the most blood flow to function properly, the _____ and _____ processes slow as people age.
    a. metabolism, excretion
    b. metabolism, absorption
    c. excretion, absorption
    d. kidneys, liver

16. Which of the following is a common reason for noncompliance by the elderly?
    a. dosing schedule is confusing
    b. difficulty understanding or remembering what the drug is
        inability to afford the drug
    d. all of the above
    e. none of the above

True or False?

17. Organ size generally increases in the elderly, as do blood flow and cardiac output.

    T   F

18. Significant cognitive impairment in the geriatric population includes loss of eyesight and loss of hearing.

    T   F

19. By the year 2050, the elderly population will increase to approximately 72 million.

    T   F

20. Common childhood conditions include infections of the skin.

    T   F

PHARMACY CALCULATION PROBLEMS

Calculate the following.

1. A normal adult requires 0.1 mcg/kg/min of remifentanil for continuous IV infusion. However, in geriatric patients, the dosage should be reduced by half. How many micrograms will a 192 lb. geriatric patient receive over 10 minutes?

2. A pediatric patient is receiving an antibiotic for an impetigo infection. The pediatrician has prescribed cephalexin 25 mg/kg q8h. The patient weighs 85 lbs. How much will the patient receive per dose?

3. Zaleplon 10 mg is usually given qhs. If a geriatric patient is prescribed half of this dose, how many milligrams will the patient receive over a 14-day period?

4. A pediatric patient has been prescribed a medication at 2 mg/kg q12h. The patient weighs 70.4 lbs. How much will the patient receive per day?

5. A geriatric patient is ordered DuoNeb (ipratropium bromide 0.5 mg/albuterol sulfate 3.0 mg) nebulizer treatments q4h. How many milligrams of albuterol sulfate is the patient receiving per day?

PTCB EXAM PRACTICE QUESTIONS

1. Adults experience a decrease in many physiological functions between the ages of:
   a. 18 and 30 years.
   b. 20 and 40 years.
   c. 30 and 50 years.
   d. 50 and 70 years.

2. Syrup of ipecac is used for:
   a. gastric lavage.
   b. whole bowel evacuation.
   c. gastric decontamination.
   d. vomiting.

3. Which of the following drugs can cause elderly patients to become dizzy, unsteady on their feet, and possibly fall if the dosage is not adjusted appropriately?
   a. benzodiazepines
   b. diuretics
   c. acetaminophen
   d. ibuprofen

4. Treatment for pediatric patients with asthma often includes a combination of:
   a. anti-inflammatory agents and bronchodilators.
   b. inhalers and syrups.
   c. bronchodilators and corticosteroids.
   d. anti-inflammatory agents and corticosteroids.

5. To help solve the problem of polypharmacy and avoid complications and adverse drug interactions, pharmacists and pharmacy technicians must record *every* medication their patients are taking and keep a current patient profile by the:
   a. "white bag method."
   b. "brown bag lunch method."
   c. "bag lunch method."
   d. "brown bag method."

ACTIVITY 37-1: Case Study—A Bad Cough

Instructions: Read the following scenario and then answer the critical thinking questions.

Mrs. Buffet is everyone's favorite customer in the grocery chain retail pharmacy where you work. She is an endearing, 78-year-old, woman whom everyone refers to as "grandma." After buying her eggs and milk, she will stop by the pharmacy and say hello even if she is not picking up any prescriptions. As the years go by, Mrs. Muffet, like a lot of people her age, forgets things all the time. The other day she admits to you about sometimes forgetting to take all of her medication as prescribed. When she misses a dose of one medication or the other, she also admits to you that she doubles up on her capsules or tablets.

Mrs. Buffet takes a total of eight prescriptions, with one of the medications being directed for her to take three times a day. Today she comes complaining of an ongoing bad and dry cough. All of the medication she takes includes an ACE inhibitor, a beta blocker, atorvastatin, stool softener, thyroid, PPI, aspirin, and an inhaler.

1. What are the concerns that are exhibited in Mrs. Buffet's case?

   _____

   _____

   _____

   _____

2. Which of the medications is most likely to cause Mrs. Buffet an ongoing bad and dry cough?

_____

_____

_____

_____

3. Do you think that Mrs. Buffet has doubled up on the medication that is causing the ongoing bad and dry cough?

_____

_____

_____

_____

4. What can you and the pharmacy team do to help Mrs. Buffet manage her medication therapy?

_____

_____

_____

_____

ACTIVITY 37-2: Case Study—Accidental Heparin Overdose in Infants

Instructions: Read the following scenario and then answer the critical thinking questions.

An infant has been prescribed heparin 1 unit/mL for an arterial line. The pediatric intensive care unit (PICU) floor nurse calls the pharmacy and orders a vial of heparin 100 units/mL. A pharmacy team member, who has been running sensitive medication orders for the past four hours, has a break from running and offers to fill the order and then take it to PICU.

The nurse from PICU administers the dose to the infant without incident. Twenty minutes later, the nurse performs a heel prick and remarks that the blood has expelled out from the heel way too thin. The nurse decides to administer a small dose of protamine sulfate to see if that will help the infant's blood to coagulate. In another 20 minutes, the nurse performs another heel prick on the infant's opposite heel and the expelled blood is thicker than when she heel pricked the infant 40 minutes ago.

The nurse calls the pharmacy and asks for the pharmacy supervisor to speak about what transpired with this order. She asks the pharmacist what strength of heparin was sent to PICU for this particular infant. The pharmacist remarks that the order was filled for a vial of heparin 100 units/mL. The nurse asks the pharmacist if she may please speak to the pharmacy team member who filled the order for this infant.

The pharmacy team member speaks with the nurse and they discuss what happened to the infant's blood when she administered the first dose of heparin to the patient. The team member next confides to the nurse that the wrong vial of heparin must have been pulled by another pharmacy team member prior to filling the order. The nurse is frustrated at this news and exclaims that she will report this incident to the pharmacy director.

1. What strength of heparin do you believe that the pharmacy team member pulled to fill the order?

_____

2. Was the PICU nurse correct with administering the protamine sulfate to the infant? Why or why not?

_____

_____

_____

_____

3. Who do you think is primarily at fault for this accidental overdose?

_____

_____

_____

4. Do you believe that fatigue was involved with the pharmacy team member safely filling this order for the infant?

_____

_____

_____

ACTIVITY 37-3: Case Study—Three Age-Related Issues

Instructions: Read the following scenario and then answer the critical thinking questions.

Mrs. Crendall and her husband have been regular customers at the retail pharmacy for over 15 years. They started coming to the pharmacy when they were in their early 60s. They both say that they have received the best care and customer service at the pharmacy, which is what keeps them coming back. Jokingly, Mrs. Crendall comments that they will be bringing in more and more business as they get older and are customers for life. Since you have been working with the Crendalls for the past five years, they have built a strong rapport and trust you with their health care needs.

Over the years, you notice that Mr. and Mrs. Crendall have experienced most of the normal things that are associated with aging. They move a little slower, cannot remember every little detail of the day, and sometimes need a little help with reaching for items on higher shelves and also bending over to reach for items on lower shelves. Their vision is also failing at different rates with both of them using bifocals to read smaller typed or written print.

They both come into the pharmacy today and would like to speak with you about three current issues they are faced with. They are both confident that the pharmacy team and you can help them with practical solutions.

The first issue they bring up with you is that even though their insurance mandates it, they can no longer cut their medication tablets in half. They no longer have the vision or the strength to precisely cut the tablets for a proper dose. The second issue is that they can no longer read the prescription labels. As the couple has so many prescriptions, they are having trouble recognizing which medication is for whom. The third issue is that for the past two months, it seems that some of their medications have changed color. What was once a green tablet last month is a pink one this month. They are very confused by the changes in color.

1. What are some solutions that you and the pharmacy team can make to assist with the Crendalls' tablet-cutting problem?

_____

_____

_____

_____

2. What solution can you suggest to the pharmacy team to help the Crendalls have an easier time recognizing their prescription labels?

_____

_____

_____

3. What will you do to assist the Crendalls with any future changes related to their medications that may be a different color(s) the next time they pick up a refill?

_____

_____

_____

_____

4. Do many pharmacies recognize the special needs of the elderly patient, as well as develop and strategize ways to assist the geriatric population with similar issues that were presented in the scenario?

_____

_____

_____

_____

ACTIVITY 37-4: Case Study—Limited Mobility

Instructions: Read the following scenario and then answer the critical thinking questions.

Jack is a 68-year-old man who gets around quite well with his wheelchair. He resisted getting the chair as long as he could, but severe knee, hip, and leg problems made it almost impossible for him to walk. Almost everyone who sees him thinks he is helpless and feels sorry for him. However, Jack does not feel that way. He is very independent, running his own errands via mass transportation, and he even teaches a swimming class for wheelchair-using seniors at the YMCA.

Jack requires a lot of ostomy supplies and orders through the ostomy and medical supply area of a pharmacy where you work. From time to time, he needs to be refitted for such things as catheters, wafers, leg bags, and "diapers." Over the years, Jack has gained some weight as he has slowed down. Jack is stubborn and refuses to get one of those "old-people electric scooters for lazy people."

With just his trusty wheelchair, Jack has managed to pick up his supplies from the pharmacy and take the bus back to his home with no problems. With his weight gain and further aging, though, Jack has had difficulty manipulating the oversized packages and boxes, and finds that he is becoming weaker, too. Although Jack really enjoys coming by the pharmacy to say hello, he finds he can no longer manage this task no matter what he does.

1. What solutions can you offer Jack to get him his ostomy supplies?

_____

_____

_____

_____

2. Do you think Jack is a good candidate for an electric scooter? Why or why not? If so, what could you do to help Jack understand that it would make life easier?

_____

_____

_____

_____

3. How can you help Jack not feel so helpless when he comes to the pharmacy?

_____

_____

_____

_____

4. What emotional impact do you think the circumstances in this scenario might have on Jack, or any older adult patient?

_____

_____

_____

_____

5. What are four condition-related barriers to medication compliance by the older adult patient?

_____

_____

_____

_____

6. What are five therapy-related barriers to medication compliance by the older adult patient?

_____

_____

_____

_____

7. What are two broad patient-related barriers to medication compliance by the older adult patient?

_____

_____

_____

_____

LAB 37-1: Pediatric Cough/Cold Medication and the FDA

Objective:

To understand why over-the-counter cough and cold medications are not recommended for infants and children under two years of age.

Pre-Lab Information:

- Review Chapter 37 in your textbook.
- Visit the FDA's website http://www.fda.gov/ForConsumers/ConsumerUpdates/ucm048682.htm.

Explanation:

Parents and pediatricians alike may have challenges to face when an infant or child has been exposed to a pathogen causing a cough and/or fever.

Activity:

Using the website (http://www.fda.gov/ForConsumers/ConsumerUpdates/ucm048682.htm), please answer the following questions.

1. What can occur if an over-the-counter product for cough or cold is given to an infant or child under two years of age?

   _____

   _____

2. What are the side effects of cough and cold medications an infant or child may face if given an over-the-counter product for cough and cold?

   _____

   _____

3. What classes of medications can cause these effects?

   _____

   _____

4. What recommendation(s) does the FDA make for parents if their child is experiencing both cough and cold symptoms?

   _____

   _____

   _____

   _____

5. What eight steps should a consumer follow to ensure that an infant or child being given an over-the-counter, cough and or cold medication is not in danger of serious side effects?

_____

_____

_____

_____

_____

Student Name: _____

Lab Partner: _____

Grade/Comments: _____

_____

_____

Student Comments: _____

_____

_____

LAB 37-2: Pediatric Dosing

Objective:

To understand the relationship between Clark's Rule and Young's Rule to accurately calculate the dose for a cough/cold medication for a pediatric patient.

Pre-Lab Information:

• Review Chapter 37 in your textbook.

Explanation:

Pediatric dosing of cough and cold medications has to be calculated with the importance of accuracy being at the forefront of the allied health professional's mindset. The two common methods used for calculating pediatric dosing of cough and cold medications are Clark's Rule and Young's Rule.

Activity:

Please refer to Chapter 37 in your textbook to use Clark's Rule and Young's Rule for the following problems.

Clark's Rule

1. A child who weighs 95 lbs. is prescribed prednisolone syrup. The normal adult dosage is 10 mg. What is the appropriate dose for this child?

2. A child who is weighing 75 lbs. is prescribed pseudoephedrine syrup as a decongestant. The normal adult dosage is 45 mg. What is the appropriate dose for this child?

Young's Rule

1. A child who is nine years old is prescribed dextromethorphan polistirex for a cough. The normal adult dose is 60 mg. What is the appropriate dose for this child?

2. A child who is six years old is prescribed acetaminophen for a fever. The normal adult dose is 500 mg. What is the appropriate dose for this child?

Student Name: _____

Lab Partner: _____

Grade/Comments: _____

_____

_____

Student Comments: _____

_____

_____

LAB 37-3: Geriatric Dosing

Objective:

To understand how a geriatric patient may not be noncompliant with his or her multiple drug regimens.

Pre-Lab Information:

• Review Chapter 37 in your textbook.

Explanation:

With 55% to 59% of the geriatric population are on more than one class of medications for various disease states and conditions, the pharmacy technician is often relied upon to assist this population with their polypharmacy needs.

Activity:

Select a team of three, which will include a "pharmacist," a "technician," and a "patient." Decide upon which team member will take on each of the roles in this activity/scenario.

Scenario:

An older adult patient comes into the pharmacy with three new prescriptions. Two of those prescriptions are for hypertension and another one is for high cholesterol. The three medications are very close in size and shape as the patient has both vision and hearing conditions as well as arthritis.

1. What steps can you take to ensure that the patient will not make his or her own medication errors and be in full compliance with his or her medications?

   _____
   _____
   _____
   _____

2. The patient tells you that his or her grandchildren come to visit him. Should this patient have safety caps for his or her vials of medications? Why or why not?

   _____
   _____
   _____

3. Does this patient take any over-the-counter medications? If so, what other assistance should you offer to the patient for better compliance?

   _____
   _____
   _____
   _____

Student Name: _____

Lab Partner: _____

Grade/Comments: _____

_____

_____

Student Comments: _____

_____

_____

CHAPTER 38
Biopharmaceuticals

After completing Chapter 38 from the textbook, you should be able to:	Related Activity in the Workbook/Lab Manual
1. Name at least two drugs developed by using recombinant DNA technology, and outline their uses.	Review Questions, PTCB Exam Practice Questions, Activity 38-1, Activity 38-2, Activity 38-3, Activity 38-4, Lab 38-1
2. Discuss the four steps in the genetic engineering process.	Review Questions, Activity 38-4, Lab 38-1
3. Explain briefly how a company gets approval for a biopharmaceutical drug from the FDA.	Review Questions, Activity 38-4, Lab 38-1
4. Discuss why biopharmaceuticals, genetic engineering, and stem cell research are important in the future of pharmacy and the practice of medicine.	Review Questions, Activity 38-1, Activity 38-2, Activity 38-3, Activity 38-4, Lab 38-1

INTRODUCTION

Biopharmacology is the branch of pharmacology that studies the use of biologically engineered drugs. Biopharmaceuticals are substances created using biotechnology. They can be proteins like antibodies, and even consist of DNA and RNA. Research is being conducted to find new therapeutic medications, or biopharmaceuticals, to treat such life-threatening diseases as AIDS, various cancers, and Parkinson's disease.

Large majorities of biopharmaceuticals are derived from existing life forms, such as plants and animals, although they are produced by means other than direct extraction from a biological source. Genetic engineering is another way to create new drugs; stem cell research also offers opportunities to discover new therapeutic treatments and is making significant strides in the development of new medications used today. As a pharmacy technician, you should be familiar with some of the concepts of biopharmacology, their impact on the pharmaceutical industry, and their role in the future of pharmacology.

REVIEW QUESTIONS

Match the following.

1. _____ allergenic
2. _____ biologics
3. _____ biopharmaceuticals
4. _____ biopharmacology
5. _____ biotechnology
6. _____ Gaucher's disease
7. _____ GMO
8. _____ Stem cells
9. _____ neutropenia
10. _____ rheumatoid arthritis
11. _____ transform
12. _____ vector

a. autoimmune disease that causes chronic inflammation of the joints

b. organism that does not itself cause disease, but spreads disease by distributing pathogens from one host to another

c. alteration of an organism itself or the cell in the genetic engineering process

d. disease in which there are an abnormal number of the white blood cells that are responsible for fighting infections

e. substances created using biotechnology

f. a substance that can cause an allergic reaction

g. use of biological substances or microorganisms to perform specific functions, such as the production of drugs, hormones, or food products

h. branch of pharmacology that studies the use of biologically engineered drugs

i. organism whose genetic material has been altered using the genetic engineering techniques known as recombinant DNA technology

j. disease in which fatty materials collect in the liver, spleen, kidneys, lungs, and brain and cause the person to be susceptible to infections

k. have a special ability to renew themselves many times through cell division, in a process called proliferation

l. a group of varied medicinal products, such as vaccines, blood products, allergenics, and proteins

True or False?

13. Genetic manufacturing is another way to create new drugs.

    T   F

14. After the successful completion of all three IND phases, the company can then file a NDA with the FDA.

    T   F

15. Erythropoietin is used for anemia for cancer therapy.

    T   F

Match the following.

16. _____ abatacept
17. _____ Humira
18. _____ anemia from cancer therapy
19. _____ etanercept
20. _____ Remicade
21. _____ breast cancer
22. _____ Gaucher's disease
23. _____ genital warts
24. _____ Pulmozyme

a. adalimumab
b. Crohn's disease
c. trastuzumab
d. Epogen
e. rheumatoid arthritis
f. Enbrel
g. cystic fibrosis
h. Cerezyme
i. Alferon N

PHARMACY CALCULATION PROBLEMS

Calculate the following.

1. A female patient who has rheumatoid arthritis has been prescribed infliximab 2.5 mg/kg for her first dose. What is the strength of her therapy if she weighs 145 lb.? On stock, you carry the medication in a vial where the concentration is 100 mg/20 mL. How much of the infliximab will you prepare for this patient?

2. Etanercept is usually dosed at 50 mg SC twice a week for three months for severe plaque psoriasis. How many grams will a patient with psoriasis receive for a three-month regimen?

3. A patient who is prescribed abatacept weighs 195 lb. According to the manufacturer's recommendation, a patient weighing less than 60 kg should receive a 500 mg dose. If a patient weighs between 60 and 100 kg, the patient should receive a 750 mg dose. If the patient weighs more than 100 kg, the patient should receive a 1,000 mg dose. What is the correct dose for this patient?

4. A patient is to receive rituximab 700 mg IV in 250 mL 0.9% sodium chloride. If the IV is to be infused at 100 mg/hr, how long will it take for the IV to be completely infused?

5. 10 mL = _____ minims.

1. Most of the biologics have a warning for a risk of contracting which highly communicable pathogen?
   a. hepatitis
   b. HIV
   c. tuberculosis
   d. influenza

2. Which of the following biotechnology drugs is used to treat breast cancer?
   a. Orencia
   b. Herceptin
   c. Humira
   d. Remicade

3. When a biopharmaceutical company has completed the preclinical phase, what does it file with the FDA?
   a. DEA
   b. ANDA
   c. BDEA
   d. INDA

4. Which of the following medications is used to treat psoriasis?
   a. adalimumab
   b. trastuzumab
   c. ustekinumab
   d. infliximab

5. The first genetically engineered drug approved by the FDA for therapeutic use was:
   a. adalimumab.
   b. recombinant human insulin.
   c. penicillin.
   d. Remicade.

ACTIVITY 38-1: Case Study—Darbepoetin Alfa

Instructions: Read the following scenario and then answer the critical thinking questions.

Mrs. Critten has had a great life. She has been married for 42 years, has four wonderful children and a miniature poodle that she loves dearly. Sometime in the past decade, during one of her annual checkups, Mrs. Critten was found to have cancer. It was a slow-growing, chronic type, but one that would, over time, cause her to easily catch infections as it progressed.

Eventually, Mrs. Critten's cancer progressed to the point where chemotherapy was considered for treatment. She weighed the pros and cons and decided to begin treatment. Treatment would not cure her condition, but it could help extend her life while maintaining a good quality of life.

Mrs. Critten experienced a few side effects common to chemotherapy patients, such as nausea and vomiting, hair loss, and anemia. She was prescribed medication for the nausea and vomiting that typically lasted a few days after each treatment, wore wigs for the increasing hair loss, and was prescribed a synthetic form of erythropoietin called darbepoetin alfa (an erythropoiesis-stimulating agent). This medication increases the number of red blood cells and is typically used for the treatment of anemia in cancer patients undergoing chemotherapy.

1. What drug form of this medicine is available?

   _____

   _____

   _____

   _____

2. What are the black-box warnings for this medication?

_____

_____

_____

_____

3. How long will Mrs. Critten's treatments with darbepoetin for anemia last?

_____

_____

_____

4. How long does it take to feel the benefits of darbepoetin?

_____

_____

_____

_____

5. Can this medication be mixed into an IV solution?

_____

_____

_____

_____

ACTIVITY 38-2: Case Study—Avonex

Instructions: Read the following scenario and then answer the critical thinking questions.

Monte Evans is a 27-year-old African-American male who enjoys volunteering at the local boys' and girls' community center. He has worked with adolescent children for many years and has served both as a counselor and a mentor for them. He also excels with planning different events for the many children whom he enjoys guiding. During his time at the center, Monte spends most of his time and energy planning energetic activities for the children.

For the past two months, Monte has been having intermittent problems such as muscle weakness, a lack of coordination, as well as a loss of the sense of touch, and pain in his muscles. Sometimes, he experiences only one of these symptoms, sometimes more than one of the symptoms, and sometimes none at all. Being confused of these recent experiences, he is baffled until he visits his doctor and is thoroughly assessed and is then diagnosed with multiple sclerosis. The doctor begins Monte's treatment for his condition with Avonex (interferon beta-1a). Monte then brings his prescription to the pharmacy to have it filled.

1. What is multiple sclerosis?

_____

_____

_____

_____

2. How is Avonex dispensed?

_____

_____

_____

_____

3. What is the route of administration and dosing frequency for Avonex?

_____

_____

_____

_____

4. After he has completed his first successful month of Avonex therapy, Monte calls your pharmacy to order a refill of his medication; however, his insurance company now requires that it has to be mailed to him. What special considerations are there to take regarding mail order delivery of Avonex?

_____

_____

_____

_____

ACTIVITY 38-3: Case Study—Etanercept

Instructions: Read the following scenario and then answer the critical thinking questions.

Mrs. Agarstier is an aging star of the theater. During her earlier years, she starred in many Off-Broadway shows—or, as she puts it, "way off Broadway." Although she did not achieve a celebrity status, it was not because she did not do her best at her craft. Mrs. Agarstier loved to act and to dance. She would rehearse for hours, day after day, polishing an already perfect routine. She would bend, stretch, and pirouette with ease and grace. When she needed to, she could perform an entire six-person scene by herself.

Mrs. Agarstier has recently developed rheumatoid arthritis. For years, she had struggled with the pain, localized in her hands and wrists. Lately, her hands have changed shape as her knuckles have protruded outward and upward and are also enlarged.

During the course of her disease, Mrs. Agarstier's nonprescribed and prescribed therapies have included analgesics, NSAIDs, cortisones, and DMARDs. Each has had its advantages and disadvantages with very minor side effects affecting Mrs. Agarstier's GI system. Now that her hands have changed shape and are very painful, Mrs. Agarstier's rheumatologist would like to start her on etanercept therapy.

1. What is rheumatoid arthritis?

_____

_____

_____

_____

2. How is etanercept dispensed?

_____

_____

_____

_____

3. For treatment of what other disease states, has the FDA also approved and indicated etanercept?

_____

_____

_____

_____

4. Etanercept, infliximab, and adalimumab belong to what drug class? List several common side effects of these drugs.

_____

_____

_____

_____

ACTIVITY 38-4: Web Research Activity—FDA and Biopharmaceuticals

Research and development of biologics have grown exponentially in the past 10–15 years. Currently, many biologics are being used to treat arthritis, diabetes, and many immune-system disorders. The many advances that are being made in this field are accompanied by the increasing debates over bioethics, ethics religion, and government regulations. This area of medicine and pharmacy services will continue to develop and grow over the course in the 21st century. Pharmacy technicians will need to become familiar with these types of therapies.

Activity:

Review Chapter 38 in your textbook.

Visit the website http://www.fda.gov/biologicsbloodvaccines/default.htm.

After reviewing the chapter in the textbook and the website, please answer the following questions regarding biopharmaceuticals and the FDA.

1. How does a biological product differ from a medication?

_____

_____

_____

_____

2. Which division of the FDA is responsible for regulating biopharmaceutical products?

_____

_____

_____

_____

3. What act do biologics fall under and why?

_____

_____

_____

_____

4. What are some of the requirements for licensing a new biological product?

_____

_____

_____

_____

LAB 38-1: Biopharmaceuticals, Genetic Engineering, and Stem Cell Research

Objective:

Review the biopharmaceutical industry and concepts of genetic engineering and stem cell research.

Pre-Lab Information:

- Review Chapter 38, "Biopharmaceuticals," in your textbook.
- Visit the following websites:
  - http://www.fda.gov/consumer/updates/genetherapy101507.html
  - http://stemcells.nih.gov/info/basics/basics1.asp
  - http://www.merck.com/product/usa/pi_circulars/f/follistim_aq_cartridge/follistim_cartridge_ppiifu.pdf

Explanation:

Genetic engineering, stem cell research, and the biopharmaceutical industry have been responsible for very exciting developments in the treatment of several human diseases. It is important for pharmacy technicians to have an understanding of how these treatments differ from other therapies. This exercise is designed to give you the opportunity to explore this promising area of medicine.

Activity:

Using the following websites, research and answer the following questions.

Human Gene Therapy

Visit http://www.fda.gov/consumer/updates/genetherapy101507.html.

1. What is a human gene therapy product?

   _____

   _____

   _____

   _____

2. How do these products work?

   _____

   _____

   _____

   _____

3. What is the potential impact of these products for consumers?

   _____

   _____

   _____

   _____

4. What is the FDA's role in regulating these products?

_____

_____

_____

5. Have any gene therapy products been approved yet?

_____

_____

_____

Stem Cells

Visit http://stemcells.nih.gov/info/basics/basics1.asp.

1. What is another term used to describe cell-based therapies?

_____

_____

2. What are the two kinds of human or animal stem cells that scientists use in research?

_____

_____

_____

3. What disease is highlighted in the website as having a very promising future treatment based on stem cells?

_____

_____

_____

Recombinant DNA

Visit http://www.merck.com/product/usa/pi_circulars/f/follistim_aq_cartridge/follistim_cartridge_ppiifu .pdf.

1. What is Follistim used to treat?

_____

_____

_____

2. Recombinant technology begins with the isolation of what?

_____
_____
_____
_____

3. What is a vector?

_____
_____
_____
_____

4. What happens to the vector before it is introduced into host cells to express the protein?

_____
_____
_____
_____

Student Name: _____
Lab Partner: _____
Grade/Comments: _____
_____
_____

Student Comments: _____
_____
_____